BIOLOGICAL APPROACHES *to* RATIONAL DRUG DESIGN

BIOLOGICAL APPROACHES *to* RATIONAL DRUG DESIGN

Edited by
David B. Weiner, Ph.D.
William V. Williams, Ph.D.

University of Pennsylvania
School of Medicine
Philadelphia, Pennsylvania

CRC Press
Taylor & Francis Group
Boca Raton London New York

CRC Press is an imprint of the
Taylor & Francis Group, an **informa** business

CRC Press
Taylor & Francis Group
6000 Broken Sound Parkway NW, Suite 300
Boca Raton, FL 33487-2742

ISBN 13: 978-0-8493-9422-5 (hbk)

Visit the Taylor & Francis Web site at
http://www.taylorandfrancis.com

and the CRC Press Web site at
http://www.crcpress.com

Library of Congress Cataloging-in-Publication Data

Biological approaches to rational drug design / edited by David B.
Weiner, William V. Williams.
p. cm. — (Pharmacology and toxicology)
Includes bibliographical references and index.
ISBN 0-8493-9422-8
1. Drugs—Design. 2. Biopharmaceutics. 3. Pharmaceutical biotechnology. I. Weiner, David B. II. Williams, William V. III. Series: Pharmacology & toxicology (Boca Raton, Fla.)
[DNLM: 1. Drug Design. QV 744 B6144 1994]
RS420.B58 1994
615′.7—dc20
DNLM/DLC
for Library of Congress 94-11157
CIP

Library of Congress Card Number 94-11157

INTRODUCTION

Rational drug design? Many would question the thesis of this book, stating that this is a goal, not a reality with today's technology. Yet, this is a question of definitions. Let's take the terms literally (from *Webster's Unabridged 20th Century Dictionary*). *Rational:* of, based on, or derived from reasoning. *Drug:* any substance used as a medicine, or in the preparation of medicines, or chemical mixtures. *Design:* to contrive; to project with an end in view; to form an idea, as a scheme. Taken together, rational drug design is simply defined as a reasoned approach to developing medicines. This does not suggest that the design process is always immediately successful, but instead that it is based on reason. By this broad definition, the age of rational drug design is clearly upon us.

A more stringent definition might also be applied: a rational approach to drug development for a disease based on understanding the molecular pathophysiology of the disease process. This could imply intervening at a critical metabolic step, perturbing a specific receptor system, or administration of a specific stimulatory/inhibitory molecule. In its purest form, rational drug design would allow the development of a specific, non-toxic drug based on the molecular and structural information of a target molecule. This is the goal many are currently striving for, with varying levels of success. However, the structural approach is not the sole approach to drug development, and is not the only rational method for drug development. Many biological and chemical approaches to therapeutic design are currently available, and the application of several complementary technologies to the drug design process is perhaps the most "rational" approach. Based on these considerations, we present *Biological Approaches to Rational Drug Design,* a companion volume to *Chemical and Structural Approaches to Rational Drug Design.* While many of the chapters utilize overlapping technologies, this broad classification highlights the predominant technology exploited by the authors. The content of the book is summarized here.

Biological Approaches to Rational Drug Design exploits an understanding of disease pathogenesis by applying a variety of biological agents to therapy. Molecular biological techniques have supplied an important array of biologically active molecules, many of which are currently in use as therapeutics. Many of the most successful of these techniques are described.

"Identifying Lead Peptides from Epitope Libraries" is written by Jamie Scott, who was the first to develop a molecular approach to screening peptide "libraries". She describes several recently developed methods of rational screening procedures for discovery of lead compounds. These utilize large libraries of oligopeptides which are developed by either chemical synthesis or molecular means. In most cases, these libraries are displayed on the surface of appropriate carriers, e.g., on beads for chemical libraries or on the surface of filamentous bacteriophage for molecular libraries. Isolation of those peptides which bind to a given "ligate" (antibody, receptor, or similar molecule) allows their sequence to be determined. This provides an initial "lead" for the drug design process, whereby the peptide is modified or structural information is derived from it, by allowing refinement of the initial structures into a higher affinity, specific ligand.

"Interleukin-1 Receptor Pathway Approaches to Drug Design," by Howard M. Einspahr, Barry C. Finzel, and Daniel E. Tracy, details the role of interleukin-1 (IL-1) in inflammatory processes. The discovery of several ligands for the high-affinity interleukin 1 receptor, including IL-1α, IL-1β, and IL-1 receptor antagonist protein (IRAP) has been of great interest as these ligands share limited amino acid sequence homology but all compete for binding to a common site. Identification of potential contact residues is detailed, with prospects for small molecule design.

"The Hematopoietic Colony-Stimulating Factors," by Kenneth Kaushansky, provides an overview of the explosion of information regarding both the clinical and molecular aspects of colony-stimulating factor (CSF)-receptor interactions. Many of the CSFs already are in widespread clinical use, and this is expected to expand as trials continue. The development of small molecule analogs and antagonists will proceed from a molecular understanding of the ligand-receptor interactions involved in signal transduction. The early studies regarding CSF-receptor interactions are described, and the structural-function relationships of these interactions are explored as pathways for rational design strategies.

"Monoclonal Antibodies: Technical Development and Therapeutic Indications" by Margaret R. Dalesandro, Martin E. Sanders, and John A. Lipani traces the history of monoclonal antibody technology from simple hybridoma methods to humanization strategies. The power of monoclonal antibody technology in developing specific ligands has been of obvious utility in many diagnostic tests. While the diagnostic use of antibodies continues to expand, the application of monoclonals as therapeutics is at a much more germinal stage. However, products are now reaching the clinic. Strategies for optimizing the clinical utility of monoclonals are described, as are many of the current therapeutic targets. The application of this powerful technology holds great promise for diagnosis and treatment in clinical practice.

"T Cell Receptor Based Therapy of Autoimmune Diseases" by Thaila Ramanujam and William V. Williams provides an overview of the molecular features of cellularly mediated autoimmune disease pathogenesis. The engagement of a specific T cell receptor by a specific antigen-MHC complex remains one of the most highly specific interactions in immunology. The recent strides made in understanding this trimolecular complex has allowed a number of strategies for inhibiting this interaction to be developed. Deletion of autoreactive T cells, blocking antigen binding to MHC, or inhibiting the interaction between T cell receptor and antigen-MHC with reagents directed at the MHC have been effective in experimental systems. The potential application of these strategies to the treatment of human autoimmune diseases is explored. These strategies offer the hope for effective, specific therapy of chronic human autoimmune diseases.

"Oligosaccharide Pharmaceuticals" by Stephen Roth and David Zopf provides insights into the roles of carbohydrates in multiple biological processes. They function in many adhesion-related phenomena, including pathogen attachment and leukocyte migration. As such, oligosaccharides and substances which interact with their receptors hold great potential as anti-infectives and immunomodulators. The current opportunities and obstacles are described in this chapter.

"Gene Therapy" by Jean Boyer and David Weiner reviews this rapidly evolving medical intervention. The application of molecular biology to the treatment of genetic diseases has already met with clinical success. In this chapter, Boyer and Weiner review the current approaches to gene delivery including the use of retroviral vectors, adenovirus vectors, Herpes virus vectors, and direct gene (DNA) injection. The experimental and clinical applications of gene therapy using these vectors have multiplied, and currently range from correction of genetic defects to treating cancer and developing vaccines. This chapter provides a succinct summary of the current strategies and opportunities for the application of gene therapy.

"Antisense Deoxynucleotides and Ribozymes" by Scott Shore and Premkumar Reddy describes the theoretical and experimental basis for nucleotide targeting technologies. The use of antisense to inhibit gene translation is already being tested in phase I clinical studies, with specific targeting of pathogenic gene expression. Ribozyme technology, which capitalizes on the ability of certain RNA molecules to catalyze RNA cleavage, is in a more embryonic stage but is rapidly evolving with specific therapeutic targets. The high level of enthusiasm for these technologies stems from their specificity and potential for targeted inhibition of pathogenic genes. This chapter reviews the relevant background and evolution of these technologies to the present, as well as detailing the technical hurdles that remain and the attractive clinical targets.

Together, these chapters provide both a broad overview of the current methodologies being applied to biological approaches to rational drug design, and in depth analyses of progress in this specific field. The reader with specific therapeutic targets in mind should be able to explore this strategy for drug development. Those with interest in specific technologies should be able to view both this volume and *Chemical and Structural Approaches to Rational Drug Design* in the broader context of the currently available technologies. The extensive reference lists provided by the authors will allow those with specific targets and technologies to explore their interests in greater depth.

David B. Weiner, Ph.D.
William V. Williams, M.D.

Pharmacology and Toxicology: Basic and Clinical Aspects

Mannfred A. Hollinger, Series Editor
University of California, Davis

Published Titles

Inflammatory Cells and Mediators in Bronchial Asthma, 1990, Devendra K. Agrawal and Robert G. Townley
Pharmacology of the Skin, 1991, Hasan Mukhtar
In Vitro *Methods of Toxicology*, 1992, Ronald R. Watson
Basis of Toxicity Testing, 1992, Donald J. Ecobichon
Human Drug Metabolism from Molecular Biology to Man, 1992, Elizabeth Jeffreys
Platelet Activating Factor Receptor: Signal Mechanisms and Molecular Biology, 1992, Shivendra D. Shukla
Biopharmaceutics of Ocular Drug Delivery, 1992, Peter Edman
Beneficial and Toxic Effects of Aspirin, 1993, Susan E. Feinman
Preclinical and Clinical Modulation of Anticancer Drugs, 1993, Kenneth D. Tew, Peter Houghton, and Janet Houghton
Peroxisome Proliferators: Unique Inducers of Drug-Metabolizing Enzymes, 1994, David E. Moody
Angiotensin II Receptors, Volume 1: Molecular Biology, Biochemistry, Pharmacology, and Clinical Perspectives, 1994, Robert R. Ruffolo, Jr.
Chemical and Structural Approaches to Rational Drug Design, 1994, David B. Weiner and William V. Williams
Biological Approaches to Rational Drug Design, 1994, David B. Weiner and William V. Williams

Forthcoming Titles

Alcohol Consumption, Cancer and Birth Defects: Mechanisms Involved in Increased Risk Associated with Drinking, Anthony J. Garro
Animal Models of Mucosal Inflammation, Timothy S. Gaginella
Brain Mechanisms and Psychotropic Drugs, A. Baskys and G. Remington
Development of Neurotransmitter Regulation and Function: A Pharmacological Approach, Christopher A. Shaw
Direct Allosteric Control of Glutamate Receptors, M. Palfreyman, I. Reynolds, and P. Skolnick
Drug Delivery Systems, V. V. Ranade
Genomic and Non-Genomic Effects of Aldosterone, Martin Wehling
Human Growth Hormone Pharmacology: Basic and Clinical Aspects, Kathleen T. Shiverick and Arlan Rosenbloom
Immunopharmaceuticals, Edward S. Kimball
Neural Control of Airways, Peter J. Barnes
Pharmacological Effects of Ethanol on the Nervous System, Richard A. Deitrich
Pharmacology in Exercise and Sport, Satu M. Somani
Pharmacology of Intestinal Secretion, Timothy S. Gaginella
Phospholipase A2 in Clinical Inflammation: Endogenous Regulation and Pathophysiological Actions, Keith B. Glaser and Peter Vadas
Placental Pharmacology, B. B. Rama Sastry
Placental Toxicology, B. B. Rama Sastry
Receptor Characterization and Regulation, Devendra K. Agrawal
Ryanodine Receptors, Vincenzo Sorrentino
Serotonin and Gastrointestinal Function, Timothy S. Gaginella and James J. Galligan
Stealth Liposomes, D. D. Lasic and F. J. Martin
Targeted Delivery of Imaging Agents, Vladimir P. Torchilin
TAXOL®: Science and Applications, Matthew Suffness
Therapeutic Modulation of Cytokines, M.W. Bodner and Brian Henderson

THE EDITORS

David B. Weiner, Ph.D., is an Assistant Professor of Pathology and Laboratory Medicine and Adjunct Assistant Professor of Medicine at the University of Pennsylvania School of Medicine and is Director of Biotechnology in the Institute for Biotechnology and Advanced Molecular Medicine at the University of Pennsylvania.

Dr. Weiner earned his B.S. in Biology from the State University of New York at Stony Brook in 1978 and obtained both M.S. and Ph.D. degrees in Developmental Biology from the University of Cincinnati in 1985. He completed postgraduate training in the Division of Immunology, Department of Pathology, at the University of Pennsylvania, in 1988.

Following his postdoctoral fellowship, Dr. Weiner was appointed in the Pathology Department at the University of Pennsylvania, then in the Wistar Institute. In 1989, Dr. Weiner was appointed as Director of Biotechnology at the Wistar Institute. He presented more than 40 invited talks at international and national meetings, and has chaired sessions at the American Society for Microbiology, Clinical Immunology Society, BioEast, GHI-Vaccines and Gene Therapy Meetings. Dr. Weiner has published over 110 peer reviewed manuscripts and 10 review chapters. He currently serves on the editorial board of *Viral Immunology*, and as Senior Editor of *DNA* and *Cell Biology*.

In 1992, Dr. Weiner was appointed the Director of Biotechnology of the newly formed Institute for Biotechnology and Advanced Molecular Medicine (IBAMM). This Institute has been developed in collaboration with the Technology Council of Greater Philadelphia and the University of Pennsylvania to foster the growth of Biotechnology in the Delaware Valley by providing expertise on critical issues to a wide range of academic and industrial interests. In 1993, he became appointed in the Department of Pathology at the University of Pennsylvania as an Assistant Professor, and as an Adjunct Assistant Professor in the Department of Medicine. He has gained international recognition for his work in the area of genetic inoculation, molecular characterization of retroviral pathogenesis, and in the characterization of human retroviral envelope and regulatory genes. His studies in genetic inoculation have led to the development of novel prophylactic and immunotherapeutic vaccines against HIV infection. His current research interests include genetic pharmaceutics, regulatory gene structure and function, as well as mechanisms of retroviral pathogenesis.

William V. Williams, M.D., is an Assistant Professor of Medicine, in the Rheumatology Division, University of Pennsylvania School of Medicine; an Assistant Professor of Medicine in Pediatrics, Children's Hospital of Philadelphia; and Head of Molecular Medicine, Biotechnology Department, Institute for Biotechnology and Advanced Molecular Medicine.

Dr. Williams received his undergraduate training from Massachusetts Institute of Technology, from 1972—1976, and was granted Sc.B. degrees in Biology and Chemistry, graduating Phi Beta Kappa. He attended Tufts University School of Medicine from 1976—1980, receiving an M.D. degree. Following his clinical training, Dr. Williams distinguished himself as an Arthritis Foundation Postdoctoral Fellow, studying mechanisms of autoimmune disease pathogenesis under the auspices of Helen Mullen, Ph.D. He then spent 2 years as a National Institutes of Health Postdoctoral Fellow, studying Molecular Immunology, at the University of Pennsylvania with Mark Greene, M.D., Ph.D. In 1988, Dr. Williams became an Assistant Professor in the Rheumatology Division, Department of Medicine, at the University of Pennsylvania. In 1989, he was appointed Assistant Professor of Medicine in Pediatrics, Children's Hospital of Philadelphia. In 1992, he was asked to head the Molecular Medicine Division of the Biotechnology Department at the Institute for Biotechnology and Advanced Molecular Medicine at the University of Pennsylvania.

Dr. Williams is a member of the American Association for the Advancement of Science, the American College of Physicians, the American College of Rheumatology, and the American

Federation for Clinical Research. He has authored over 100 papers, and has been the recipient of several research grants. He serves as a Senior Editor for the journal *Antibody*.

Dr. Williams has gained international recognition for his work in the development of biologically active peptides based on antibody structure. His research interests include molecular analysis of ligand-receptor interactions (particularly antibody-receptor interactions), molecular mechanisms of immunoregulation, molecular diagnostics, and rational drug design.

CONTRIBUTORS

Jean Boyer
Department of Pathology
University of Pennsylvania
Philadelphia, Pennsylvania

Margaret R. Dalesandro
Centocor, Inc.
Malvern, Pennsylvania

Howard M. Einspahr
Bristol-Myers Squibb Pharmaceutical Research Institute
Princeton, New Jersey

Barry C. Finzel
The Upjohn Company
Kalamazoo, Michigan

Kenneth Kaushansky
Associate Professor of Medicine
Division of Hematology
University of Washington
Seattle, Washington

John A. Lipani
Smith Kline Beeham Pharmaceuticals
King of Prussia, Pennsylvania

Thaila Ramanujam
Santa Cruz, California

E. Premkumar Reddy
The Fels Institute
Philadelphia, Pennsylvania

Stephen Roth
Neose Pharmaceuticals, Inc.
Horsham, Pennsylvania

Martin E. Sanders
Centocor, Inc.
Malvern, Pennsylvania

Jamie K. Scott
Institute of Molecular Biology and Biochemistry and Department of Chemistry
Simon Fraser University
Burnaby, British Columbia
Canada

Scott K. Shore
The Fels Institute
Philadelphia, Pennsylvania

Daniel E. Tracey
BASF Bioresearch Corporation
Cambridge, Massachusetts

David B. Weiner
Assistant Professor
Department of Pathology and Laboratory Medicine
University of Pennsylvania School of Medicine
Philadelphia, Pennsylvania

William V. Williams
Assistant Professor
Rheumatology Division
University of Pennsylvania
School of Medicine
Philadelphia, Pennsylvania

David Zopf
Neose Pharmaceuticals, Inc.
Horsham, Pennsylvania

ACKNOWLEDGMENTS

The editors would like to acknowledge support received from the Institute of Biotechnology and Advanced Molecular Medicine, the National Institutes of Health for DBW and WVW during the editing of this book, and the contributions of all the authors. We also would like to acknowledge the following people for their inspiration and support over the years: Elof Carlson, Carolyn Trunca, Henry Wortis, and Helen Mullen; our wives, Abby I. Phillipson and Lorraine M. Williams, and our children, Rebecca, Lindsey, Elizabeth, Ron, Chris, and Jon, for their forebearance and understanding.

TABLE OF CONTENTS

Chapter 1

IDENTIFYING LEAD PEPTIDES FROM EPITOPE LIBRARIES

Jamie K. Scott

CONTENTS

I. INTRODUCTION

Commonly, the first step in the process of drug development is the identification of *lead compounds*. These compounds, often having moderate affinity for the target receptor, are identified after extensive screenings using receptor-binding or biological assays, and are then modified to possess pharmacologically useful properties. *Epitope libraries* promise to make the strategy of lead compound discovery more fruitful by both increasing the scale of search and by decreasing the screening time. Epitope libraries comprise hundreds of millions of

0-8493-9422-8/94/$0.00+$.50

different short peptides, and are so named to emphasize that each peptide represents a potential binding determinant *(epitope)* that is recognized by an antibody, receptor, or other binding molecule *(ligate)*. These vast collections of peptides can be produced by chemical synthesis or by recombinant DNA technology. The peptides in *synthetic peptide libraries* are of two forms.[1-4] Peptides can be attached to solid supports, which allows the identification of peptide ligands by their ability to bind, and thus immobilize, a target ligate bearing a fluorescent, radioactive, or enzymatically derived signal.[1,4] Alternatively, libraries of free synthetic peptides have been developed.[2,3] Peptide ligands are identified from these latter libraries by their ability to block binding of a known ligand to its ligate or to affect activity in a bioassay.

In *fusion protein libraries*,[5-14] the "peptides" are actually peptide sequences that are expressed as part of a fusion protein. Each peptide sequence in a library is physically associated with the nucleic acid sequence encoding it. This allows the peptides in fusion protein libraries to be screened at the protein level, but generated and replicated at the nucleic acid level. Thus, fusion proteins bearing ligand sequences can be enriched by binding immobilized ligate, then amplified by growth in bacterial cells. The sequences of peptide ligands borne by fusion proteins can then be identified by means of simple molecular biological techniques.

As the peptides in both synthetic and fusion protein libraries are relatively short, a large portion of the surface area of the ligands identified from screening bears information relevant to the structure and chemistry of binding. This feature makes the peptide ligands derived from these libraries ideal lead compounds for structural analysis, modeling, and further modification. The purposes of this chapter are to describe the current synthetic and fusion protein libraries in use, to assess the relative advantages and disadvantages of these emerging technologies, and to outline the challenges facing future epitope library development and use. First, the role of peptides in the process of drug discovery, and in understanding protein recognition in general will be discussed.

II. IDENTIFYING LEAD COMPOUNDS FROM EPITOPE LIBRARIES

A. PEPTIDES AS LEAD COMPOUNDS

In the pharmaceutical industry, the discovery of lead compounds typically requires the screening of tens of thousands to millions of compounds with receptor-binding assays and takes about 2 years. Lead compounds, often having moderate affinity for the target receptor as well as poor pharmacologic properties, are then modified into pharmacologically useful agents. As with many lead compounds, peptides are poor candidates as final drug products. Peptides tend to be vulnerable to proteolytic attack, unable to cross the blood-brain barrier readily, and can be highly immunogenic. However, the structural and chemical information available from peptides can be applied to the design of non-peptide pharmaceuticals, making peptides potential lead compounds.

In most cases peptide ligands are derived by dint of "rational design". For example, Greene and coworkers utilized a monoclonal antibody (MAb) that recognizes the cellular receptor of reovirus type 3 and acts to inhibit virally induced cellular proliferation. Constrained peptides that block the receptor's activity were designed based on the hypothesis that a particular complementarity-determining region (CDR) of the MAb was involved in binding the cellular receptor.[15] This success proved that the CDR hypothesis was correct, and allowed a model to be built based on the structure of this region in the MAb along with the constrained peptides bearing the CDR sequence. The model in turn was used to design, synthesize, and confirm the structure of a nonpeptide ligand produced by organic synthesis.[16] This relatively small organic compound chemically and sterically mimics key amino acid side chains of the CDR model, and exhibits the biological activity of the MAb and CDR peptides. Moreover, the analog possesses chemical properties associated with good pharmacologic activity (i.e., small molecular weight, conformational rigidity, solubility, and resistance to proteolysis). This is one instance in which a viable drug candidate, via a peptide intermediate, was designed based on the activity of a protein epitope.

In contrast to this, lead peptides may be discovered in the same way that many lead compounds are found: by the "irrational design" of blind screening. The major advantages of screening epitope libraries, rather than the more conventional "gemisches", such as fungal extracts, used by drug companies, are that (1) many more potential ligands are screened *en bloc*, (2) screening involves the purification or direct synthesis of lead peptides as well as their detection, and (3) because epitope libraries are synthesized directly or made from expression vectors, the context of the molecular variability being screened can be controlled and thus optimized. By this approach, lead peptides could be identified in 2 weeks instead of 2 years using straightforward molecular biological and chemical tools.

B. EPITOPES, MIMOTOPES, AND THE REQUIREMENTS FOR BINDING

Besides the example cited above, there are many instances in which a protein-binding ligate will recognize both a contiguous sequence in the context of a larger protein, called a *continuous epitope*, as well as a short peptide comprising the same sequence (e.g., References 17 and 18). This testifies to the importance of forming noncovalent interactions between a few *critical residues* in an epitope and the ligate binding site. For many protein epitopes, where about 15 to 20 residues form the interface between antigen and antibody, only a small subset of these contacts involve the noncovalent interactions crucial for binding.[19-21] This concept, in part, underlies the strategy of using vast libraries of peptides to find ligands for protein-binding ligates that do not recognize continuous epitopes when presented as short peptide fragments, as well as for ligates that recognize nonprotein targets. Such peptides, called *mimotopes*,[1] are usually thought of as short sequences that chemically mimic epitopes on folded proteins. This type of epitope, termed an *assembled epitope*, is formed from a discontinuous sequence whose residues are brought into proximity by protein folding; thus, protein folding is necessary for the integrity of assembled epitopes. The mimotope concept can be extended to include peptides that mimic the chemistry and structure of *constrained continuous epitopes*, whose binding activity also depends upon protein folding, as well as *nonproteinaceous epitopes*. Thus, for the purposes of this chapter, *the term mimotope will be used to designate a ligand that functionally mimics the binding activity of another unrelated or poorly related ligand.*

For the sake of clarity, the term mimotope should be contrasted with the terms analog, ligand, and mimetic.[22] *Analogs* are structurally and/or chemically homologous compounds with similar ligate-binding function. The term *ligand* refers to any compound that binds a macromolecule, but does not address its structure. *Mimetics* (agonists or antagonists) are ligands that either stimulate or diminish the activity of a receptor without regard for chemical structure. Thus, a mimotope can be thought of as a ligand having similar binding activity to native ligand, but a nonhomologous structure. This concept is important to drug design, as the most valuable lead peptides are often those which provide unexpected solutions to the problem of ligate binding. Such peptides provide unique insights into the requirements for binding ligate.

As the exact forces governing protein recognition are generally not well understood, the sequence of a mimotope may be difficult to deduce *a priori*. They may better be found by blindly screening vast peptide libraries with a ligate. Other residue clusters in the binding site may be available for binding, but are not in contact with the native ligand. These would also be involved in the screening process. Thus, epitope library screening may turn up *epitope fingerprints* comprising mimotopes that bind ligate using the same chemistry as native ligand, as well as those that use different chemistries to bind other residue clusters within or near the binding site.

The purpose of the epitope libraries and their screening approaches described in the sections below are aimed at two goals: (1) to test the performance of epitope libraries by assessing whether sequences are found that are related to the unconstrained, short peptide sequences known to bind a ligate; and (2) more significantly, to identify unanticipated peptide ligands by screening these vast peptide libraries. For many ligates, success in achieving this second goal will depend upon the ability to obtain mimotopes for ligates that normally recognize assembled, constrained continuous, or nonproteinaceous epitopes.

III. SYNTHETIC PEPTIDE LIBRARIES

The earliest synthetic peptide libraries, first pioneered by Mario Geysen, identified continuous epitopes using *peptide scans* of proteins.[23] These are relatively small collections of short peptides sharing overlapping sequences corresponding to the sequence of a protein antigen (e.g., for a protein of 100 residues, 96 separate pentapeptides, covering residues 1-5, 2-6, 3-7, ..., and 96-100) that are each made separately and tested for binding. Three general results were obtained from performing peptide scans with a number of MAbs as well as polyclonal sera. First, some of the antibodies in an antibody response to a protein typically recognize a few epitopes in a peptide scan; in these cases four to six residues are critical to binding. Second, only about 10 to 15% of all MAbs screened in peptide scans recognize short peptide epitopes.[23] Thus, Geysen and others concluded that most antibodies in a response recognize assembled epitopes not present in peptide scans. Assuming that a few critical residues are also involved in binding assembled epitopes, Geysen and colleagues devised the *mimotope strategy* as a way of identifying short peptides whose residues mimicked those of an assembled epitope.[1] I will call this novel strategy *multistep screening*, as it can be used to find the sequences of continuous epitopes as well,[2,3] and so that the reader can discriminate it from other *en bloc* approaches to screening.

A. MULTISTEP SCREENING WITH LIBRARIES OF PIN-BOUND PEPTIDES

Multistep screening involves an iterative process for deducing the sequence of a peptide ligand. Hundreds of mixed peptide pools of limited diversity are synthesized and screened for binding to a ligate. The peptide pools that bind ligate best are then used to direct the synthesis of a new set of peptide pools of even less diversity. These are tested for binding, and the process of synthesis and screening is repeated until a set of single peptides is attained.

In the system developed by Geysen et al.,[1] each peptide pool is synthesized on a separate polyethylene pin and tested for binding to ligate. The length of each peptide is five to seven residues, and the amino acid composition at each position is either *fixed*, i.e., comprising a single amino acid at that position, or *randomized*, i.e., synthesized with a mixture of all 20 amino acids so that all residues occur with equal frequency at that position. In the example below defining a hexapeptide epitope, two positions, say the third and fourth, are chosen as fixed and the remaining four are synthesized as randomized positions; 400 (20^2) pools are made, each having a different combination of amino acids at the fixed positions (**XXAAXX, XXACXX, XXADXX, ..., XXYVXX, XXYWXX, XXYYXX**)*. These mixed peptide pools are each tested for binding to ligate, and the pools with the highest signals are chosen for the next screening step. For each peptide mixture chosen, say **XXADXX**, 40 smaller peptide pools are synthesized; 20 in which position 2 is fixed (**XAADXX, ..., XYADXX**), and 20 in which position 5 is fixed (**XXADAX, ..., XXADYX**). These peptide pools are tested for binding, and the tightest binding pools are selected and used to direct a third round of synthesis and selection. In these 40 syntheses, the second through fifth positions are specified by the previous round, to be for example, **KADY**; every amino acid in the first position is fixed and

* Amino acids denoted by Ala, A; Cys, C; Asp, D; Glu, E; Phe, F; Gly, G; His, H; Ile, I; Lys, K; Leu, L; Met, M; Asn, N; Pro, P; Gln, Q; Arg, R; Ser, S; Thr, T; Val, V; Trp, W; Tyr, Y; any of the 20 natural L-amino acids, X.

the sixth is randomized, or conversely the sixth position is fixed in 20 ways and the first is randomized. The peptide mixtures are tested for binding, with the fixed positions having the tightest binding being used to define the sequence of the final product. Thus, the sequence of hexapeptide ligands are deduced after three rounds of synthesis and binding. At present, about 1 μmol of peptide can be synthesized on each pin. Chemistry has been developed to allow removal of peptide from the pins, giving free peptide mixtures.[24]

There are two published instances in which mimotope peptides have been found.[1,25] The first case involves a MAb that binds the VP1 capsid protein of the foot and mouth disease virus type A_{10}.[1] The sequence **WQMGHS** gave the highest activity; this sequence is not present in the VP1 protein. This lead peptide was then studies in a series of replacement studies where D- and nonnatural amino acids were introduced into the chain (see Section V). In a second study, a Bence Jones light chain dimer and its corresponding immunoglobulin G (IgG) were screened in a series of "extension" studies, in which a series of progressively longer peptides containing L-, D- and nonnatural amino acids were tested.[25] Two nonrelated sequences that bound the dimer were identified and shown by preliminary X-ray crystallographic studies to bind the cleft that other antigens were known to bind. The IgG also recognized the peptides, but had different preferences for related peptides in the series.

These are the only published cases in which true mimotopes have been successfully identified from synthetic peptide libraries. In most cases, however, tight-binding mimotopes are not found.[23a] Instead, a wide variety of weak-binding peptides is found, rather than a few closely related, tight-binding sequences. Interestingly, the outcome of screening may change depending upon which positions are chosen as fixed in the first step of this strategy. For this reason, Geysen's group now begins screening with hexapeptide mixtures comprising all five possible combinations of adjacent residues, such that 2000 peptide mixtures (instead of 400) with two fixed residues are used in the first step of screening.[58]

There are several potential disadvantages of this approach. The first has to do with the screening strategy itself, which relies on the overall signal obtained from a peptide pool. The signal in a given pool may be relatively strong because of a large number of weak-binding peptides, or the signal may be weak yet represent a few tight-binding peptides; this is especially true for the initial peptide pools where there are over 100,000 different species. Secondly, not more than about six randomized residues can be screened by this strategy, since the maximum capacity of each pin is 1 mmol of peptide (or about 15 pmol of each different 6-mer). Finally, there may be significant differences in the behavior of peptides in the immobilized vs. free form that affect their interaction with ligate.

B. MULTISTEP SCREENING WITH LIBRARIES OF FREE PEPTIDES

Houghten and coworkers have devised a novel means of using libraries of free peptides in a multistep screening strategy.[2] They previously developed a "teabag" approach to multiple peptide synthesis.[26] Peptides are synthesized by standard t-Boc chemistry on a resin support confined in teabags, which can be transferred between reaction mixtures. Each teabag ultimately contains a different peptide. In each step of peptide synthesis, the teabags are distributed among reaction mixtures, with each mixture adding a different protected amino acid. After multiple rounds of synthesis, the completed peptides are cleaved from the beads and the side chain protecting groups are removed. This synthetic approach uses straightforward reaction conditions, for only a single amino acid is added to the peptides in any given reaction. Relatively large reactions can be carried out using up to 250 g of beads (equivalent to 225 mmol of peptide).

This multiple peptide synthesis strategy was modified to make pools of free hexapeptides that could be screened by a multistep strategy.[2] The initial set of hexapeptide pools comprised fixed residues at the first and second positions, and randomized ones at the C-terminal four positions. The randomized positions are synthesized first and the fixed ones last, since peptide synthesis proceeds from C- to N-terminus. All of the amino acids (except Cys) were added at the sixth position by splitting the beads evenly between 19 bags and reacting each of the bags with a different amino acid. The beads were removed from the bags and mixed together, then split evenly between 19 reactions for addition at the fifth randomized position, and this was repeated for the randomized residues occurring at the fourth and third positions. For the synthesis of fixed residues at the first and second fixed positions, the beads were split among 400 teabags and the two designated amino acids were added consecutively. About two billion resin particles are present in the 400 g of resin used in the synthesis of this library. Thus, most or all of the 52 million hexapeptides possible from this synthesis strategy are present in the library, as on average, each peptide in the library is synthesized on 19 resin particles. The completed hexapeptides were deprotected and cleaved from the beads, providing a maximum concentration of each peptide in a pool at about 100 n*M*. Each peptide pool was tested for its ability to block the binding of a ligate to its target, then, as with the screening strategy described above, the best peptide pools were used to direct the synthesis of the 20 peptide pools having fixed residues at the third position. These pools were tested and after three further rounds of synthesis and screening, the remaining three positions of the peptide were determined. A total of 480 syntheses were required for this screening.

Houghten's group has obtained impressive results by using free peptides for screening, as the activity of free peptide is detected by its ability to *block* binding of test ligand to a target ligate. This allows for the use of bioassays in which the ligate for screening the peptide library is not purified or even known in some cases. The sequences of the peptide pools that are most effective at blocking the assay signal are used in determining the next round of synthesis. Peptides were identified that are known to bind two different MAbs. Moreover, the N-terminal sequences of Met- and Leu-enkephalin were identified by an assay in which the binding of a radiolabeled Met-enkephalin analog to crude membrane preparations from rat brain was blocked in the presence of active peptide mixtures.[2,3] Two different peptides that block the growth of the Gram-positive pathogen *Staphylococcus aureus* were deduced by testing peptide pools for their ability to inhibit bacterial growth. Tables 1A and 1B show the development of the peptides from two different starting pools (**RRXXXX** and **FRXXXX**) that significantly inhibited bacterial growth. This result points up an interesting facet of multistep screening approaches, in that more than one peptide mixture in the initial library may react with ligate (in this case an unknown ligate on bacterial cells).

Unlike the other peptide library screening strategies described in this review, this approach has the unique advantage of using free peptides, obviating the need for purified, or even characterized, ligate for screening. Peptide ligands can be identified from the inhibition of bioassay activity, assuming that a single binding specificity, or a set of related binding specificities, is responsible for activity (e.g., a MAb rather than polyclonal antibodies is used for screening). With free peptides, there is also no danger of potential differences in affinity arising between a peptide's bound and free forms. A large amount of peptide can be synthesized, depending on the amount of beads used for synthesis.

As was mentioned in the preceeding section the multistep screening strategy itself poses two potential problems that may especially affect the initial peptide pools: (1) the number of peptides contributing to a given signal from a peptide pool may vary, thus leading to falsely high or low signals, and (2) there may be different outcomes depending on which positions in the sequence are initially fixed. Furthermore, if a synthetic strategy is used in which the position of the two initial fixed amino acids is different from the N-terminus, then many more separate syntheses in teabags must be used than the 480 used to make this library. For instance, if a hexapeptide library were made in which the two C-terminal residues are fixed, 32,400 teabags would have to be used. A potential disadvantage of using free peptides is that bias may occur because of the absence of peptides that are poorly soluble or insoluble, whereas resin-bound peptides may remain soluble, depending on the nature of the linker arm attaching them to the support.

TABLE 1A
Pathway of Identifying the Antimicrobial Peptide RRWWCX

Peptide Mixture	IC$_{50}$ (mg/ml)	Peptide Mixture	IC$_{50}$ (µg/ml)
2nd Screen		**4th Screen**	
Ac-RRXXXX-NH_2	450	Ac-RRWWXX-NH_2	32
Ac-RRWXXX-NH_2	216	Ac-RRWWCX-NH_2	8.7
Ac-RRYXXX-NH_2	239	Ac-RRWWWX-NH_2	9.9
Ac-RRRXXX-NH_2	275	Ac-RRWWRX-NH_2	9.9
Ac-RRHXXX-NH_2	286	Ac-RRWWFX-NH_2	12
Ac-RRCXXX-NH_2	338	Ac-RRWWIX-NH_2	14
3rd Screen		**5th Screen**	
Ac-RRWXXX-NH_2	273	Ac-RRWWCX-NH_2	8.7
Ac-RRWWXX-NH_2	36	Ac-RRWWCR-NH_2	3.4
Ac-RRWFXX-NH_2	58	Ac-RRWWCW-NH_2	4.1
Ac-RRWRXX-NH_2	77	Ac-RRWWCV-NH_2	4.9
Ac-RRWCXX-NH_2	88	Ac-RRWWCY-NH_2	5.4
Ac-RRWLXX-NH_2	178	Ac-RRWWCK-NH_2	5.5

TABLE 1B
Pathway of Identifying the Antimicrobial Peptide FRWLLX

Peptide Mixture	IC$_{50}$ (mg/ml)	Peptide Mixture	IC$_{50}$ (µg/ml)
2nd Screen		**4th Screen**	
AC-FRXXXX-NH_2	1730	Ac-FRWLXX-NH_2	111
Ac-FRWXXX-NH_2	459	Ac-FRWLCX-NH_2	12
Ac-FRLXXX-NH_2	526	Ac-FRWLWX-NH_2	13
Ac-FRFXXX-NH_2	559	Ac-FRWLLX-NH_2	19
Ac-FRMXXX-NH_2	676	Ac-FRWLRX-NH_2	24
Ac-FRHXXX-NH_2	758	Ac-FRWLFX-NH_2	33
3rd Screen		**5th Screen**	
Ac-FRWXXX-NH_2	459	Ac-FRWLLX-NH_2	19
Ac-FRWWXX-NH_2	67	Ac-FRWLLF-NH_2	11
Ac-FRWLXX-NH_2	111	Ac-FRWLLR-NH_2	13
Ac-FRWMXX-NH_2	135	Ac-FRWLLW-NH_2	14
Ac-FRWCXX-NH_2	145	Ac-FRWLLC-NH_2	15
Ac-FRWRXX-NH_2	155	Ac-FRWLLL-NH_2	18

C. SELECTIDE LIBRARIES

Selectide libraries were devised by Lam and coworkers.[4] In this elegant approach, each peptide sequence is displayed on a separate bead, allowing millions of peptides to be screened *en bloc* for binding to ligate. The original library consisted of about 2 million beads, with each bead displaying 50 to 200 pmol of a single pentapeptide sequence. The peptides in this library were synthesized by the same approach described for the free peptide libraries, except that only randomized positions (consisting of the common amino acids except Cys) were made. The beads were divided into 19 vessels and in each, a different amino acid addition was carried out using standard Fmoc chemistry. The beads were removed, mixed, divided into 19 new aliquots and put through another round of synthesis. At the end of five cycles a library of 2 million beads, comprising 81% of the 2.5 million pentapeptides possible (19^5), was ready for screening.

Screening involves reacting the beads with ligate in a volume of about 20 ml, washing, and then reacting with a second "detection" antibody, that binds to the ligate and is linked to either a fluorescent tag or an enzyme. In the latter case, the enzyme is incubated with a precipitable

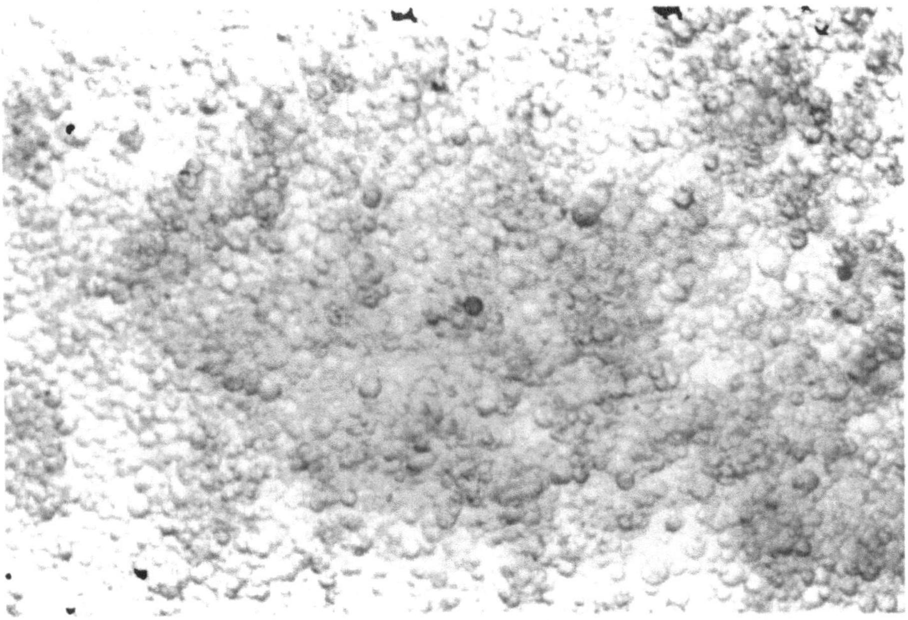

FIGURE 1. Positively reacting beads as viewed from a dissecting microscope. (Kindly provided by K. Lam, University of Arizona, Tucson.)

substrate that colors positive beads. After washing, the beads are added to 21 microtiter plates (about 500 beads per well) and scanned by microscope to find fluorescent or colored beads (the beads are about 100 μm in diameter). Figure 1 shows a photograph of the positive (colored) beads on a background of negative (colorless) beads. A single positive bead is removed using micromanipulators (which are somewhat like microtweezers), then washed and directly sequenced. About three beads can be sequenced per day using an automated sequencer.

The efficacy of affinity selection (i.e., the ability to identify the tightest-binding peptides present in a library) can be assessed in several ways. First, the occurrence of a *consensus sequence* among independent beads indicates that affinity selection by ligate has occurred. The most important residues for binding are revealed by comparing the sequences of peptide ligands from a given *consensus group.* Highly selected residues that are critical for binding are conserved among peptides in a consensus group, while other residues may vary. Consensus sequences can be synthesized as free peptides, and their relative affinity for ligate compared with that of a known ligand. Both sequence comparisons and binding studies are important for determining the optimal conditions for affinity selection. Binding studies are also necessary for deciding if the affinity and selectivity of peptides isolated with biologically important ligates is strong enough to permit their use as probes, antigens, or mimetics.

The pentapeptide library described above was screened with two ligates, the β-endorphin-binding MAb 3-E7 and streptavidin. These ligates are known to bind short, unconstrained peptides and have previously been used to identify peptides from other libraries.[6,7,27] In each case, beads bearing the correct consensus sequences were identified.[4,28] Using MAb 3-E7 under optimal conditions, about 200 beads of varying color intensity were identified.[59]

The main advantage of this approach, and all *en bloc* screening strategies, is that each peptide in the library is given an equal chance at binding. A further advantage of this system is that, once the library is made, library screening takes a day. A portion of the peptides on a bead can be cleaved off and used for testing, allowing the remainder to be used for sequencing, which may aid in limiting the number of beads chosen for sequencing.

The selectide library is limited to about two million peptides because, for most purposes, a 200-ml reaction volume and 4000 microtiter wells are the largest workable sizes for screening. One disadvantage of this approach is that the microscopic screening procedure is fairly labor intensive, while sequencing a large number of clones takes a considerable amount of time. As mentioned above, potential problems come from bias in the representation of peptides that may arise during synthesis and in the presentation of peptide by immobilization.

D. ADVANTAGES/DISADVANTAGES OF SYNTHETIC PEPTIDE LIBRARIES

Synthetic peptide libraries have several advantages for ligand screening. Of greatest importance, unnatural amino acids, including those creating branched polypeptide chains, can be used in a synthetic library. This allows for the engineering of *local* constraints into peptide structures.[29,30] Compared with the more complex fusion protein libraries described in the following section, libraries of free peptides or peptides linked to a chemically neutral, homogeneous carrier are less likely to produce biases in the presentation of peptide for binding. Moreover, the free peptide library strategy offers the added option of screening based on bioassay activities. This enables the use of unpurified or very complex ligates, such as crude extracts, membrane preparations, and living cells, for screening.

A major disadvantage in the use of synthetic peptide libraries is the limitation in the length of the peptides. At this time it is difficult to synthesize libraries of peptides of more than 15 residues. The synthesis of *globally* constrained peptides[29,30] in which variable regions form part of a larger structural framework, is prohibited due to this length restriction; however, there may be alternative ways of imposing global constraints on short peptides that would be amenable to the synthesis of peptide libraries. Most of the synthetic peptide libraries exclude Cys residues because of the threat of forming *inter*molecular rather than *intra*molecular disulfide bridges; yet this strategy is often used in nature for constraining small, biologically active peptides.

Although each of the amino acids in the mixed pools is added with good overall efficiency at any step, small inherent biases may exist that reduce the efficiency of addition of particular amino acids at the N-termini of a small population of peptide sequences. Such small biases may cause certain peptides or groups of related peptides to be missing or under-represented in a library. This raises an important point. It is extremely difficult to determine if small, unexpected biases are present in a library, whether of synthetic or fusion protein origin, and thus to assess the true representation of peptide sequences. Instead, only gross estimates of representation can be made based on (1) the amount of peptide made (in the case of the pin and free peptide strategies), (2) how many beads were used (in the free peptide and selectide strategies), (3) the composition of amino acids at a randomized position in a sequence (all strategies), or (4) sequencing a number of fusion protein clones or beads bearing a single peptide each (the selectide strategy). Similar drawbacks exist with the fusion protein libraries, as will be discussed below.

IV. FUSION PROTEIN LIBRARIES

The "random peptides" in fusion protein libraries actually comprise regions of randomized sequences *(variable regions)* that have been engineered into a larger protein. In contrast to synthetic peptide libraries, where random peptide sequences are generated directly from chemical synthesis, the randomized peptides in fusion protein libraries are produced by bacterial cells that have been transformed with vector DNA bearing *degenerate* nucleotide sequences encoding random peptide sequences. These degenerate sequences are chemically synthesized as oligonucleotides with mixtures of nucleotides at the randomized positions. The oligonucleotides are then spliced into the fusion protein gene located on the vector DNA. The design of the cloning vehicle is such that each unique fusion protein is physically associated with the nucleic acid encoding it. As described below, the fusion proteins used in these libraries include (1) coat proteins of filamentous bacteriophage, which are encoded by a phage or phagemid genome,[5-12] (2) a *lac* repressor protein, which binds directly to the plasmid encoding it,[13] and (3) a plasmid-encoded bacterial surface receptor for phage λ.[14]

As with selectide libraries, the peptides in fusion protein libraries are screened *en bloc*. Rather than selectively labeling peptide ligands, however, ligate binding is used to physically isolate fusion protein/nucleic complexes in the form of phage, repressor-bound plasmid, and bacteria by affinity purification *(panning)*. In panning strategies, fusion proteins bearing peptide ligands bind to immobilized ligate, then the vast majority of fusion proteins bearing nonbinding peptide sequences are removed by extensive washing. Thus, the fusion proteins that have survived washing by binding immobilized ligate are selectively enriched. The bound fusion proteins are released from the ligate and are amplified in bacterial cells by virtue of their associated nucleic acid sequences. This strategy of selective enrichment followed by amplification can be repeated until a pure population of binding peptides is attained. Moreover, the conditions of enrichment can be modified through the course of repeated pannings to force binding peptides to compete with each other for ligate, thus encouraging selection of the best binders. Selected peptide sequences are obtained by the isolation and sequencing of DNA in the region encoding the peptide, and amplified fusion protein clones can be directly tested for binding to ligate. When binding peptides are successfully identified from screening a library, their sequences are often homologous, forming a consensus group. As with selectide screening, panning selects different peptides bearing particular critical binding residues, with sequence variation at other positions. Consensus sequence information can be used to direct the synthesis of free peptides, which can be tested directly for binding and bioactivity. The peptides identified from such experiments are the ultimate products for testing as lead compounds.

Fusion protein libraries offer a means of building variable regions into the framework of a larger constrained peptide, thus imposing structural restrictions on the variable region sequences. This section on fusion protein libraries includes discussions of the potential for these systems to express properly folded proteins, as well as multimeric proteins. This feature of structural design has bearing on the final section of this review, which discusses the design of peptide libraries with the goal of producing mimotopes that better imitate assembled, constrained continuous and nonproteinaceous epitopes.

A. FILAMENTOUS PHAGE LIBRARIES

The randomized sequences in phage libraries are fused to a coat protein of a bacterial virus, allowing the peptides to be displayed on the viral surface. Two proteins have been used as vehicles for displaying these peptides, a *minor coat protein pIII* and the *major coat protein pVIII*.[31] In both fusion systems, the variable regions are placed at the N-terminus of the coat protein, or a few residues from it. In general, the termini of proteins are more flexible than most other parts of proteins and are exposed to solvent. Therefore, termini are more likely to tolerate the insertion of foreign peptides and to present them for recognition. Furthermore, insertions at protein termini are less likely to be structurally influenced by the coat protein than if they were located further within the sequence. Foreign sequences ranging from short peptides to relatively large protein domains, such as antibody Fabs, have been expressed on both pIII[5-7,9,11,12,31-38] and pVIII.[8,10,36-41]

The minor coat protein pIII folds into two domains. The C-terminal domain interacts with viral coat proteins and is required for viral assembly, whereas the N-terminal two thirds of the protein forms a knob-like domain that projects away from the virions, and functions to infect male *Escherichia coli* cells by binding to F pili. Foreign sequences have been successfully displayed at or near the N-terminus of mature pIII,[5-7,9,11,12,33-38] as well as in the hinge region, located between the two domains of pIII.[31,32] As shown in Figure 2A, recombinant phage bearing foreign sequences in pIII are multivalent with regard to the peptide epitope they display, as pIII occurs in four to five closely apposed copies at one tip of the virion. (For simplicity's sake, only a single copy of pIII is shown, rather than the four to five copies that are actually present on the virion.)

Alternatively, the major coat protein pVIII can be used to display foreign sequences. When insertions of over five residues are introduced near the N-terminus of pVIII, phage assembly is disrupted.[39] This can be overcome by supplying both wild-type and recombinant pVIII for viral assembly via a *phagemid* expression system.[8,10,36-41] Recombinant pVIII is encoded on a phagemid, a plasmid that also encodes the intergenic region of filamentous phage, which includes the origins of replication and the morphogenetic signal *mos*.[31] Wild-type pVIII and other proteins involved in viral replication and morphogenesis are supplied by "helper phage", so that phagemid DNA encoding the recombinant coat protein is copied into single strands and packaged into viral coats. Figure 2B shows that multiple copies of recombinant pVIII mix with wild-type pVIII to form the viral coat, which surrounds the phagemid genome encoding the recombinant fusion protein. In contrast to the clustered fusion proteins displayed by pIII, each pVIII-based fusion protein is probably locally monovalent, since fusion products are most likely surrounded by wild-type pVIII to maintain virion stability. Phagemid approaches have also been used to make pIII-based libraries of larger domain proteins, such as human growth hormone,[34,42] antibody binding domains,[35-37] and alkaline phosphatase,[35-37] which are displayed as one or fewer copies per phage.

Whether displayed as part of a pIII or a pVIII protein, the variable region borne by each phage clone in a library comprises a different amino acid sequence. To make a phage library (detailed procedures in Reference 43), a mixture of oligonucleotides, called a *degenerate oligonucleotide*, is synthesized by using single nucleotides at positions encoding the invariant portions of the sequence and mixed nucleotides at residues encoding the variable region. Each randomized amino acid in the variable region is encoded by a *degenerate codon*, represented by either **NNK** or **NNS**, which includes all four nucleotides (**N**) in the first and second positions, and G and T (**K**) or G and C (**S**) in the third. All 20 amino acids and one stop codon are encoded by the 32 different codons represented by **NNK** or **NNS**. As shown in the example in Figure 3, the variable regions are flanked by invariant regions in the degenerate oligonucleotide to allow cloning into the vector DNA. The degenerate oligonucleotides are cloned (either directly, or after polymerase chain reaction [PCR] amplification and digestion with restriction endonucleases) into the appropriate sites in the coat protein genes of the phage or a phagemid vector. Ligated product is introduced into bacterial cells by electroporation with an efficiency of about 10^9 transformants per microgram of covalently closed DNA. Phage are propagated by the transformed cells, then collected and purified.

The number of phage clones in a library is crucial to its utility. For instance, a library containing all possible hexapeptides would consist of 64 million (20^6) different six-amino acid sequences and would be encoded by about one billion (32^6) different hexa-codons. Thus, a hexapeptide library that includes all possible six-amino acid sequences must contain well over a billion phage clones. Libraries of up to 200-300 million independent clones have been constructed, with a workable library probably having an upper limit of ten billion clones. Six residues is the maximum length of a variable region if all possible sequences are to be screened. Given the same number of clones in the library, a longer variable region, such as a 15-mer, will represent a larger fraction of the total number of hexapeptides than a short, say hexamer, variable region.

Figure 4 shows an example of a typical panning experiment[33] (detailed procedures in Reference 43). Biotinylated ligate is reacted with a library. Phage-bearing peptide ligands are then affinity purified by immobilizing phage: biotinylated ligate complexes on plates coated with streptavidin, washing away free phage and eluting the bound phage with acid. The eluted phage are amplified by growth in bacterial cells and then used in subsequent rounds of panning to further enrich for binding phage. Phage clones can be amplified, isolated, and tested for binding to ligate. The amino acid sequence of the epitope region can be deduced from sequencing the single-stranded DNA from virions. The occurrence of consensus

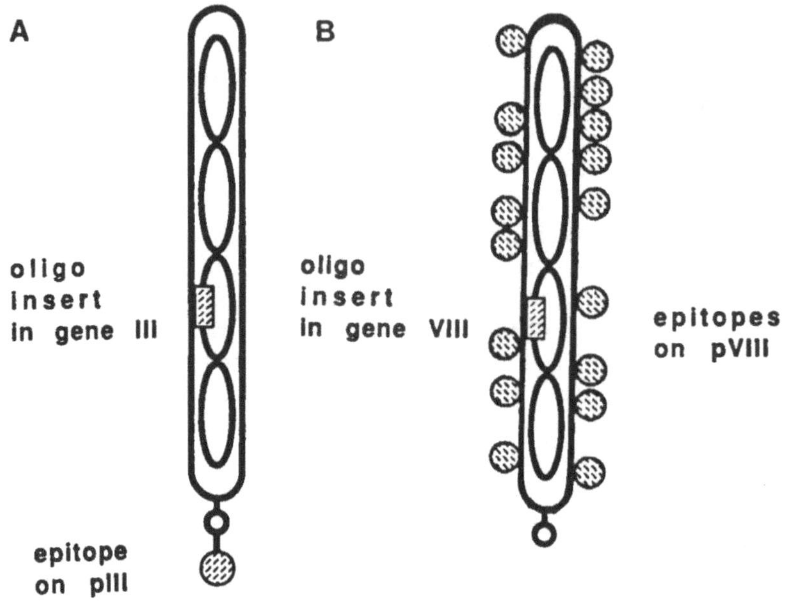

FIGURE 2. Filamentous bacteriophage displaying peptide epitopes fused to the minor viral coat protein pIII (A) and the major coat protein pVIII (B). Also shown is the single-stranded DNA genome of the phage, which bears an oligonucleotide insert encoding the displayed epitope. (Kindly provided by G.P. Smith and copied with permission from Reference 38).

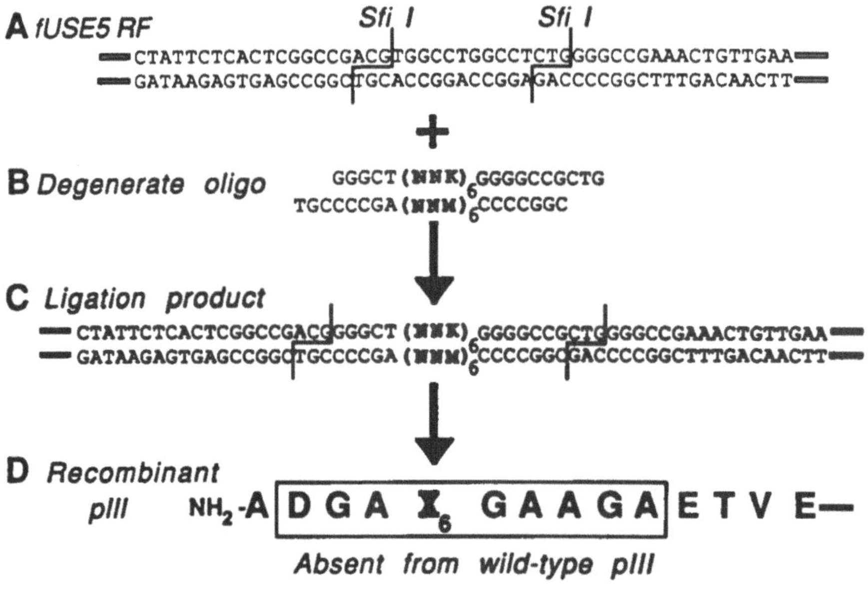

FIGURE 3. Construction of a recombinant viral genome bearing epitope-encoding degenerate oligonucleotide inserts in pIII. The DNA of the fUSE5 vector (A) is cleaved with SfiI then ligated with a similarly cleaved, double-stranded oligonucleotide bearing degenerate (NNK) codons (B) to form a recombinant genome (C). The amino acid sequence of mature recombinant pIII, starting at the N-terminus of the pIII fusion product (D). (Adapted from Reference 5 and copied with permission from Reference 38.)

sequences among independent phage clones indicates selective enrichment of ligate-binding phage from the library.

Work with eight different phage libraries has been described.[5-12] The variable regions displayed by five of these libraries include random, unconstrained hexapeptides,[5,6]

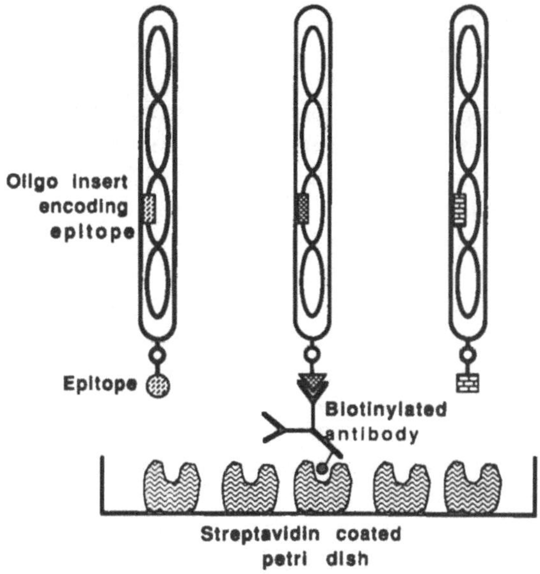

FIGURE 4. Panning, a method of purifying phage that bind ligate. Three phage clones are shown, each bearing a different peptide sequence fused to pIII. Phage from a library are reacted with biotinylated ligate, then immobilized on a streptavidin-coated plate and extensively washed to remove unbound or weakly binding phage. The bound phage are eluted from the plate in acid, and base is added to neutralize the eluates. The phage are concentrated, used to infect cells, and propagated. The resulting amplified phage can be partially purified and used in further rounds of panning, or cloned, sequenced in the epitope region and tested for binding to ligate. (Copied with permission from References 38 and 43.)

octapeptides,[8,9] and pentapeptides.[7] Three other libraries display disulfide-bridged loops constraining variable regions of four,[11] six,[12] and nine[10] residues. These libraries have been used to identify different consensus groups whose peptides bind six MAbs,[5,6,8,10,11,44] a peptide-binding cellular receptor,[12] and two ligates that recognize nonproteinaceous ligands: streptavidin[7,11] (which binds biotin) and the plant lectin concanavalin A (Con A),[9,45] (which binds mannosyl residues). The MAbs and the cellular receptor were especially useful for testing the efficacy of library screening, because the consensus sequences they identified corresponded to the continuous epitopes on native protein ligands that these ligates recognize.

Phage libraries can be fairly well purified compared with other fusion protein libraries, making them less complex reagents. The phage are resistant to a variety of conditions, including heat, proteolytic degradation, and low pH.[31] In addition, the viral coat protects the single-stranded genome from attack by nucleases. The phage expression system is also excellent for displaying properly folded proteins, even multimeric ones.[34,37,41] For instance, antibody libraries displaying Fab have been constructed in which the heavy chain variable domain ($V_H + C_{H1}$) is fused with pIII or pVIII and encoded by a phagemid.[35,41] The light chain variable domain ($V_L + C_L$) is also encoded on the phagemid and, after synthesis, is secreted into the periplasmic space, where it associates with the coat protein-borne V_H to make phage-displayed Fab.

The variable regions of phage-displayed peptide libraries are encoded by degenerate codons that do not represent the amino acids equally. Although the bias toward overrepresenting certain amino acids (such as Leu, Ser, and Arg) is lessened compared with an NNN degenerate codon, there still remain multiple codons for several amino acids and only one for others. Moreover, amber stop codons (a signal for terminating translation) are introduced in the variable region by NNK and NNS degenerate codons. The problem of chain termination can be overcome by growing the phage in an amber suppressor strain of bacteria, in which amber suppressor tRNAs read amber stop codons and add a specific amino acid to the polypeptide chain, so that its extension is not terminated.[35,42] Another potential problem with this system is biased representation of certain peptide sequences or classes due to biological selection. For instance, a given peptide may prevent its fusion coat protein from crossing the cell's inner membrane, interfere with the process of infection or uncoating, or disrupt assembly of the viral coat. So far, such problems have not been detected. As mentioned above, however, significant but proportionally small biases would be difficult if not impossible to detect in this or any large library.

B. THE *lac* REPRESSOR PROTEIN LIBRARY

Fusion protein libraries using the *lac* repressor protein are also called *peptides-on-plasmid* libraries. A library of this type was made of random dodecapeptides that were engineered at the C-terminus of the *lac* repressor protein, LacI.[13] After synthesis within the cell, the repressor protein fusion product binds to the plasmid encoding it by virtue of two *lac O* sites (which are the binding sites for the *lac* repressor) present on the plasmid (Figure 5). Optimal library construction depends on the production of similar amounts of plasmid and protein within each cell, so that neither is in the unbound state in the library. Expression of the *lacI* fusion gene is controlled by the *araB* promoter, which is, in turn, both positively and negatively regulated by the AraC protein, also encoded by the plasmid. Thus, the ratio of plasmid to fusion protein can be controlled by the *araB* promoter, which is repressed in the presence of glucose in the growth medium, and induced by L-arabinose.

A library was made of about 550 million clones bearing a random dodecapeptide fused to the C-terminus of the *lac* repressor. Bacterial cells were transformed with recombinant plasmid bearing a degenerate region composed of 12 contiguous NNK codons located at the C-terminus-encoding region of *lac I*. The cells were grown under conditions that optimized the repressor:plasmid ratio, then lysed, centrifuged, and the crude supernatant washed and concentrated. These partially purified lysates were screened with magnetic beads that had been coated with ligate. In this case, the ligate used was MAb D32.39, which binds the C-terminal region of a 13-residue opioid peptide. The lysate:bead reactions were washed extensively. The bound plasmid was eluted and purified by phenol extraction and ethanol precipitation, and used to transform cells. Lysates made from these cells were used in a second round of panning, extraction, precipitation, and transformation. After four rounds, the transformed cells were cloned and infected with helper phage, which allowed for the production of virions bearing single-stranded copies of the plasmid (which is actually a phagemid) for sequencing. Phagemid DNA was sequenced in the peptide region, revealing a six to seven-residue consensus sequence that was similar to the C-terminal region of the opioid peptide.

This library is unique for two important reasons. First, it is a fusion protein library with a C-terminal variable region, which is useful for screening with ligates that recognize epitopes comprising C-terminal sequences. Second, this is the closest version of a "stripped down" fusion protein library system available. This system draws library design closer to Tuerk and Gold's suggestion of peptide libraries that covalently link a translated product with the nucleic acid encoding it.[46]

There are several possible disadvantages to using libraries of peptides- or proteins-on-plasmids. As with all fusion protein libraries, there is bias that may be introduced in this particular biological system. There may be considerable binding of peptides in a library to bacterial cellular constituents, which would make them unavailable for screening, or there may be peptides that block binding of the *lac*-fusion to the repressor sites on the plasmid. The problem of protein folding is of concern, as foreign proteins that are not secreted often aggregate within the bacterial cell, forming inclusion bodies. This is in part due to the reducing environment of the cell, which prevents disulfide bridge formation. Finally, panning must be restricted to conditions that both prevent the degradation of plasmid DNA and favor binding of the repressor protein to the plasmid, with the protein to plasmid ratio optimized to yield mainly bound complex.

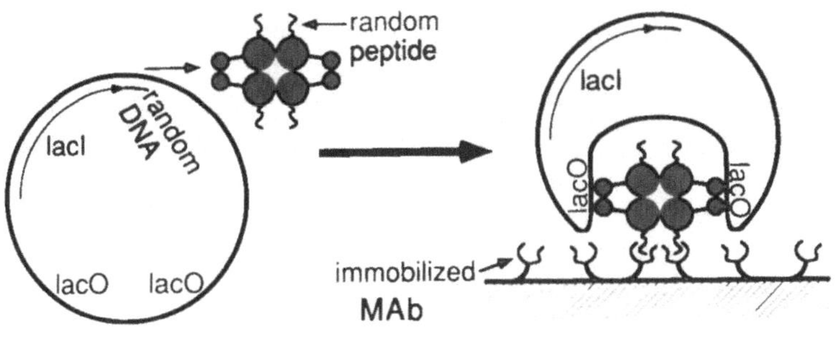

FIGURE 5. Design of the peptides-on-plasmids library. The library plasmid carries the *lacI* gene with a variable region fused to its 3′ end. The *lacI* repressor-peptide fusion produced by the recombinant gene binds the *lacO* sites on the same plasmid that encodes it. After lysis of cells containing the random library, those plasmid-repressor-variable region complexes that specifically bind an immobilized MAb are enriched by affinity purification. Transformation of *E. coli* with recovered plasmids amplifies these DNAs, allowing additional rounds of panning or sequencing of isolated clones. (Adapted from Reference 13; kindly provided by P. Schatz, Affymax Research Institute, Palo Alto.)

C. THE PHAGE λ RECEPTOR LIBRARY

The receptor for phage λ, the product of the *lamB* gene, has been used to construct a library of peptides displayed on the surface of *E. coli* cells.[14] The λ receptor spans the outer membrane of the cell a number of times, functioning both in the diffusion of maltose and maltodextrins through the outer membrane, as well as in λ infection. Three sites, corresponding to surface exposed loops on the protein, have been identified as regions that can accept inserts of foreign amino acid sequences.[47] Site LamB153 is known to accept sequences of up to 55-60 residues,[48] including the C3 epitope of poliovirus.[49] This was chosen as the site of insertion of the variable region for this library.[14] Variable regions were constructed by ligating together multiple oligonucleotide units, each encoding 11 amino acids, 9 of which are randomized. Depending on its orientation in the ligated product, each oligonucleotide unit bore either the sequence **(VNN)$_9$**, where **V** equally represents **A, C,** and **G,** or its complement, **(NNB)$_9$**, where **B** represents **T, C,** and **G.** Thus, a mixture of oligonucleotides encoding **LEX$_9$LE,** was ligated to produce fragments of different lengths encoding the amino acid sequence **LEX$_9$LEX$_9$** ..., where each **X$_9$** is encoded by **(VNN)$_9$** or **(NNB)$_9$**. The single stop codon possible from this codon usage scheme is suppressed by growth in an amber suppressor bacterial strain, so that even very long variable regions are translated. The fragments were ligated into a plasmid bearing the *lamB* gene, and a library of two million clones was generated by transformation. The recombinant plasmid isolated from library clones bore from 1 to 20 oligonucleotide units, corresponding to variable regions that ranged from 9 to 180 amino acids in length. Library size is limited to about 10 billion clones, considering that cells can be concentrated for screening to about a billion per milliliter, and at least 100 copies of each clone should be present for effective screening; this number of cells (one trillion) represents about 2 l of library cells grown to early stationary phase.

This library of cells was screened for λ receptor variants that would bind iron oxide. Expression of the receptor was induced by incubating cells in log-phase growth with isopropyl-β-D-thiogalactoside (IPTG). The induced cells were then washed and reacted with iron oxide. A magnet was placed on the outer wall of the culture tube to immobilize the iron oxide and adherent cells, and the liquid and nonadhering cells were removed by aspiration. The magnet was then removed and the remaining cells were diluted and plated. Established colonies were grown in liquid culture to log phase growth, induced by IPTG and subjected to further enrichment.

After five rounds of enrichment, seven of ten clones isolated bore identical variable regions comprising six oligonucleotide units. This sequence was also found in a second, independent enrichment experiment. Cells harboring plasmid pSB1972, which encodes this sequence, aggregated in the presence of iron oxide. To identify which of the six oligonucleotide units encode residues that recognize iron oxide, a library comprised of *shuffled* oligonucleotides was made. This involved excising and isolating the oligonucleotide units from the *lamB* gene of pSB1972, then mixing them with a large excess of the random oligonucleotide units used to make the original library. These were religated with the plasmid vector and used to transform cells. Iron oxide-binding clones were isolated by magnetic panning in the presence of iron oxide. Their variable regions were analyzed, and clones were tested for their ability to bind iron oxide or its components, Fe_2O_3 and Fe_3O_4. The clones from the shuffled library that contained oligonucleotide units from pSB1972 and bound iron oxide bore the same pSB1972-derived oligonucleotide unit in the same sense orientation and mostly in the same position within the variable region as in pSB1972 (at the N-terminal end of this region). All of these clones had the same metal oxide-binding specificities as cells harboring pSB1972, recognizing mixed iron oxide and pure Fe_2O_3, binding weakly to Fe_3O_4, and not at all to Cr_2O_3. An iron oxide-binding clone was also discovered from the shuffled library that had no sequences in common with pSB1972; this clone bound only mixed iron oxide and none of the pure metal oxides tested. Thus, sequences that differ in their iron oxide-binding specificities were isolated and partially identified from λ receptor libraries.

This unique system offers an elegant approach to library screening; bacterial cells are simply grown, washed, and screened. Possible problems involved with the library include biological biases, which exclude sequences that are incompatible with expression of the receptor protein, as well as biases imposed by the codon usage strategy. Four residues are excluded by the degenerate codon **VNN**; this and the overrepresentation of many residues by both **VNN** and **NNB** are magnified, since each oligonucleotide unit in a variable region encodes a single codon orientation (**VNN** or **NNB**) nine consecutive times. Although long oligonucleotides can be cloned into the *lamB* gene, it is not clear that larger domains would fold properly when both N- and C-termini are spliced into a surface-exposed loop of the fusion protein.

D. ADVANTAGES/DISADVANTAGES OF FUSION PROTEIN LIBRARIES

The fusion protein libraries have several advantages to their use. First, panning conditions can be controlled to select pools of the tightest-binding peptide ligands in a library. Second, although libraries are difficult to construct, once made, they can be amplified for hundreds of uses. Third, fusion protein libraries and the epitope sequences identified from them are obtained from straightforward methods requiring standard molecular biology facilities, as opposed to the limited access most investigators have to most types of synthetic peptide library. Finally, the phage libraries have been particularly successful at displaying properly folded foreign protein domains, allowing larger framework regions that constrain variable regions to be designed and expressed. The other fusion protein libraries have not been extensively tested in this respect.

Problems that are inherent in these systems include biases favoring the overrepresentation of certain amino acids in library variable regions caused by degenerate codons, and biases that are peculiar to the protein expression system of each library type. Compared with synthetic peptide libraries, a major drawback of fusion protein libraries is their inability to incorporate unnatural, modified, or branched amino acids into the epitope region. As opposed to free peptide libraries, each epitope region is physically attached to a larger, complex entity, which may affect its affinity for ligate.

V. THE OVERALL PERFORMANCE OF EPITOPE LIBRARIES

Table 2 shows the published results obtained from screening the synthetic peptide and fusion protein libraries. Most of the protein-binding ligates used for screening were known in advance to bind linear epitopes on their normal ligands as well as short peptides comprising these sequences. In every case the same or nearly identical sequences to those of the native epitopes were determined from a group of consensus peptides obtained from screening peptide libraries. These results were obtained regardless of whether synthetic peptides or fusion proteins were screened.

There are two instances in which the same ligates were used to screen both synthetic peptide libraries and phage libraries. Three libraries, the selectide library[4] and two phage libraries[7,11] were screened with streptavidin, and all isolated the consensus sequence **HPQ.** Moreover, three synthetic peptide[2,4,28,50] and two phage libraries[6,11,27] were screened with the β-endorphin-binding MAb 3-E7, and all isolated the consensus sequence **YGGF.** The most inhibitory peptide identified from a free hexapeptide library had the sequence **YGGFMT,** with an IC_{50} of 3.2 n*M*.[50] This sequence matches that of the β-endorphin used to prepare MAb 3-E7. However, many other peptides, including the mixed sequence pools **YGGFIX, YGGFMX,** and **YGGFLX** had IC_{50}s within a threefold range of this activity. The strongest binding peptides found from the pentapeptide library formed the consensus sequence **YG(G/A)(F/L/M/W),** whereas those from the octapeptide library generated **YG(A/G)(L/W).** One of the phage libraries screened[11] displayed a constrained hexapeptide variable region with the sequence **XCX_4CX.** Interestingly, the **YGGF** consensus was isolated from this constrained library, even though MAb 3-E7 is known to prefer this sequence positioned at an N-terminus. In a similar study, an octapeptide selectide library that lacked Phe residues was screened with MAb 3-E7 as well as a pentapeptide library that included Phe.[28] Taken together, these results show that pools of the best binding peptides will be isolated from a library, given the particular chemical and structural limitations imposed by its variable region. A phage library displaying a hexapeptide variable region at the N-terminus of pIII was also screened with this ligate, and in the first attempt, only the lower affinity consensus sequence **YGG** was identified.[6] However, when the panning conditions used to screen this phage library were improved to select stronger-binding peptides, the **YGGFL** consensus sequence was identified among the enriched clones.[27] Thus, the comparative tests performed so far show that there is little, if any, difference in the sequence or affinity of the consensus peptides isolated from phage and synthetic peptide libraries when similar variable regions are screened.

In two cases, peptide ligands were found for ligates that recognize nonproteinaceous determinants,[9,45] and only in five cases were mimotopes identified for protein-binding ligates.[1,5,10,25] As will be described in the following section, three of the five mimotopes are disulfide-constrained peptides; the remaining two bore non-natural amino acids. Thus, the current epitope libraries have been most useful for finding peptide ligands of ligates that recognize linear epitopes on proteins, and sometimes of ligates that recognize nonproteinaceous ligands. Unfortunately, there is no published record of screening experiments that were negative.

Our unpublished work, in which about 50 ligates have been used to screen a hexapeptide library, corroborates this trend. Table 3 shows results (including unpublished findings) from screenings with some of these ligates in terms of whether a consensus sequence was identified and whether binding of phage-borne consensus peptides to ligate was relatively weak or strong. Based on phage-binding assays, fairly tight-binding peptides (class I) were always found for ligates that were known to bind a linear epitope or a peptide. These consensus sequences are similar or identical to the corresponding linear epitopes in the native proteins. The ligates that recognize nonproteinaceous ligands mostly isolate fairly weak-binding peptides

TABLE 2
Results of Screening with Peptide Libraries

Library Type	Displayed Epitope	Ligate	Ligand	Consensus Sequences	Refs.
		Synthetic Peptides			
Peptides-on-pins	Pentapeptide	MAb	Assembled epitope	WQMGHS	1
		B-JP[a]	Unknown	QfHpβA[b]	24
		B-JP	Unknown	VβAwMhβAH	
Free peptides	Hexa-octapeptide	MAb	Peptide	YGGFM	45
		MAb	Linear epitope	DVPDY	2
		Receptor	Peptide	YGGFL	3
		Bacteria	Unknown	RRWWC	2
		Bacteria	Unknown	FRWLL	3
Peptides-on-beads	Pentapeptide	MAb	Peptide	YGGFL	4
	Octapeptide	MAb	Peptide	YGG/AW/L	27
	Pentapeptide	Streptavidin	Biotin	HPQ	4
		Fusion Proteins			
Phage libraries					
pIII	Hexapeptide	2 MAbs	Linear epitope	DFL	5
		Con A	MaM[c]	YPY	38
		MAb	Linear epitope	RHSVV/I	37
	Hexapeptide	MAb	Peptide	YGGFL	6
	Octapeptide	Con A	MaM	YPY	9
	Pentadecapeptide	Streptavidin	Biotin	HPQ	7
	Disulfide-bridged hexapeptide	Receptor	Linear epitope	RGD	12
	Disulfide-bridged, discontinuous hexapeptide	MAb	Linear epitope	YGGF	11
		Streptavidin	Biotin	HPQF	
pVIII	Nonapeptide	MAb	Linear epitope	SND/E	8
	Disulfide-bridged nonapeptide	MAb	Assembled epitope	GSXF	10
				YDX_4W	10
lac repressor	Dodecapeptide	MAb	Linear epitope	RQFKV	13
λ receptor	9-180 residues	Iron oxide	Fe_2O_3	RRTVKHHVN	14

[a] Bence-Jones protein (light chain dimer).
[b] Lower case letters indicate D-amino acids; βA is β-Ala.
[c] Methyl alpha-D-mannopyranoside.

(class II) or do not identify a consensus sequence at all (class III). The best examples showing this are the independent screenings performed with Con A and two closely related lectins that have the same sugar-binding specificity as Con A.[45] Although peptide ligands sharing a consensus sequence were identified with Con A, no such peptides were isolated when the hexapeptide library was screened with either of the two closely related lectins. This indicates that peptide ligands cannot be routinely found for even closely related, nonprotein-binding ligates. Similarly, peptide ligands were found only about a third of the time when the library was screened with MAbs and receptors that recognize assembled or conformation-dependent epitopes.

That relatively tight-binding peptides are always found when libraries of unconstrained peptides are screened with peptide-binding ligates shows that the correct combinations of critical binding residues are present and can be isolated from these libraries. The contrasting result, that peptide ligands are often not found for ligates that recognize assembled, constrained linear and nonproteinaceous epitopes, indicates

TABLE 3
Results of Screening a Hexapeptide Phage Library

Class I Sequences — specific sequence motif and positive binding on ELISA
- 3 myohemerythrin-binding MAbs (A, M, and I)[a,c]
- 2 anti-influenza HA-related peptide MAbs (2GD8 and 17/9)[a]
- S-protein of RNAse[b]
- Streptavidin
- Concanavalin A

Class II Sequences — specific sequence motif but weak/no binding on ELISA
- Anti-gp120 RP loop MAb (28G12)[b,c]
- 2 human chorionic gonadotropin-binding MAbs (13 and 14)[a]
- Polyclonal rheumatoid factor (IgG)
- Polyclonal anti-70-kDa protein Ab (snRNP)[c]
- Polyclonal anti-A protein Ab (snRNP)[c]
- FK 506-binding protein (FKBP)
- Cyclophilin

Class III Sequences — no sequence motif and weak/no binding on ELISA
- Anti-progesterone MAb (DB3)
- 2 human chorionic gonadotropin-binding MAbs (18 and 35)
- Anti-lysozyme MAb (HyHEL10)[c]
- Anti-cytochrome c MAb (E8)
- Interleukin-2 receptor (α-subunit; IL2R-α)
- Epidermal growth factor receptor (EGFR)
- Nerve growth factor receptor (NGFR)
- Insulin

[a] These ligates isolated sequences that were related or identical to sequences on the immunogen.

[b] These ligates isolated sequences that bore no resemblence to the immunogen (mimotopes).

[c] MAb 28G12 isolated a hexapeptide mimotope that shares no homology with an antigenic peptide bearing the native epitope; K_I is ~10 m*M* (M. Gefter, personal communication).

Ligate Sources: MAbs: I, A, and M (G. Fieser and I. Wilson); 17/9 and 2GD8 (U. Schulze-Gahmen); 28G12 (M. Gefter); HyHEL 5, 8, 9, and 10 (S. Smith-Gill); 13, 14, 18, and 35 (V. Stevens); OKB7 (W. Lernhardt); DB3 (J. Arevalo). Polyclonal Abs, rheumatoid factors (M. Mannik); anti-snRNP Abs (Y. Takeda). Other ligates: S-protein (J.M. Scholtz); FKBP and cyclophilin (J. Liu); IL2R-α (W. Greene); EGFR (M. Das); NGFR (D. Santi).

that peptides mimicking these epitopes (i.e., mimotopes) are mostly missing from these libraries. To bind effectively, mimotopes must encompass characteristics beyond having the correct binding residues, otherwise they would have been identified from the unconstrained peptide libraries.

VI. DESIGNING NEW EPITOPE LIBRARIES

How can epitope libraries be improved to include better mimotopes? To successfully mimic natural epitopes, the peptides in epitope libraries can take advantage of the three aspects of binding: (1) close-range noncovalent interactions, such as hydrogen bonding, salt bridging, and van der Waals forces; (2) three-dimensional steric fit; and (3) entropic considerations, which include changes in the degrees of freedom of the ligand, ligate, and solvent upon binding. The unconstrained peptide libraries that have been screened thus far mostly ignore aspects (2) and (3), in that unconstrained peptides can take on a multitude of structures and thus carry a high entropic cost. This last section explores how epitope libraries might be designed to better address these other aspects of binding.

A. ARE THERE STRUCTURAL PREFERENCES FOR EPITOPES?

The binding strength of a peptide ligand has often been improved by imposing constraints on the peptide's structure. For example, Williams et al.[15] showed that affinity of the CDR-derived peptide for the cellular receptor for reovirus could be improved by circularizing the peptide with disulfide bridges. Similarly, many peptides have been chemically modified to produce tighter binding analogs by introducing local and long-range constraints via non-natural amino acids. Thus, as the entropic cost of binding is diminished for correctly constrained residues, many ligates may have *preference* for peptides whose mobility is restricted by structural frameworks.

Mimotopes have been identified for a MAb by multistep screening of pin-bound peptides.[1] Peptide binding was further improved by introducing β-Ala, which increased the flexibility of the peptide backbone. A Bence-Jones light chain dimer was screened with pin-bound peptides containing L-amino acids, D-amino acids, which favor turns in peptides, as well as β-Ala.[24] The peptides **V(β-Ala)wMh(β-Ala)H** and **QfHp(β-Ala)** (where lower case letters in bold indicate D-amino acids) bound the same cavity of the dimer, and thus can be considered functional mimotopes. Thus, the antigenicity of the peptides was improved by altering local constraints in the peptide backbone.

Mimotopes have also been identified from a constrained epitope library. Luzzago and coworkers have prepared a library that displays near the N-terminus of pVIII a nine-residue variable region flanked on either side by Cys.[10] Many of the peptides in this library were constrained by disulfide bridges, as five of six randomly chosen phage clones tested had disulfide bonds (there are no Cys residues in pVIII so the oxidative state of Cys residues can be tested by titration). This disulfide-constrained library was screened with MAb H107, which recognizes an assembled epitope on recombinant human H ferritin. Two different, constrained consensus sequences were identified, **YDX$_4$W** and **GSXF**. Ferritin residues Tyr40, Phe41, Asp92, Trp93, and Ser95 are most likely part of the epitope, as the crystal structure of ferritin shows these residues to be in close proximity to each other.[51] Furthermore, replacement of Asp92 and Ser95 selectively ablates ferritin binding by MAb H107, but not by other ferritin-binding MAbs. Free synthetic peptide was tested for binding to the MAb. In an inhibition enzyme-linked immunosorbent assay (ELISA), 50 pmol of a constrained synthetic peptide bearing the **YDX$_4$W** consensus sequence inhibited MAb H107 binding to the same degree as 0.14 pmol of ferritin, showing that a mimotope peptide can bind ligate with significant affinity relative to native antigen.

In a similar vein, Scott and Smith screened a phage library displaying a hexapeptide variable region with a MAb that recognizes short, unconstrained peptides bearing the sequence **DFL.**[5] Among the clones isolated were three constrained peptides consisting of tetrapeptides flanked by Cys residues. Interestingly, one of the sequences, **CRFVWC,** was a constrained mimotope sequence, as it bore no resemblance to the native epitope. Disulfide bridging was probably important for binding as this sequence was not found among the other, non-cysteine-containing sequences isolated in the screening. Phage bearing this constrained mimotope bound the MAb with similar affinity to phage bearing the disulfide-constrained **DFL** recognition sequence. Moreover, the mimotope was one of a few peptides isolated that did not bind another MAb that also recognizes the **DFL** epitope. This indicates that this mimotope bound its ligate highly specifically, using different chemical properties than those of the constrained **DFL**-containing peptides that both MAbs recognized.

Constrained libraries have also been used to find continuous epitopes with higher affinity than the corresponding linear peptide epitope. O'Neil et al. used a phage library to show that peptide binding may be improved by imposing structural constraints on critical binding residues.[12] This library expresses disulfide-looped hexapeptides of the sequence **CX$_6$C.** Screening was performed with the platelet glycoprotein IIb/IIIa an integrin that binds the consensus sequence **RGD,** and which is known to bind a cyclic peptide bearing this sequence. Peptides containing **RGD**, as well as **KGD**, were identified from the library, synthesized and tested in the reduced and oxidized states for binding to the receptor. The cyclized peptides were found to bind more tightly than the linear ones, indicating that affinity was improved by the simple constraints imposed by disulfide bridging. Thus, constrained peptides libraries have been shown to identify mimotopes as well as peptides that bind ligate as well as, or better than, their nonconstrained counterparts. Importantly, both of the cyclic peptides blocked receptor binding at less than one tenth the concentration of a "rationally designed" constrained peptide inhibitor also bearing the **RGD** sequence. This shows that unforeseen improvements in the chemistry of binding can be obtained when rationally designed constraints are incorporated into peptide libraries.

B. DESIGNING CONSTRAINED EPITOPE LIBRARIES

In general two approaches can be used to bias a variable region in favor of a particular class of structures. Local constraints on the peptide backbone come from residues that are positioned within or *internal* to a variable region. In contrast, global constraints result from covalent bonds or noncovalent interactions occurring outside or *external* to a variable region, which impose structural bias on a variable region via the regions surrounding it. Folding of a protein domain is usually required for the formation of global constraints arising from noncovalent interactions.

1. Chemically Synthesized, Constrained Epitope Libraries

Synthetic peptide libraries have the unique advantage of incorporating non-natural amino acids, which allows a finer scale of diversity in local structure and chemistry to be introduced into a variable region. The importance of local constraints to binding can be assessed by incorporating residues that rigidify the peptide backbone to varying degrees. The contribution of side chain chemistry to binding can be exhaustively studied using the large number of residues with different functionalities available. Furthermore, it may be possible to develop libraries of peptide mimics that display side chains from a nonpeptide backbone (such as β turn mimics; Reference 52). Such libraries would circumvent some of the problems inherent in designing nonpeptide analogs from peptide ligands.

Recently, a strategy has been proposed for constructing large libraries of synthetic peptides, with each peptide directly linked to a nucleic acid tag.[53] For each residue addition to the growing peptide chain, whether it be a natural or a non-natural amino acid, a "codon" specific to that residue would also be attached as a linked oligonucleotide. Thus, each unique peptide in the library would be linked to an oligonucleotide specifying its sequence. The linked peptide/oligonucleotide library would be used for *en bloc* screening, and the oligonucleotide of the bound ligands could then be PCR-amplified, cloned, and sequenced. In contrast with Tuerk and Gold's proposal,[46] the linked oligonucleotide would not be directly translated to produce peptides, but would rather serve as an amplifiable code for the peptide sequence. Since this code would not be restricted to nature's genetic code, many different non-natural amino acids could be encoded, increasing the diversity of local constraints and chemistries within a library.

The design of global constraints into synthetic peptide libraries is problematic, as intermolecular, rather than intramolecular, bonds and interactions may arise between closely spaced peptides on a resin. This is why most of the synthetic peptide libraries constructed so far have avoided incorporating Cys into their variable regions.[2-4] Moreover, only relatively simple constraints may be used, such as simple disulfide bridges or limited hydrogen bonding, because synthetic peptide libraries are limited to about 20 residues in length. Thus, for a six-residue long variable region, only about 14 positions could be used in designing global constraints on the variable region. These length limitations may eventually be overcome, allowing constrained domains to be formed from longer peptides. For instance, it is now possible to synthesize small proteins by chemically "ligating" shorter peptide segments together.[54] Using this approach, free peptide variable regions may eventually be grafted into long flanking regions that would fold into a constrained domain structure.

2. Constrained Epitope Libraries on Fusion Proteins

In fusion protein libraries, complex domains constraining a variable region can be easily designed, since there is relatively little limitation on the length of the inserted region. Libraries of constrained domains are likely to fold into stable structures if they are expressed on fusion proteins that are secreted or exposed on the bacterial surface. Furthermore, secreted fusion proteins allow disulfide bond constraints to be included in library design without creating problems from intermolecular bridging. Thus, fusion protein libraries may be designed to display potential binding residues in the context of longer variable regions, simple constrained structures, or small folded domains comprising discontinuous variable regions, with the goal of more closely mimicking the epitopes on folded proteins.

In contrast to synthetic peptide libraries, constrained epitope libraries borne by fusion proteins encompass less chemical diversity, as well as less diversity of local constraints. This may eventually be overcome by developing a means of incorporating unnatural amino acids into the polypeptide chain during *in vivo* synthesis. Mutant tRNAs that recognize stop codons or redundant amino acid codons (such as Ser codons) may be developed that can be charged with non-natural amino acids, thus allowing them to be incorporated into the polypeptide chain during synthesis. Ellman and coworkers have made progress toward this goal by devising means of adding non-natural amino acids to proteins that are synthesized by an *in vitro* translation system.[55] They have modified a yeast suppressor tRNA to carry non-natural amino acids. These amino acids are added to the polypeptide chain wherever the corresponding mRNA encodes the appropriate stop codon.

In theory, fusion protein systems also offer the possibility of constructing libraries of multimeric proteins, with each subunit having a different variable region, such that there is selection at the protein level for subunit pairs that form stable associations. As a case in point, the genes encoding most antibody phage libraries are chosen at random from large pools of cloned heavy and light chain cDNAs (e.g., References 35 and 41). Because a single light chain variable domain and a single heavy chain variable domain are cloned into a cell at random, many of the heavy-light chain pairs may not form stable enough associations to produce viable antibodies. These poor light:heavy chain associations may cause the variable domains of many clones in an antibody phage library to be unstable, resulting in poor antigen binding sites. With a system like peptides-on-plasmids,[13] it may be possible to link each heavy chain and each light chain directly to the DNA encoding them, so that two separate fusion libraries are made. These libraries may then be mixed to allow each heavy chain and each light chain to search each respective library to find a partner with which to form a stable association. This would allow domains whose variable regions associate only with particular other domains to "find" their complements from within a library, thus permitting the formation of stable assembled epitopes (or, in the case of antibody libraries, stable idiotypes). These multimeric domains could then be purified from the single domains that did not find a partner. Libraries of domains, such as antibody light and heavy chains, that would associate to form stable associations would be difficult to construct with either the phage or the λ receptor systems, but may eventually be possible from a system in which free peptides or proteins are directly linked to the nucleic acids encoding them (as suggested by Reference 46). One could envision the construction not only of libraries of binding sites, as with antibodies, from this approach, but also of libraries of assembled epitopes, as are found in nature.

3. Future Uses of Epitope Libraries

There are several potential ways in which epitope libraries could be used to screen for binding activity, besides the straightforward experiments mentioned already. First, peptides that specifically bind "ligate A", but not its closely related counterpart, "ligate B", could be isolated from *blocking experiments,* in which ligate A is either immobilized or labeled, and ligate B is present in excess in solution. Ligate B, being in relative excess, will competitively block any of the peptides it recognizes from binding to ligate A. Thus, only peptides that are not recognized by ligate B will be able to bind ligate A.

In a second type of experiment, sequences that are targets for specific modification could be identified from epitope libraries. A library may be specifically modified *en bloc* by, for example, specific proteolytic cleavage, phosphorylation or glycosylation, or "activated" by cofactor or metal binding. The library of modified peptides could then screened by ligate (e.g., recognizing cleaved peptide, phosphorylated or glycosylated residues, or bound metal) for binding to specific peptide sequences.

In a third type of experiment, complementary pairs of binding sequences could be identified by screening two libraries (or two aliquots of the same library) against one another. In these *library-against-library* screenings, one library, "library A", would be immobilized, and the other, "library B", screened against it. The enriched sequences from library B would then be immobilized, and library A would be screened on it. Repeated rounds of complementary panning on progressively enriched phage would result in two pools of complementary binding peptides. Single clones from either pool could be immobilized and the binding complements isolated in a final round of screening. Thus, library-against-library screening mimics the process of evolution, with selection acting at the level of molecular recognition. This approach would allow one to probe the question of how a ligand might compensate for small changes in a binding site. For instance, a library of mutagenized receptor could be screened against a library of mutagenized hormone to find pairs that bind each other in unanticipated ways and with high affinity. Similarly, a pool of tight-binding "marker" peptides for monoclonal species in a given antibody response could be isolated by screening an antibody library against a peptide library. Such peptides could then be screened for immunogenic or antigenic activity. On a more basic level, libraries of different constrained peptides may be screened against each other to discover recognition motifs for particular secondary structure interactions. The structural and chemical information derived from complementary peptide pairs may be used to predict regions of potential complementary interaction between larger proteins, and thus may aid in the design of ligands for macromolecules.

C. IMPLICATIONS FOR DRUG DESIGN AND THE UNDERSTANDING OF MOLECULAR RECOGNITION

Constrained libraries could yield information that cannot be obtained from screening unconstrained peptide libraries. Through consensus sequences, both types of library give information about the chemistry of binding, since critical binding residues are highly conserved among peptides defining a consensus group. However, the structure of the constrained variable region gives additional information about the three-dimensional arrangements of the critical binding residues that are accepted by the binding site. Compared with unconstrained peptides, the relatively limited number of configurations possible with constrained peptides simplifies solution structure determination of binding peptides from CD and NMR spectroscopy. The conformations of bound constrained peptides can be studied by techniques such as X-ray crystallography or isotope-edited NMR.[56] For these reasons, constrained peptides provide more information for making highly refined models of a peptide epitope. Such models can be used in designing non-peptide analogs having good pharmacologic qualities, allowing further modification, testing, and refinement on the way toward a suitable therapeutic compound (e.g., Reference 51).

Synthetic peptide libraries, synthetic nonpeptide libraries, and fusion protein libraries could play important roles in the discovery of lead compounds for a variety of ligates in the future. A plausible scenario of screening for lead compounds might use a variety of fusion protein libraries, each of which displays a variable region in the context of a particular structural bias to define a structural and chemical starting point for further refinement. Synthetic libraries comprising shorter peptides whose general structure and chemistry fit the conserved (selected) regions of the best peptides isolated from the fusion protein libraries would then be screened. Non-natural amino acids whose side chain chemistries are subtly different from the chemistries of the critical residues could be used to augment binding chemistry and mimetic bioactivity. Non-natural amino acids with constrained backbones could be used to optimize local rigidity for the epitope, while cystine and non-natural amino acids that form covalent bridges could be used to optimize the degree of global constraint around the epitope. Synthetic libraries of non-amino acids may also be used to these ends.

What will the general structural requirements for binding turn out to be? If binding to native epitopes involves rigid structures with strict three-dimensional requirements for binding (i.e., a lock and key mechanism of binding), then even a wide range of constrained epitope libraries may not be able to encompass the amount of structural variation necessary for finding good lead peptides. On the other hand, if binding involves flexible but defined structures (as with an induced fit mechanism), then well-designed constrained libraries may yield peptide ligands for a wide range of ligates. The general trends found from crystallographic studies of protein antigen:antibody complexes indicate that side chain as well as some main chain movement accompanies most binding interactions of this type (see Reference 57 for a review of this topic). Thus, at least some induced fit is involved in most protein antigen:antibody interactions. In addition, differences in the affinity and fit of ligand to ligate may have implications for antagonistic vs. agonistic properties of a mimetic lead.[29]

Most likely, some libraries will give higher yields of peptide ligands in general, or will be better suited to certain types of ligates. The *quality* of libraries, i.e., the frequency with which ligates find peptide ligands, may be related to the overall constraints imposed on the peptides in the different libraries. Moreover, synthetic libraries will allow side chain functionality, as well as local and global constraints, to vary beyond those found in nature. Epitope library studies should prove increasingly valuable for the identification of peptides suitable for use as lead peptides. In addition, these studies will most certainly advance our general understanding of the forces behind molecular recognition.

NOTE ADDED IN PROOF

See the latest review of peptide libraries in *Curr. Opinion Biotechnol.*, xx, xx, 1994.

ACKNOWLEDGMENTS

This work was supported by National Institutes of Health grants GM41478 (G.P. Smith) and GM13772 (J.K.S.), U.S. Army grant DAAL03-92-G-0178 (G.P.S.), the Molecular Biology Program and the Departments of Biological Sciences and Medicine, University of Missouri, the Protos Division of Chiron Corporation, Terrapin Technologies, Incorporated, and especially by James R. and Lois M. Dayhoff. Thanks to Elizabeth Getzoff, Victoria Roberts, Maurice Boissinot, and Richard Houghten for comments on this manuscript, and to George Smith, Kit Lam, and Peter Schatz for figures. Stanley Brown, Ron Barrett, Robert Ladner, Kit Lam, Mario Geysen, Mike Kahn, Ron Hoess, Richard Houghten, Peter Schatz, Riccardo Cortese, and Alessandra Luzzago are gratefully acknowledged for sharing their unpublished data and manuscripts, as well as personal insights in this area.

REFERENCES

1. **Geysen, H.M., Rodda, S.J., and Mason, T.J.,** *A priori* delineation of a peptide which mimics a discontinuous antigenic determinant, *Mol. Immunol.*, 23, 709, 1986.
2. **Houghten, R.A., Pinilla, C., Blondelle, S.E., Appel, J.R., Dooley, C.T., and Cuervo, J.H.,** Generation and use of synthetic peptide combinatorial libraries for basic research and drug discovery, *Nature*, 354, 84, 1991.
3. **Houghten, R.A., Appel, J.R., Blondelle, S.E., Cuervo, J.H., Dooley, C.T., and Pinilla, C.,** The use of synthetic peptide combinatorial libraries for the identification of bioactive peptides, *Bio Tech.*, 13, 412, 1992.
4. **Lam, K.S., Salmon, S.E., Hersh, E.M., Hruby, V.J., Kazmierski, W.M., and Knapp, R.J.,** A new synthetic peptide library for identifying ligand-binding activity, *Nature*, 354, 82, 1991.
5. **Scott, J.K. and Smith, G.P.,** Searching for peptide ligands with an epitope library, *Science*, 249, 386, 1990.
6. **Cwirla, S.E., Peters, E.A., Barrett, R.W., and Dower, W.J.,** Peptides on phage: a vast library of peptides for identifying ligands, *Proc. Natl. Acad. Sci. U.S.A.*, 87, 6378, 1990.
7. **Devlin, J.J., Panganiban, L.C., and Devlin, P.E.,** Random peptide libraries: a source of specific protein binding molecules, *Science*, 249, 404, 1991.
8. **Felici, F., Castagnoli, L., Musacchio, A., Jappelli, R., and Cesareni, G.,** Selection of antibody ligands from a large library of oligopeptides expressed on a multivalent exposition vector, *J. Mol. Biol.*, 222, 301, 1991.
9. **Oldenberg, K.R., Loganathan, D., Goldstein, I.J., Schultz, P.G., and Gallop, M.A.,** Peptide ligands for a sugar-binding protein isolated from a random peptide library, *Proc. Natl. Acad. Sci. U.S.A.*, 89, 5393, 1992.
10. **Luzzago, A., Felici, F., Tramontano, A., Pessi, A., and Cortese, R.,** Mimicking of discontinuous epitopes by phage-displayed peptides. I. Epitope mapping of human H ferritin using a phage library of constrained peptides, *Gene*, 128, 51, 1993.
11. **McLafferty, M.A., Kent, R.B., Ladner, R.C., and Markland, W.,** M13 bacteriophage displaying disulfide-constrained micro-proteins, *Gene*, 128, 29, 1993.
12. **O'Neil, K.T., Hoess, R.H., Jackson, S.A., Ramachandran, N., Mousa, S.A., and DeGrado, W.F.,** Identification of gpIIb/IIIa-binding peptides using a conformationally constrained phage peptide library, *Protein* 14, 509, 1992.
13. **Cull, M.G., Miller, J.F., and Schatz, P.J.,** Screening for receptor ligands using large libraries of peptides linked to the C terminus of the *lac* repressor, *Proc. Natl. Acad. Sci. U.S.A.*, 89, 1865, 1992.
14. **Brown, S.,** Engineered iron oxide adhesion mutants of the λ-receptor, *Proc. Natl. Acad. Sci. U.S.A.*, 89, 8651, 1992.
15. **Williams, W.V., Kieber-Emmons, T., VonFeldt, J., Greene, M.I., and Weiner, D.B.,** Design of bioactive peptides based on antibody hypervariable region structures, *J. Biol. Chem.*, 266, 5182, 1991.
16. **Saragovi, H.U., Fitzpatrick, D., Raktabutr, A., Nakanishi, H., Hahn, M., and Greene, M.I.,** Design and synthesis of a mimetic from an antibody complementarity-determining region, *Science*, 253, 792, 1991.
17. **Geysen, H.M., Tainer, J.A., Rodda, S.J., Mason, T.J., Alexander, H., Getzoff, E.D., and Lerner, R.A.,** Chemistry of antibody binding to a protein, *Science*, 235, 1184, 1987.
18. **Wilson, I.A., Niman, H.L., Houghten, R.A., Cherenson, A.R., Connolly, M.L., and Lerner, R.A.,** The structure of an antigenic determinant in a protein, *Cell*, 37, 767, 1984.
19. **Van Regenmortel, M.H.V.,** Structural and functional approaches to the study of protein antigenicity, *Immunol. Today*, 10, 266, 1989.
20. **Getzoff, E.D., Tainer, J.A., Lerner, R.A., and Geysen, H.M.,** The chemistry and mechanism of antibody binding to protein antigens, *Adv. Immunol.*, 43, 1, 1988.
21. **Laver, W.G., Air, G.M., Webster, R.G., and Smith-Gill, S.J.,** Epitopes on protein antigens: misconceptions and realities, *Cell*, 61, 553, 1990.
22. **Stenesh, J.,** *Dictionary of Biochemistry and Molecular Biology*, 2nd ed., John Wiley & Sons, New York, 1989.
23. **Geysen, H.M., Rodda, S.J., Mason, T.J., Tribbick G., and Schoofs, P.G.,** Strategies for epitope analysis using peptide synthesis, *J. Immunol. Methods*, 102, 259, 1987.

23a. **Geysen, H.M.,** personal communication.

24. **Maeji, N.J., Bray, A.M., and Geysen, H.M.,** Multi-pin peptide synthesis strategy for T cell determinant analysis, *J. Immunol. Methods*, 134, 23, 1990.
25. **Tribbick, G., Edmundson, A.B., Mason, T.J., and Geysen, H.M.,** Similar binding properties of peptide ligands for a human immunoglobulin and its light chain dimer, *Mol. Immunol.*, 26, 625, 1989.
26. **Houghten, R.A.,** General method for the rapid solid-phase synthesis of large numbers of peptides: specificity of antigen-antibody interaction at the level of individual amino acids, *Proc. Natl. Acad. Sci. U.S.A.*, 82, 5131, 1985.
27. **Barrett, R.W., Cwirla, S.E., Ackerman, M.S., Olson, A.M., Peters, E.A., and Dower, W.J.,** Selective enrichment and characterization of high affinity ligands from collections of random peptides on filamentous phage, *Anal. Biochem.*, 204, 357, 1992.

28. **Lam, K.S., Hruby, V.J., Lebl, M., Knapp, R.J., Kazmierski, W.M., Hersh, E.M., and Salmon, S.E.,** The chemical synthesis of large random peptide libraries and their use for the discovery of ligands for macromolecular acceptors, *Bioorg. Med. Chem. Lett.*, 3, 419, 1993.
29. **Hruby, V.J., Al-Obeidi, F., and Kazmierski, W.,** Emerging approaches in the molecular design of receptor-selective peptide ligands: conformational, topographical and dynamic considerations, *Biochem. J.*, 268, 249, 1990.
30. **Rizo, J. and Gierasch, L.M.,** Constrained peptides: models of bioactive peptides and protein substructures, *Annu. Rev. Biochem.*, 61, 387, 1992.
31. **Model, P. and Russel, M.,** Filamentous bacteriophage, in *The Bacteriophages*, Vol. 2, Calendar, R, Ed., Plenum Press, New York, 1988, chap. 6.
32. **Smith, G.P.,** Filamentous fusion phage: novel expression vectors that display cloned antigens on the surface of the virion, *Science*, 228, 1315, 1985.
33. **Parmley, S.F. and Smith, G.P.,** Antibody-selectable filamentous fd phage vectors: affinity purification of target genes, *Gene*, 73, 305, 1988.
34. **Bass, S., Greene, R., and Wells, J.A.,** Hormone phage: an enrichment method for variant proteins with altered binding properties, *Proteins Struct. Funct. Genet.*, 8, 309, 1990.
35. **Barbas, C.F., Kang, A.S., Lerner, R.A., and Benkovic, S.J.,** Assembly of combinatorial antibody libraries on phage surfaces: the gene III site, *Proc. Natl. Acad. Sci. U.S.A.*, 88, 7978, 1991.
36. **Smith, G.P.,** Surface presentation of protein epitopes using bacteriophage expression systems, *Curr. Opin. Biotechnol.*, 2, 668, 1991.
37. **Birnbaum, S. and Mosbach, K.,** Peptide screening, *Curr. Opin. Biotechnol.*, 3, 49, 1992.
38. **Scott, J.K.,** Discovering peptide ligands using epitope libraries, *Trends Biochem. Sci.*, 17, 241, 1992.
39. **Greenwood, J., Willis, A.E., and Perham, R.N.,** Multiple display of foreign peptides on a filamentous bacteriophage: peptides from *Plasmodium falciparum* circumsporozoite protein as antigens, *J. Mol. Biol.*, 220, 821, 1991.
40. **Il'ichev, A.A., Minenkova, O.O., Tat'kov, S.I., Karpyshev, N.N., Eroshkin, A.M., Ofitserov, V.I., Akimenko, A.A., Petrenko, V.A., and Sandakhchiev, L.S.,** *Mol. Biol. (Moscow)*, 24, 530, 1990.
41. **Kang, A.S., Barbas, C.F., Janda, K.D., Benkovic, S.J., and Lerner, R.A.,** Linkage of recognition and replication functions by assembling combinatorial antibody Fab libraries along phage surfaces, *Proc. Natl. Acad. Sci. U.S.A.*, 88, 4363, 1991.
42. **Lowman, H.B., Bass, S.H., Simpson, N., and Wells, J.A.,** Selecting high-affinity binding proteins by monovalent phage display, *Biochemistry*, 30, 10832, 1991.
43. **Smith, G.P. and Scott, J.K.,** Libraries of peptides and proteins displayed on filamentous phage, in *Meth. Enzymol.*, 217, 228, 1993.
44. **Stephen, C.W. and Lane, D.P.,** The mutant conformation of p53: precise epitope mapping using a filamentous phage epitope library, *J. Mol. Biol.*, 225, 577, 1992.
45. **Scott, J.K., Loganathan, D., Easley, R.B., Gong, X., and Goldstein, I.J.,** A family of concanavalin A-binding peptides from a hexapeptide epitope library, *Proc. Natl. Acad. Sci. U.S.A.*, 89, 5398, 1992.
46. **Tuerk, C. and Gold, L.,** Systematic evolution of ligands by exponential enrichment: RNA ligands to bacteriophage T4 DNA polymerase, *Science*, 249, 505, 1990.
47. **Hofnung, M.,** Expression of foreign polypeptides at the Escherichia coli cell surface, in *Meth. Cell Biol.*, Vol. 34, Tartakoff, A.M., Ed., Academic Press, Orlando, 1991, 77.
48. **Charbit, A., Molla, A., Saurin, W., and Hofnung, M.,** Versatility of a vector for expressing foreign polypeptides at the surface of Gram-bacteria, *Gene*, 70, 181, 1988.
49. **Charbit, A., Boulain, J.-C., Ryter, A., and Hofnung, M.,** Probing the topology of a bacterial membrane protein by genetic insertion of a foreign epitope. Expression at the cell surface, *EMBO J.*, 5, 3029, 1986.
50. **Pinilla, C., Appel, J.R., and Houghten, R.A.,** Synthetic peptide combinatorial libraries: the identification of the antigenic determinant of β-endorphin recognized by mAb 3E7, Gene, 128, 71, 1993.
51. **Lawson, D.M., Artymiuk, P.J., Yewdall, S.J., Smith, J.M.A., Livingstone, J.C., Treffry, A., Luzzago, A., Levi, S., Arosio, P., Cesareni, G., Thomas, C.D., Shaw, W.V., and Harrison, P.M.,** Solving the structure of human H ferritin by genetically engineering intermolecular crystal contacts, *Nature*, 349, 541, 1991.
52. **Ball, J.B. and Alewood, P.F.,** Conformational constraints: nonpeptide β-turn mimics, *J. Mol. Recognition*, 3, 55, 1990.
53. **Brenner, S. and Lerner, R.A.,** Encoded combinatorial chemistry, *Proc. Natl. Acad. Sci. U.S.A.*, 89, 5381, 1992.
54. **Schnolzer, M. and Kent, S.B.H.,** Constructing proteins by dovetailing unprotected synthetic peptides: backbone-engineered HIV protease, *Science*, 256, 221, 1992.
55. **Ellman, J.A., Mendel, D., and Schultz, P.G.,** Site-specific incorporation of novel backbone structures into proteins, *Science*, 255, 197, 1992.

56. **Fesik, S.W., Luly, J.R., Erickson, J.W., Abad-Zapatero, C., and Zuiderweg, E.R.P.,** Conformations of enzyme-bound ligands by isotope-edited 2D NMR techniques, in *Frontiers of NMR in Molecular Biology*, Alan R. Liss, New York, 1990, 51.
57. **Davies, D.R., Sheriff, S., and Padlan, E.A.,** Antibody-antigen complexes, *J. Biol. Chem.*, 263, 10541, 1988.
58. **Rodda, S.,** *Pinnacles, the Chiron Mimotope Newslett.*, 2(2) 1992.
59. **Lam, K.S.,** personal communication.

Chapter 2

INTERLEUKIN-1 RECEPTOR PATHWAY APPROACHES TO DRUG DESIGN

Howard M. Einspahr, Barry C. Finzel, and Daniel E. Tracey

CONTENTS

I. INTRODUCTION

Of all the known cytokines that regulate cell function and intracellular communication, interleukin-1 (IL-1) has received the most attention (see References 1 to 3 for extensive reviews of IL-1). Part of the reason for this is historical, but part is the suspected prominence of IL-1 in the pathology associated with inflammation, microbial infection, and autoimmune disease. The interaction of IL-1 with specific cellular receptors represents an attractive therapeutic target. This chapter will address the structural basis for IL-1 activity and various experimental approaches for IL-1-based drug design and therapeutic intervention.

A. IL-1 BIOLOGY

Interleukin-1 is actually a general term for the products of two separate genes.[4] These genes code for 30-kDa proteins that are processed to the mature 17-kDa forms called IL-1α and IL-1β. With few exceptions, IL-1α and IL-1β are equipotent in IL-1 assays and interact identically with cell surface IL-1 receptors. However, these two proteins are only about 25% identical in amino acid sequence. With the exception of some epidermal cells and some brain neurons, cells from healthy individuals do not produce IL-1. As shown in Figure 1, during microbial infections, stress, trauma, and a variety of diseases, IL-1 can be produced by many

0-8493-9422-8/94/$0.00+$.50

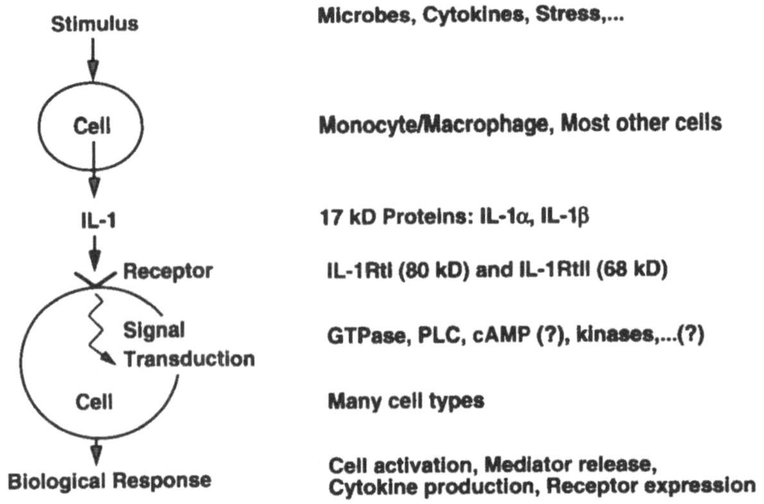

FIGURE 1. Overview of interleukin-1 production and receptor-mediated biological responses.

different cell types. The monocyte-macrophage lineage is generally considered to be the major source of IL-1 in inflammatory lesions, although all mammalian cells, with the exception of erythrocytes, are capable of synthesizing IL-1. Monocytes can be stimulated with viruses, bacteria, bacterial lipopolysaccharides, immune complexes, complement components, and a variety of cytokines, including IL-1 itself, to produce IL-1. Within a few hours IL-1 is produced and some of this cytokine, especially IL-1β, can be released by the cells.

When released from monocytes or other cells, IL-1 can act locally on a variety of cell types or systemically in the brain, liver, and other tissues. As shown in Figure 2, IL-1 bioactivities can be classified, broadly speaking, as immunological (acting on T and B lymphocytes, natural killer [NK] cells and macrophages), neurological (acting on the hypothalamus or other brain regions), and inflammatory (acting on fibroblasts, endothelial cells, neutrophils, macrophages, chondrocytes, osteoclasts, and hepatocytes). The inflammatory group of activities is the most relevant to current strategies to inhibit IL-1 for therapeutic reasons.

B. IL-1 IN DISEASE

There are many diseases in which IL-1 has been implicated as a possible mediator of disease pathology. Notable among these are septic shock and rheumatoid arthritis (RA). Bacterial sepsis can lead directly or indirectly to monocyte-macrophage stimulation and the explosive release of tumor necrosis factor-α (TNF-α) and IL-1β into the circulation.[5] These cytokines may then activate endothelial cells and vascular smooth muscle cells to cause hypotension, edema, and cardiovascular collapse. Many activities of IL-1 may play a strong role in RA as well. These activities include endothelial cell stimulation to promote leukocyte adherence; chondrocyte stimulation to produce prostaglandins, proteoglycan degrading enzymes, and metalloproteinases such as collagenase; fibroblast stimulation to proliferate and produce prostaglandins, collagen, and collagenase; osteoclast stimulation, perhaps indirectly through osteoblast induction of IL-6, to cause bone resorption; and T lymphocyte stimulation to proliferate and produce IL-2 and IL-2 receptors (Figure 2). Some of these proinflammatory activities of IL-1 may be partially offset by the production of anti-inflammatory glucocorticoids or acute-phase reactants.

Rheumatoid arthritis patients have levels of IL-1 in their blood plasma that correlate with disease severity.[6] Explants of synovial cells from RA patients contain IL-1 mRNA[7] and IL-1 proteins are released into the supernatants of cultured RA synovial cells.[8] Moreover, synovial fluid from RA patients often contains high levels of IL-1. In experimental animal models, administration of IL-1 by bolus injection or slow-release infusion induced inflammation and cartilage erosion in normal joints and

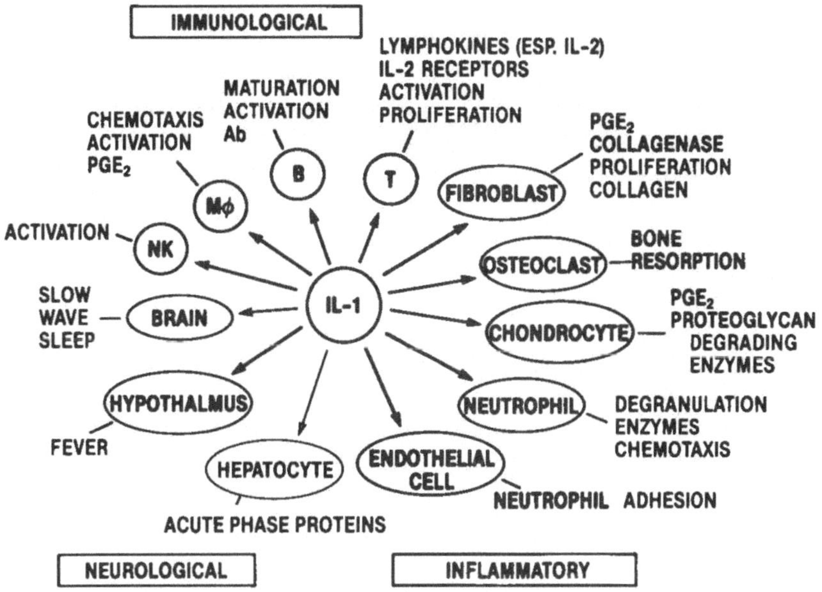

FIGURE 2. Interleukin-1 bioactivities.

exacerbated the onset and severity of arthritis lesions in animals with experimentally induced arthritis.[9,10] These findings, together with a striking correlation between the known bioactivities of IL-1 and the pathophysiology of RA, suggest that inhibition of IL-1 is a good mechanistic target for development of a therapeutic agent for the treatment of RA.

C. IL-1 RECEPTORS AND SIGNAL TRANSDUCTION

All of the known bioactivities of IL-1 are thought to be initiated by binding of the IL-1 molecules to high-affinity cell surface receptors (Figure 1). Two distinct classes of IL-1 receptors have been identified on various cell types.[11-16] The most common is the 80-kDa type I IL-1 receptor (IL-1RtI), found on stimulated T lymphocytes, fibroblasts, endothelial cells, and chondrocytes. It binds IL-1 with a K_d of about 50 p*M*.[17-19] Some cells, such as B lymphocytes, macrophages, and neutrophils, bear 68-kDa type II IL-1 receptors (IL-1RtII), which bind IL-1 with a K_d of about 200 to 300 p*M*.[20-23] Some cells that bear IL-1RtII also bear a low number of IL-1RtI and the question whether IL-1RtII are even biologically functional remains unanswered.[15] One important characteristic of IL-1-responsive cells is the low number (10 to 1000) of receptors per cell on most cell types.[24,25] Downregulation of IL-1R expression on some cells occurs after IL-1 binding or treatment with transforming growth factor-β.[26,27] Conversely, upregulation of IL-1R expression has been observed in fibroblasts treated with platelet-derived growth factor or with prostaglandin E_2.[28,29]

The extracellular portion of the IL-1RtI contains three domains, each reminiscent of an immunoglobulin domain and including an intrachain disulfide bridge.[18] A soluble form of the IL-1RtI, which comprises the three extracellular domains, retains the ability to bind IL-1 with an affinity comparable to that of the cellular receptor.[30] A short transmembrane region and a 213-amino acid cytoplasmic tail complete the human IL-1RtI. There is currently no information on the tertiary structure of IL-1 receptors, so one can only speculate on how the various domains are organized to create an IL-1 binding site. The human IL-1RtI is glycosylated and there are suggestions that the carbohydrate contributes to IL-1 binding.[31]

The human IL-1RtII also has three extracellular domains, but is genetically distinct from the IL-1RtI.[22] The two receptors share only 28% homology in the extracellular portions. The major structural difference is the very short cytoplasmic tail (26 amino acids) in the IL-1RtII, raising the speculation that this receptor may not be able to transduce a signal to the cell after IL-1 binding. The murine IL-1RtI and IL-1RtII appear to be structurally and functionally very similar to their human counterparts and are similarly distributed among certain cell types.

As was stated above, although IL-1 receptors appear to bind IL-1α and IL-1β with comparable affinities, some studies have demonstrated that these ligands may interact in different ways with IL-1 receptors. For example, in one pair of studies on IL-1RtI-bearing cells, IL-1α and IL-1β were equipotent on fibroblasts, but IL-1α was 100-fold more potent than IL-1β on T cells.[32] Furthermore, certain antibodies to the IL-1RtI preferentially inhibited the binding of IL-1β as compared with IL-1α to IL-1RtI.[33] With IL-1RtII on B cell lines, some studies have shown preferential binding of IL-1β as compared with IL-1α,[34] while others have shown the opposite effect with other B cell lines.[15]

An interesting difference between IL-1RtI and IL-1RtII is that only the former are rapidly internalized within the cell after binding IL-1.[20] Moreover, the IL-1 remains intact after internalization and the complex between IL-1 and IL-1RtI appears in the nuclear compartment after a few hours.[35] The relationship between internalization of IL-1 and signal transduction events remains obscure. One of the earliest events after IL-1 binding to the IL-1RtI is the serine/threonine phosphorylation of the cytoplasmic tail of the IL-1RtI.[36] Some of the signal transduction events in some IL-1-responsive cells have been defined, but there remains much uncertainty and some controversy about the specific elements in these pathways. Although some studies have implicated cyclic AMP increases in IL-1 signal transduction via G-protein activation of adenylate cyclase,[37] others have not been able to confirm these observations. There is evidence with T cells for activation of a phospholipase via a GTPase, which becomes activated within 1 min of IL-1 binding to its receptor.[38] Subsequently, it is likely that the phospholipase releases diacylglycerol from phospholipids and the diacylglycerol activates a protein kinase, but probably not the cyclic AMP- or calcium-dependent protein kinases. Evidence has been recently presented that IL-β signal transduction uses the sphingomyelin pathway, involving sphingomyelinase generation of ceramide and stimulation by ceramide of a specialized serine-threonine protein kinase.[129] A number of proteins are phosphorylated following IL-1 signaling, including hsp27 in T cells.[39] Whether IL-1 initiates the same signal transduction pathways in all IL-1-responsive cells or utilizes cell type-specific pathways is not known.

D. IL-1 RECEPTOR ANTAGONIST PROTEIN (IRAP)

Naturally occurring IL-1 inhibitors were simultaneously discovered by two groups during the mid-1980s. Seckinger et al. described an IL-1 inhibitor in febrile human urine that blocked the ability of IL-1 to bind to IL-1 receptors.[40] Arend's group described an IL-1 inhibitor in the supernatant of immune complex-stimulated human monocytes which blocked IL-1-mediated thymocyte proliferation.[41] We began to try to isolate the latter factor from human monocyte culture supernatants and found that addition of granulocyte-macrophage colony stimulating factor (GM-CSF) to the monocyte cultures greatly enhanced the production of IL-1 inhibitory activity. Similar activities were generated in the supernatants of the human monocytic cell lines THP-1 and U937, the former after differentiation with phorbol myristate acetate (PMA) and the latter after PMA-induced differentiation and stimulation with GM-CSF. The proteins from all three sources were purified by gel filtration and ion-exchange chromatography to yield homogeneous preparations of proteins with an apparent M_r of about 25 kDa. Amino acid sequencing of peptides derived from these three sources yielded sequences that were used to construct oligonucleotide pools, which were then used to isolate a cDNA clone from a U937 cDNA library coding for a 177-amino acid protein.[42] The sequence predicted a 152-amino acid mature protein flanked by a 25-amino acid leader sequence. The cDNA for the mature protein was expressed in *Escherichia coli* and recombinant protein was purified and characterized.[42] The protein was called IL-1 receptor antagonist protein (IRAP), which turned out to be identical to the factors identified by Seckinger et al.[40] and Arend et al.,[41] and to a protein, IL-1ra, cloned from human monocytes.[43]

Recombinant mature human IRAP (rhIRAP) is 17 kDa in size, but appears to run at about 20 kDa on SDS-PAGE. It has one N-linked glycosylation site at Asn 84. Four forms of glycosylated native IRAP were isolated from THP-1 cells, all of which shared the same amino acid core, but differed in the extent of glycosylation.[44] Interestingly, the amino acid sequence of IRAP is homologous with IL-1α and IL-1β, having 18% identity with human IL-1α and 26% with human IL-1β. It appears that the IRAP gene has evolutionarily diverged from a common precursor gene that also gave rise to IL-1α and IL-1β.[45] IRAP appears not to be constitutively produced by monocytes-macrophages, but can be induced with lipopolysaccharides (LPS), immobilized immune complexes (or IgG), GM-CSF, or IL-3.[46,47] Thus, IRAP appears to be a naturally occurring IL-1 inhibitor, the evolutionary selection for which may relate to its ability to inhibit the inflammatory and tissue destructive activities of IL-1 in pathological situations.

Throughout the isolation and cloning of IRAP, two assays were used to measure IL-1 inhibition: an IL-1 bioassay using murine T cell lines and an IL-1 receptor-binding competition assay. Native and recombinant IRAP inhibited both assays, confirming that IRAP's mode of action is to compete for IL-1 binding to IL-1 receptors. Receptor-binding competition studies,[26] such as those shown in Figure 3 with displacement of ^{125}I-rhIL-1α binding to IL-1RtI on murine LBRM-33-1A5 T cells, showed that IRAP (native or recombinant) bound specifically to IL-1 receptors with an affinity very close to that of IL-1α or IL-1β (K_i values for IL-1α, IL-1β, and IRAP were 22, 43, and 88 p*M*, respectively). By contrast, rhIRAP bound very poorly to IL-1RtII on murine bone marrow cells (presumably granulocytes), as shown in Figure 4. The inhibition constants (K_i) for IL-1α, IL-1β, and IRAP were 200, 2700, and 320,000 p*M*, respectively. Thus, rhIRAP binds to both IL-1RtI and IL-1RtII, but the relative affinity for the murine IL-1RtII is about 3000-fold lower than for the murine IL-1RtI. The apparent affinity of rhIRAP for the murine IL-1RtI is only two- to fourfold lower than for IL-1 ligands, however.

The biological activities of IRAP *in vitro* and *in vivo* are consistent with the conclusions from the receptor-binding studies: namely, that IRAP is a competitive antagonist of IL-1 at the level of the IL-1 receptor. We have shown that rhIRAP inhibits induction of murine thymocyte proliferation by treatment with IL-1 and mitogen, the induction of IL-2 by similar treatment with IL-1 and mitogen in murine LBRM-33-1A5 T cells, and the adhesion of human neutrophils and eosinophils to IL-1-stimulated human endothelial cells.[42] In all cases, the inhibition by rhIRAP was dose related and achieved complete inhibition of IL-1 activity at the higher concentrations used. The amounts of rhIRAP necessary for 50% inhibition varied significantly among these assays, however, despite the fact that they all are driven by the IL-1RtI. The molar ratios of IRAP to IL-1 necessary for 50% inhibition were about 7 to 10:1 for the thymocyte and endothelial cell assays, but about 200:1 for the LBRM-33-1A5 assay. By comparison, the molar ratio for 50% inhibition of IL-1 binding to the IL-1RtI was about 4:1. The reason for the need for higher ratios of IRAP to IL-1 in the LBRM-33-1A5 assay probably relates to the low percentage of receptors that are required for triggering a response in that cell line. The LBRM-33-1A5 cells are about 30-fold more sensitive to IL-1 than thymocytes in the respective bioassays. IRAP would need to occupy the majority (probably greater than 90%) of the IL-1 receptors on LBRM-33-1A5 cells in order to block the triggering of a sufficient number of receptors by IL-1 to achieve a biological response. In addition to these assays, we have shown that rhIRAP can completely and specifically inhibit the activity of IL-1α and IL-1β on fibroblasts, chondrocytes, and human T cells *in vitro*. We have tested rhIRAP in assays for non-IL-1 cytokines, such as IL-2 and IFN-γ, but have never seen any inhibition. These observations suggest that IRAP may be specific for IL-1 receptors and IL-1-mediated biological activities. It should also be noted that throughout the course of these studies, no IL-1-like agonist activities of rhIRAP have ever been observed.

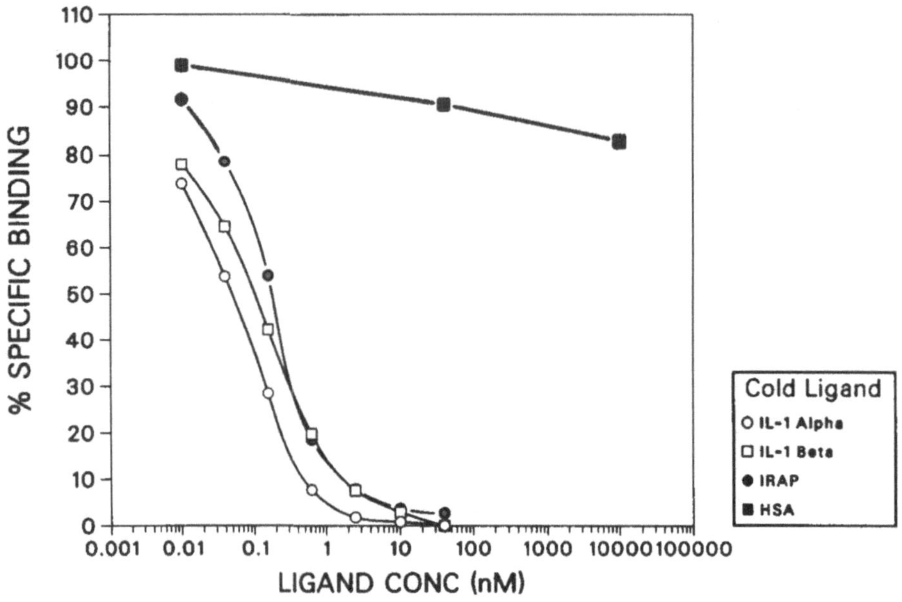

FIGURE 3. Receptor-binding competition study with murine LBRM-33-1A5 cells (IL-1RtI-bearing) and ^{125}I-IL-1α.

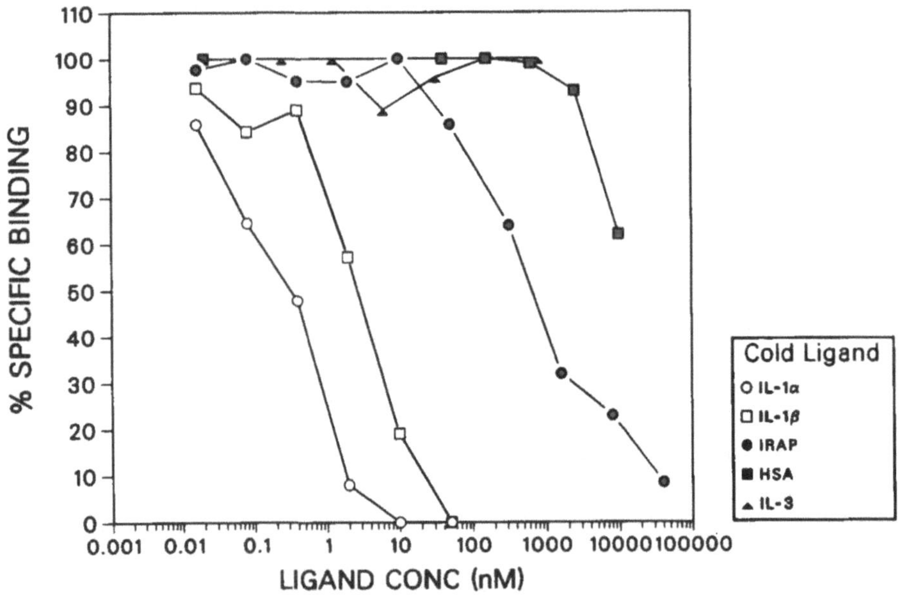

FIGURE 4. Receptor-binding competition study with murine bone marrow cells (IL-1RtI-bearing) and ^{125}I-IL-1α.

We also wanted to demonstrate that IRAP could inhibit IL-1 activities *in vivo*. Two distinct IL-1 assays in mice were utilized: the induction of blood neutrophilia and the induction of serum corticosterone 3 h after subcutaneous injection of 50 or 500 ng of rhIL-1α.[42] With the higher dose of IL-1, simultaneous injection of IRAP potently inhibited corticosterone induction (complete inhibition by 30 mg/mouse rhIRAP), but not inhibit neutrophilia (even at a dose of 300 mg/mouse). However, dose-related inhibition of neutrophilia was achieved with 300 to 1000 mg/mouse rhIRAP using the lower dose of IL-1.[48] The molar ratio of rhIRAP relative to IL-1 required for 50% inhibition of neutrophilia was about 1000-fold higher than for inhibition of corticosterone. Although it is tempting to speculate from these results that the corticosterone response is mediated by IL-1RtI in the brain and neutrophilia is mediated by IL-1RtII on bone marrow cells, others have demonstrated that IL-1-induced neutrophilia in mice is inhibited by antibodies to the IL-1RtI.[49] It is possible that the quantitative differences in IRAP potencies in these two assays reflect the pharmacokinetics or tissue accessibilities of rhIRAP as compared with rhIL-1α *in vivo*. Nonetheless, rhIRAP was able to inhibit IL-1 activities *in vivo*, at least in mice. Other studies with IRAP have substantiated these results in other IL-1-driven models *in vitro* and *in vivo* and have extended them to a variety of inflammation models in animals (reviewed in References 1 and 50). The clinical utility of IRAP or IL-1ra in septic shock, rheumatoid arthritis, inflammatory bowel disease, and other inflammatory diseases remains to be demonstrated.

II. IL-1 INHIBITION STRATEGIES

Under the assumptions that IL-1 agonists exacerbate a variety of disease conditions and that moderation of IL-1 activity would be of therapeutic benefit in these circumstances, a number of possible intervention strategies present themselves. They fall roughly into two categories: those that aim to reduce the effective concentration of active IL-1 species at the site of action and those that attempt to intervene directly in the interactions of IL-1 with its receptors to eliminate or retard IL-1 signal transduction. Several of the strategies in the first category propose to develop agents that would disable the IL-1 molecule by, for example, chemical modification or by use of monoclonal antibodies to the agonist or by use of a soluble form of a receptor. Other strategies in the first category propose to reduce the production of active IL-1 molecules and one of the more popular of these targets is the protease that processes the IL-1β precursor.[51] Among the strategies in the latter category are those proposing to develop agents that bind to IL-1 receptors and prevent agonist binding or signal transduction, and the soundness of such strategies is seemingly underscored by the existence of naturally occurring IL-1 receptor antagonists.[42]

Several of the strategies in both categories incorporate the inherent specificity of the interactions of IL-1 agonists with receptors and, as specificity is one of the most prized attributes of a therapeutic agent, these strategies are especially attractive to those involved in drug discovery. The need to incorporate this specificity into bioassays with which to screen for discovery and guide drug development was recognized and fulfilled from the very beginning. The need for more detailed chemical and structural information about the nature of IL-1 receptor interactions with which to select from among appropriate strategies and guide drug design was also recognized early, and the first of the relevant proteins available to us for structure study was a recombinant version of processed human IL-1β.[52]

III. IL-1 STRUCTURE

The nearly simultaneous appearance of IL-1β protein in the crystallographic laboratories of several pharmaceutical companies sparked a flurry of crystallographic effort and produced at least four independent crystallographic determinations of the structure of the human IL-1β molecule, all based on the same tetragonal crystal form, all at about the same resolution,[53-57] a structure determination of murine IL-1β,[58] as well as a solution structure of the human IL-1β molecule by nuclear magnetic resonance (NMR).[59] The four independent crystal structures of human IL-1β are essentially the same; only minor differences distinguish them from each other[60] or from the NMR structure.[61] All concur in an IL-1β molecule composed primarily of β strands, 12 of them in all, joined by 11 loops and assembled antiparallel into a compact structure (Figure 5). The centerpiece of this structure is a six-stranded β barrel, which is capped at one end by the other six strands in a pseudo-threefold symmetric arrangement about the axis of the barrel. In this structure, the β strands represent the girders internal to the

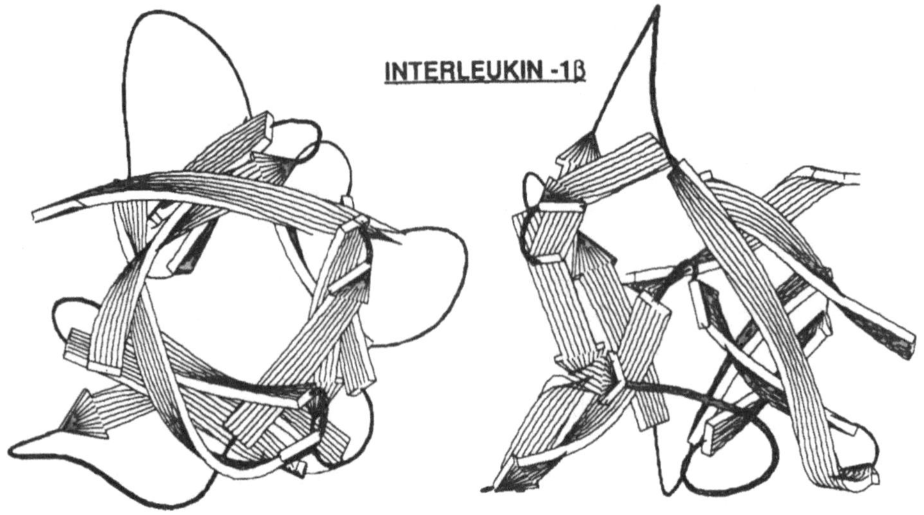

FIGURE 5. Schematic representation of the structure of human interleukin-1β. The arrows denote the position and orientation of β strands. The view at left is down the axis of the barrel. In the right view, this axis is turned horizontal and lies in the plane of the page.

molecule and they are arranged to present the loops on the surface of the molecule and open to the external environment.

A topological homologue of the IL-1β structure had been encountered previously in the crystal structure of a Kunitz-type serine protease inhibitor from legume seeds, soybean trypsin inhibitor, in complex with trypsin,[62] and analysis of the topology of the inhibitor had recognized the pseudo-threefold symmetry of the fold.[63] A second structure of a legume seed protease inhibitor, this one from the seeds of *Erythrina caffra* (Figure 6) and not complexed with protease, confirms the structural similarities between these two groups of proteins.[64]

Structure determinations of IL-1α, in its processed form, followed shortly after those of IL-1β and confirmed expectations, based on modest similarities in sequence (about 25% identity), that the two IL-1 agonist forms would be similar in structure.[65,66] In fact, with one notable exception, IL-1α is topologically identical to IL-1β in that there is a one-to-one structural correspondence between the β strands and loops in IL-1β and β strands and loops in IL-1α. The exception is an extra β strand in IL-1α formed by an extension of the N-terminus relative to IL-1β that folds down along the side of the barrel and forms β sheet-type hydrogen bond interactions with portions of two of the loops (Figure 7). There are, of course, significant structural differences between IL-1α and IL-1β in the compositions and conformations of the loops. The similarities in folding topology between the two agonists, however, combined with the expectation that the IL-1 receptor antagonist molecule would have a homologous structure,[42-45] have led us, with apologies to soybean trypsin inhibitor advocates, to come to think of this pseudo-threefold symmetric β structure, with a six-stranded β barrel capped at one end, as the interleukin-1 fold. Because of its occurrence in two such diverse protein families as the interleukins-1 and the legume seed serine protease inhibitors (Kunitz), we conclude that the interleukin-1 fold represents a special structural arrangement adaptable by nature to a wide variety of biological uses.

This conclusion has been underscored by the results of structure determinations that showed that the acidic and basic forms of fibroblast growth factor, each with weak (about 10%) sequence similarities to IL-1β, both have the interleukin-1 folding topology,[67-69] as do a serine proteinase-amylase inhibitor from wheat germ[70] and the hisactophilin from *Dictyostelium discoideum*,[71] and by a detailed analysis of the patterns of structure in the interleukin-1, or β-trefoil, fold.[72]

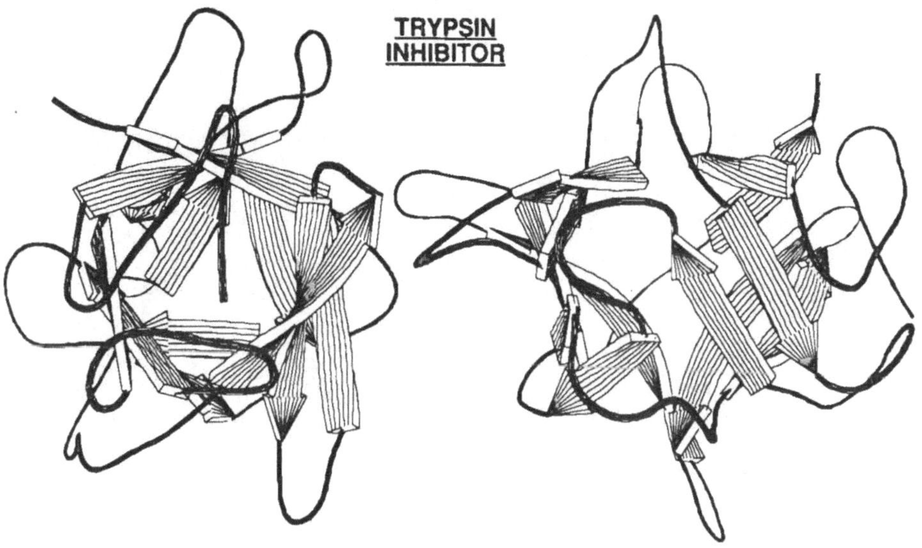

FIGURE 6. The structure of the trypsin inhibitor from seeds of *Erythrina caffra*.

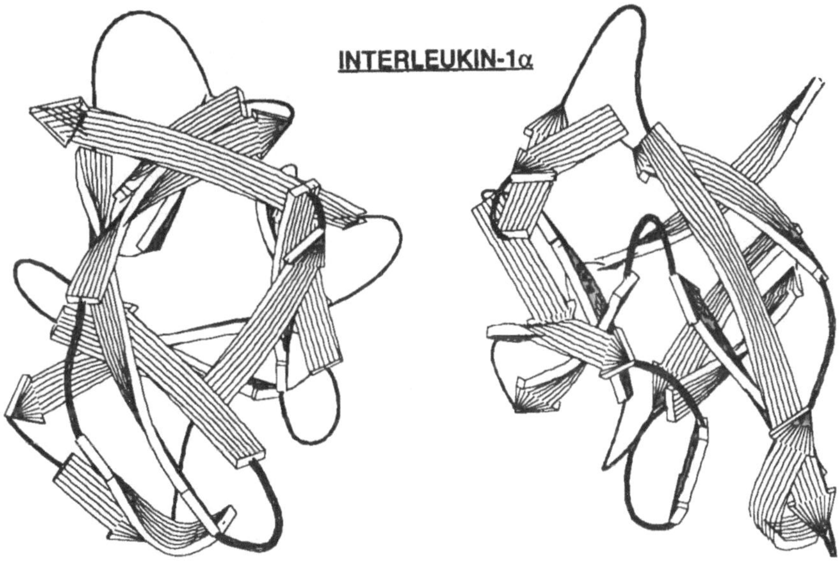

FIGURE 7. The structure of human interleukin-1α.

But a parallel, and perhaps more important, conclusion must also be acknowledged. If molecules of such diverse biological purposes as the legume seed protease inhibitors, mammalian IL-1 cytokines, and fibroblast growth factors share a common β strand architecture, then it must be the loops connecting the strands, and the chemical and conformational structures of those loops, that distinguish these proteins one from another, determine their interactions with their environments and their receptors, express their specificities, and provide their activities. In the case of the fibroblast growth factor structures (Figure 8), these external loops are in general less extensive than their counterparts in the IL-1s or other homologues and, as a result, the fibroblast growth factors appear to approach more closely ideal threefold molecular symmetry than do their homologues. Thus, while these molecules

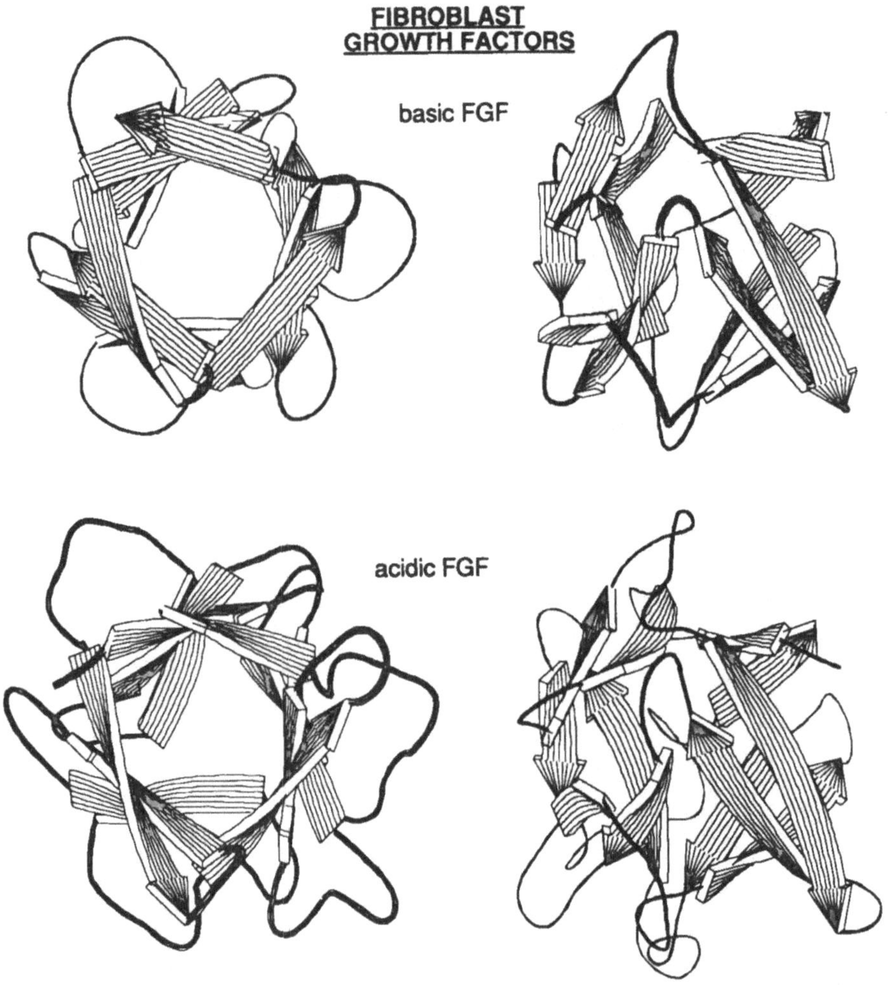

FIGURE 8. The structures of two forms of human fibroblast growth factor, basic and acidic.

may show some fundamental similarities, it is their differences that are likely to hold the keys to understanding of receptor binding, specificity, and activity.

IV. IL-1 MOLECULAR INTERPRETATIONS

Experimental efforts to identify those parts of the IL-1 molecules critical for function were initiated as soon as the molecular nature of these agents was established. This work began well before the structures of these molecules were determined, and its start is approximately contemporary with the successful cloning of IL-1α and -β. As more became known about the IL-1 system and its receptors, it became clear that there were two key features to IL-1 function, receptor binding and stimulation of IL-1 responses. A number of different techniques were used to probe for regions of the IL-1 molecule crucial for function. They include mutagenesis techniques, peptide fragment techniques, chemical modification techniques, and techniques based on the use of monoclonal antibodies.

Some of the earliest work involved heterologous expression of N- and C-terminal truncations of IL-1 to identify the minimum lengths required for activity.[73-80] These studies showed that truncations, natural or artificial, of up to three or four residues could be tolerated from either end of the processed forms of IL-1α and -β, and that somewhat more extensive truncations could be made to the N-terminus of processed IL-1α, before activity was extinguished. The structures of IL-1α and IL-1β provide a structural rationale for some, but not all, of these findings. As seen in Figures 5 and 7, both N- and C-termini in these molecules are staves in the six-stranded β barrels that are core structural features, and successive truncations of termini in these molecules quickly begin to remove residues and hydrogen bonds critical to the stability of β barrel structure. The exception is the N-terminus of IL-1α, which includes some 15 residues prior to the first in the barrel and which experiments show accomodates more extensive truncation.

A logical extension of these truncation studies hypothesized that sequences crucial to IL-1 function could be identified by preparing those peptides and testing them in available assays. Peptides for use in these studies could be obtained by proteolysis of IL-1 samples, by recombinant methods, or by direct peptide synthesis. Some expectation that an approach of this type might provide useful results for IL-1 came from the successes of a similar approach targeting basic fibroblast growth factor.[81] The analysis of IL-1 subpeptides for biological activity proved to be one of the more popular modes of study of IL-1 for several years; a number of subpeptides were identified in early studies and a variety of activities were ascribed to them.[82-89] In general, however, further study has shown the specific activities of these subpeptides to be too weak to be exploited for practical use (for example, Reference 90), and none of these subpeptides has led to the development of a therapeutic antagonist of IL-1 activity. In fact, more systematic approaches have led to disappointing conclusions.[91,92] In the former,[91] overlapping synthetic octapeptides, corresponding to all elements of the IL-1β sequence exposed on the surface of the molecule, were tested for receptor-binding activity in a radiolabeled IL-1α competition assay and no binding was found even at up to 100-fold excess of peptide over radioligand. In the latter study,[92] the structure of IL-1β was used to design a series of subpeptides meant to emulate the loops on the surface of the molecule, maximizing the likelihood of maintaining similar tertiary structure and minimizing hydrophobicity (Figure 9). Thirteen peptides were designed, synthesized, and tested in IL-1β and IL-1α receptor-binding assays, a T cell activation assay, and against a battery of monoclonal antibodies to IL-1β. In no case was a peptide identified that competed effectively for receptor binding or expressed IL-1β activity.

Mutagenesis studies that target individual residues in IL-1 have also proved to be a popular tactic for searching for the sequences critical to function. A variety of target residues have been analyzed by this method, in which mutants with different residues replacing the target residue are expressed, purified, and tested in receptor-binding and activity assays.[93-99] Some of these mutant proteins proved to be important in structural studies of IL-1β by NMR.[93,97] As was the case with peptide fragment analyses, a variety of activities have been ascribed to mutant proteins discovered in these studies, but activities of mutants are generally weak and none has so far led to development of a therapeutic antagonist of IL-1 activity. A number of these studies have been very informative, however.[100-105] As a specific example, mutation of the arginine at position 11 in the sequence of processed IL-1β to glycine is reported to reduce the bioactivity of the IL-1β mutant, allowing it to bind to receptors with about the same affinity as wild-type, but diminishing its signal transduction capability by about 100-fold.[106] We have found similar results for this mutant,[107] whose properties suggest that receptor binding and signal transduction are at least to some extent separate and distinct properties of the IL-1β molecule.

Similarly detailed, residue-specific information has been obtained from chemical modification studies of the interleukins-1. In these studies, reactive residues near the molecular surface and exposed to solution are treated with reagents that covalently modify these residues. Studies of this kind have pointed out the importance of specific cysteine, lysine, and arginine residues to the receptor-binding and biological properties of mature IL-1β and IL-1α.[108-113]

Antibodies, monoclonal and polyclonal, neutralizing or non-neutralizing, to IL-1 molecules have played a major role in evaluations and interpretations of peptide studies and

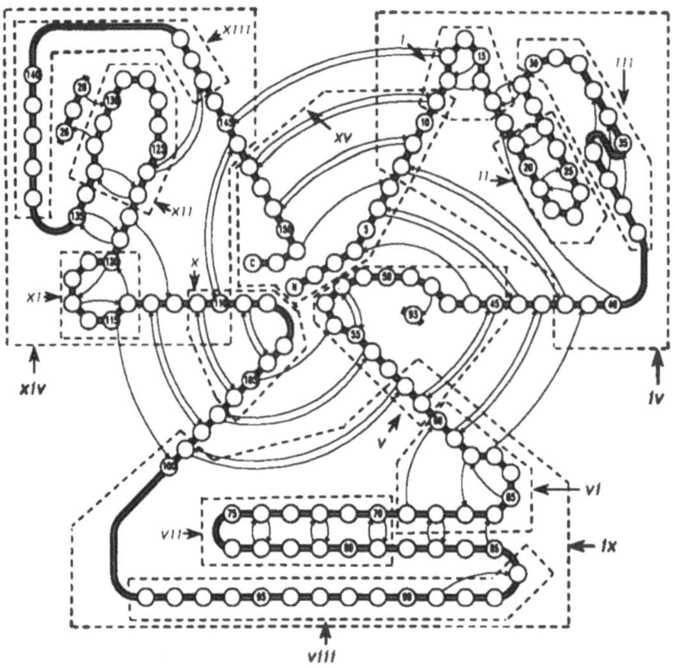

FIGURE 9. Schematic representation of the structure of IL-1β, emphasizing the relationships between residues (circles) that interact through backbone hydrogen bonds (arrows). The dashed lines isolate polypeptide segments, primarily exposed surface loops, that were tested for activity.

mutational studies. This role has been recently reviewed.[114] Antibodies have also proved important in probing the role of IL-1 in disease conditions (for example, Reference 115).

Recently, mutagenesis studies have been used to distinguish IL-1β residues crucial for type I receptor binding, but not for type II receptor binding.[116] Seven residues widely separated in sequence were found that, when replaced by other amino acid residues, resulted in greater than 100-fold reductions in competitive binding to type I receptors. These residues cluster on the surface of the molecule near the N-terminal side of the rim of the β barrel and represent about 400 Å^2 of the accessible surface of the molecule. Expectations that receptor-binding sites on IL-1 molecules would be discontinuous and would involve significant tracts of molecular surface area had been raised by some of the peptide fragment studies cited above and by studies of surface areas occluded in protein-protein interactions.[117,118] Of more significance here is the confirmation of suspicions that binding sites for different receptors on IL-1 molecules might be different. This is a precious, but imperfect glimpse of the interaction of IL-1β with the type I receptor; it suggests much more must be known of the structure and variety of possible ligand-receptor interactions before we will be able to fully understand the IL-1 system.

V. IRAP STRUCTURE

Speculations on the nature of differences and similarities between structures of IL-1β, IL-1α, and the receptor antagonist protein followed closely on reports of the primary structure of IRAP.[42-45] The sequence of IRAP, when aligned with sequences of IL-1β and IL-1α, is identical to those sequences in 26% and 18% of amino acid positions, respectively (Figure 10). The higher observed similarity to the IL-1β sequence led to immediate assumptions that IRAP more closely resembles this form of IL-1. Only 17 amino acids are conserved in all three sequences. These residues are found in conserved elements of secondary structure and are apparently more important to the homologous folding of these molecules than to the conservation

```
IL-1β                          APVRS LNCTLRDSQQ KSLVMSGPYE LKALHLQGQD MEQQVVFSMS
IRAP                      RPSGRKSSKM QAFRIWDVNQ KTFYLR NNQ LVAGYLQGPN VNLEEKIDVV
IL-1α           SSPFSFLSN VKYNFMRIIK YEFILNDALN QSIIRANDQY LTAAALH  N LDEAVKFDMG

IL-1β           FVQGEESNDK IPVALGLKEK NLYLSCVLKD DKPTLQLESV D PKNYPKKK MEKRFVFNKI
IRAP            PI      EP HALFLGIHGG KMCLSCVKSG DETRLQLEAV NITDLSENRK QDKRFAFIRS
IL-1α           AYKSSKDDAK ITVILRISKT QLYVTAQDE  DQPVLLKEMP EIPKTITG   SETNLLFFWE

IL-1β           EINNKLEFES AQFPNWYISI SQAENMPVFL GGTK GGQDI TDFTMQFVSS
IRAP            DSGPTTSFES AACPGWFLCI AMEADQPVSL TNMPDEGVMV IKFYFQEDE
IL-1α           THGTKNYFTS VAHPNLFIAI KQ  DYWVCL AGG  PP SI TDFQILENQA
```

IRAP *vs* IL-1β
26% amino acid conservation

IRAP *vs* IL-1α
18% amino acid conservation

FIGURE 10. Optimum alignment of sequences of interleukins-1α, -1β, and IRAP.

of any surface characteristic that we would expect to find among molecules that bind a common receptor. No clearly conserved portion of the IL-1 sequence can be identified as important to function by comparison of the sequences alone.

The availability of sequence data has led naturally to efforts to devise models for the structure of IRAP. Using the backbone conformation of IL-1β as a template on which to build, models of IRAP have been proposed that have all the gross structural characteristics of IL-1β.[119,120] Homology modeling experiments of this sort can often be an aid in identifying parts of a structure that must be different for the reason that the sequence of the homologous protein cannot be mapped conservatively onto the known structure. Most of the IRAP sequence can be mapped onto IL-1β without difficulty, again suggesting that the two structures are quite similar.

Detailed experimental characterization of the IRAP structure has also been initiated. NMR has been used to show that IRAP has a secondary structure consistent with its assignment as a member of the interleukin-1 fold, and that the sequence alignment used in homology modeling efforts[119,120] was correct.[121,122] Hydrogen bond relationships defined by heteronuclear three-dimensional NMR spectroscopy confirm that the structure has the twelve β strands homologous to IL-1β, and two short helical segments in the loops joining β3 to β4 and β7 to β8 (using here and elsewhere the IL-1β secondary structure designation[42]).

Our own efforts to determine the structure of IRAP by use of X-ray crystallographic techniques have met with success recently.[123] Crystals can be grown from samples of purified human IRAP[42] at 4°C from solutions of PEG 4000 buffered at pH 7.0.[124] These crystals belong to space group $P4_32_12$, with cell dimensions a = b = 72.46 Å, c = 114.4 Å, and two molecules per asymmetric unit. Persistent attempts to solve this structure by molecular replacement failed, whether with trial models based on complete or truncated models of IL-1β or IL-1α or with models of IRAP derived from homology modeling.[119,120] We have identified two heavy atom derivatives of this crystal form, one obtained by soaking native crystals in a solution of 5 m*M* $Au(CN)_2$, the other in 5 m*M* $(CH_3)_3PbCl$. While heavy atom substituents in both these derivatives occupy the same binding site in IRAP crystals, isomorphous and anomalous differences in structure factor amplitudes observed in these two derivatives are sufficient to calculate 4.0 Å phases. The resulting electron density, flattened in areas of disordered solvent,[125] can be readily interpreted. We have finished construction of

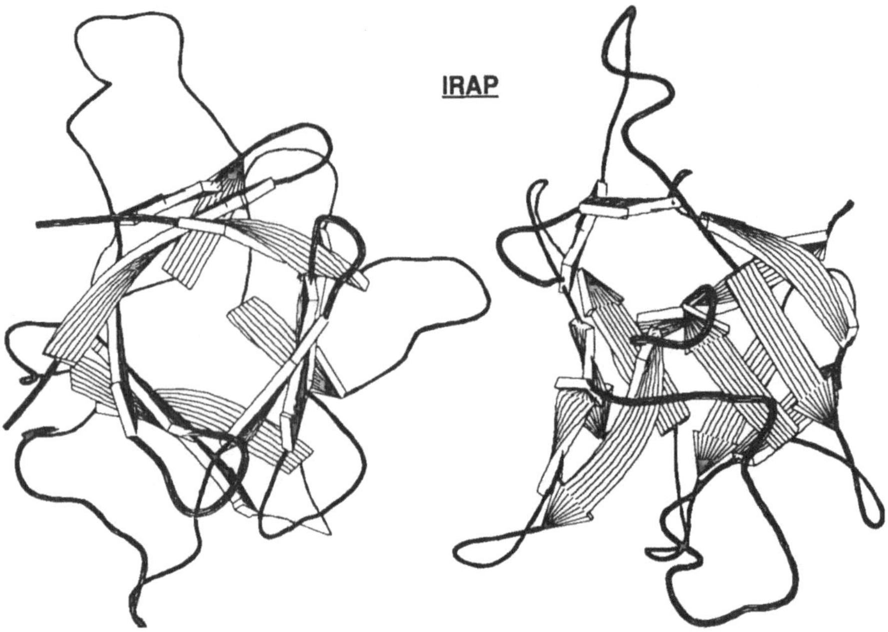

FIGURE 11. The structure of human IRAP.

models for each of the two molecules in the asymmetric unit. Though these results must be considered preliminary while refinement continues, the models offer the first complete view of the IRAP structure.

A schematic illustration of the IRAP structure is shown in Figure 11 so the arrangement of β strands may be compared to those in the other IL-1 molecules. Secondary structure identifications derived from our model agree very closely with those obtained by NMR for IRAP in solution. All 12 β strands characteristic of molecules in this structural class are found as arranged in IL-1β. Loops dominate the molecule surface. Agonist and antagonist molecules are most different on one hemispheric face of the molecule. The conformation of loops joining strands β4 to β5, β7 to β8, and β11 to β12 are quite different in IRAP, and all these loops converge to form the one face of the molecule that diverges strongly from the same face on IL-1β. In contrast, loops joining strands β2 to β3, β3 to β4, and β5 to β6 show only small differences, while the remainder of the loops and the exposed portion of the β barrel are nearly identical to IL-1β in backbone conformation. The backbone conformation of some, but not all, of the region of IL-1β that bears the site proposed to bind to IL-1 receptors[116] is conservatively replicated in IRAP, and this is equally true for IL-1α. On the other hand, none of the amino acids in positions suggested as crucial to receptor-binding efficacy in IL-1β are conserved among all three IL-1 ligand molecules.

The most conspicuous difference in the structures arises from the truncation of six residues from the loop joining β strands β4 and β5 in the antagonist protein. It has been claimed[82-84] that a peptide fragment from IL-1β including much of this loop (EESNDKI) possesses immunostimulatory properties. While both IL-1α and IL-1β utilize the same number of residues in completing this loop, our structural data show that the conformation of this loop is quite different in the two structures. IL-1β adopts a novel configuration for this loop,[42] probably necessitated by the presence of an interfering proline residue at position 57 (using the numbering for the mature, fully processed molecule). This loop possesses quite a different arrangement in IL-1α,[65] that of the much more commonly encountered twisted beta pair. In

IRAP,[123] this loop appears to be truncated to a much shorter twisted beta pair. It is difficult to envision an important role for this loop in receptor binding or signal transduction in light of such striking differences in structure among the three homologues.

It has been reported that a point mutation in IRAP (Lys 145 to Asp) changes the antagonist into a weak agonist.[126] This observation complicates our understanding of the IL-1 system, because the point of mutation is outside of the region identified as the discontinuous binding site of IL-1β.[116] This suggests that either a larger binding site is required for signal transduction than previously believed, or that a different binding site on IRAP, one not structurally homologous to the binding site on IL-1β, is used in interactions between the antagonist and receptor.

VI. IL-1 RECEPTOR STUDIES

As described in the introduction above, two different kinds of IL-1 receptors have so far been characterized, one the predominant IL-1 receptor on the surfaces of T lymphocytes and fibroblasts, the other predominating on B cells and monocytes. The receptors, both of which seem to interact to a greater or lesser degree with the three known IL-1 ligands, are separate gene products.[12] The T cell or type I receptor of about 80 kDa is a concatenation of three similar extracellular domains that bear some resemblance to immunoglobulin-like domains, and this concatenation is attached through a short transmembrane segment to an intracellular domain of about 200 residues.[18,19] The B cell or type II receptor of 68 kDa also is a concatenation of three extracellular immunoglobulin-like domains attached through a short transmembrane segment to an intracellular domain, but in this case the inner domain of about 30 residues is drastically truncated relative to that of the type I receptor.[22] The function of one or both of these receptors is to bind IL-1 ligand and signal this binding intracellularly. Because of differences in intracellular domains, it is not inconceivable that the two types of receptor feed into different signal transduction pathways. It is also possible that the type II receptor, with its truncated intracellular domain, plays no role in signal transduction at all.

The diverse variety of activities displayed by the three IL-1 molecules has already been described. The fact that a sizeable part of the surface of IL-1β, when altered by mutation, eliminates binding to type I receptor without materially affecting binding to type II receptor suggests that different receptors may bind to different parts of a ligand.[116] One is led to consider the possibility that each ligand-receptor pair is itself unique, and that, with three known ligands and two known receptors, the number of such unique pair-wise interactions could be as many as six. While the tools of molecular biology and biochemistry are critically important in defining ligand-receptor interactions, they are not sufficient in themselves to provide the information required for drug design. Structural studies are required, and both X-ray crystallographic and NMR techniques can provide important information.

We have begun to attack the problem of getting structural information about IL-1 ligand-receptor interactions by crystallographic methods. The extracellular portion of the mouse receptor type I, truncated near the beginning transmembrane segment, has been expressed in insect cells by infection with baculovirus, purified, and provided to us for crystallization experiments.[127] Samples of this protein mixed with human IRAP have produced very small crystals in the form of hexagonal plates or tablets in crystallization trials.[128] When IRAP ligand is eliminated, an apparent second form occurs in which crystals appear as very small tetragonal bipyramids or octahedra. In neither case have we been able so far to obtain crystal specimens large enough for crystallographic purposes. We hope, however, that continued experimentation will lead to the protein samples and crystals needed to determine the structures of IL-1 ligand-receptor complexes and provide the structural detail needed to exploit the IL-1 system for therapeutic purposes.

VII. CONCLUSIONS

A large body of evidence points to a pathogenic role of IL-1 in inflammatory diseases such as septic shock, rheumatoid arthritis, and inflammatory bowel disease. A drug that blocks IL-1 activities would be extremely useful in treating these diseases. The pathways involved in IL-1 binding to its receptors and the subsequent signal transduction events present many potential opportunities for drug design. However, at the present time, the signal transduction pathways in the various IL-1-responsive cells are not well defined, and certainly no molecular targets unique to the IL-1 signal transduction pathways, other than the IL-1 receptors, have been reported as yet. The scope of IL-1 receptor pathway approaches to drug design is thus effectively limited to the interactions of ligands directly with IL-1 receptors. Since there is no direct evidence that the IL-1RtII actually tranduces a signal to cells, the most reasonable first candidate for drug targeting becomes the IL-1RtI and its interaction with IL-1 ligands. To this end, IRAP and the IL-1α and IL-1β ligands are invaluable tools with which to probe and model the structural bases of interactions with IL-1RtI. The use of IRAP directly as a therapeutic agent is being tested clinically in a large number of diseases. However, the use of this protein as a therapeutic agent is limited to parenteral administration. An orally active, small molecule IL-1 receptor antagonist of comparable affinity to IRAP would be the preferred drug.

The design of a small molecule that acts as an IL-1 receptor antagonist will require much more detailed structural characterizations of the interactions of IL-1 ligands with IL-1 receptors. Initial studies in our laboratory suggest that crystallization of soluble IL-1 receptor-ligand complexes is an achievable goal. What is needed to determine the structure of such a receptor-ligand complex, we believe, is a dedicated effort by a team with molecular biology, protein chemistry, and crystallography capabilities to optimize the preparation of component proteins for crystallographic success.

A broad surface region of IL-1β has been proposed as the receptor binding site, based on mutation and other studies.[116] Our structure determination of IRAP shows that the backbone conformation of some, but not all, of this discontinuous region has a counterpart in IRAP, and the same is true for IL-1α. This rough similarity in backbone structure is not reflected in sequence similarities, however; none of the amino acids in positions suggested as crucial to receptor binding in IL-1β are conserved among all three IL-1 ligand molecules. Clearly, there remain significant questions about the identity and extent of a receptor-binding epitope. In fact, some of the data on fine specificity of IL-1 ligand binding suggest that IL-1α and IL-1β may not share a common receptor-binding epitope at all. The corresponding epitope on the IL-1 receptor is completely undefined, so that, in any case, structure-based design of an IL-1 receptor antagonist continues to present significant challenges.

There remains the possibility that multiple epitopes on IL-1 agonist ligands may be necessary for function. The strong similarities in the tertiary structures of agonist and antagonist ligands, coupled with the observations that (1) IRAP binds to IL-1RtI with high affinity, (2) IRAP competitively inhibits IL-1 binding, (3) the complex of IRAP and IL-1RtI is not internalized in cells, and (4) IRAP does not activate transduction of an IL-1-like signal to cells, support the notion that there may be distinct receptor-binding and signal-transduction epitopes on IL-1 agonist ligands. It is possible that either internalization of the receptor-ligand complex or signal transduction or both are initiated by colocalization or binding of the complex with an accessory molecule in the membrane, and this is consistent with our current understanding of the signal transduction pathways used by the IL-1 system (see, for example, Reference 129). Although evidence is limited, this theory seems to explain the available data. It also offers the possibility that agents might be designed to interfere with this second epitope and block the interactions between the IL-1 receptor-ligand complex and its signal transduction apparatus.

In conclusion, structure determinations of the IL-1 ligand molecules, IL-1α, IL-1β, and IRAP, have provided a glimpse of the structural bases for the interactions of these ligands with IL-1 receptors. As knowledge of the structures of IL-1 receptors is obtained, structure-based design of IL-1 receptor antagonists will become a feasible and reasonable approach to the discovery of novel anti-inflammatory drugs.

ACKNOWLEDGMENTS

We thank our many colleagues and former colleagues at the Upjohn Company who have worked with us to study the interleukin-1 system and its role in disease. We also thank P. M. Allred and M. L. Adams of the Upjohn Corporate Technical Library for their unstinting help in accessing the interleukin-1 literature.

REFERENCES

1. **Dinarello, C.A.,** Interleukin-1 and interleukin-1 antagonism, *Blood,* 77, 1627, 1991.
2. **Dinarello, C.A.,** Interleukin-1 and its biologically related cytokines, *Adv. Immunol.,* 44, 153, 1989.
3. **Oppenheim, J.J., Kovacs, E.J., Matsushima, K., and Durum, S.J.,** There is more than one interleukin-1, *Immunol. Today,* 7, 45, 1986.
4. **March, C.J., Mosley, B., Larsen, A., Cerretti, D.P., Braedt, G., Price, V., Gillis, S., Henney, C.S., Kronheim, S.R., Grabstein, K., Conlon, P.T., Hopp, T.P., and Cosman, D.,** Cloning, sequence and expression of two distinct human interleukin-1 complementary DNAs, *Nature,* 315, 641, 1985.
5. **Cannon, J.G., Tompkins, R.G., Gelfand, J.A., Michie, H.R., Stanford, G.G., van der Meer, J.W.M., Endres, S., Lonnemann, G., Corsetti, J., Chernow, B., Wilmore, D.W., Wolff, S.W., and Dinarello, C.A.,** Circulating interleukin-1 and tumor necrosis factor in septic shock and experimental endotoxin fever, *J. Infect. Dis.,* 161, 79, 1990.
6. **Eastgate, J.A., Symons, J.A., Wood, N.C., Grinlinton, F.M., di Giovine, F.S., and Duff, G.W.,** Correlation of plasma interleukin 1 levels with disease activity in rheumatoid arthritis, *Lancet,* 2, 706, 1988.
7. **Firestein, G.S., Alvaro-Gracia, J.M., and Maki, R.,** Quantitative analysis of cytokine gene expression in rheumatoid arthritis, *J. Immunol.,* 144, 3347, 1990.
8. **Wood, D.D., Ihrie, E.J., Dinarello, C.A., and Cohen, P.L.,** Isolation of an interleukin 1-like factor from human joint effusions, *Arthritis Rheum.,* 29, 975, 1983.
9. **Chandrasekar, S., Harvey, A.K., Hrubey, P.S., and Bendele, A.M.,** Arthritis induced by interleukin-1 is dependent on the site and frequency of intraarticular injection, *Clin. Immunol. Immunopathol.,* 55, 382, 1990.
10. **Staite, N.D., Richard, K.A., Aspar, D.G., Franz, K.A., and Galinet, L.A.,** Induction of an acute erosive monoarticular arthritis in mice by interleukin-1 and methylated bovine serum albumin, *Arthritis Rheum.,* 33, 253, 1990.
11. **Dower, S.K. and Sims, J.E.,** Structure and function of murine and human IL-1 receptors, in *Cellular and Molecular Mechanisms of Inflammation,* Vol. 1, Gimbrone, Micael, A., Ed., Academic Press, New York, 1990, 137.
12. **Chizzonite, R., Truitt, T., Kilian, P.L., Stern, A.S., Nunes, P., Parker, K.P., Kaffka, K.L., Chua, A.O., Lugg, D.K., and Gubler, U.,** Two high-affinity interleukin 1 receptors represent separate gene products, *Proc. Natl. Acad. Sci. U.S.A.,* 86, 8029, 1989.
13. **Bomsztyk, K., Sims, J.E., Stanton, T.H., Slack, J., McMahan, C.J., Valentine, M.A., and Dower, S.K.,** Evidence for different interleukin 1 receptors in murine B- and T-cell lines, *Proc. Natl. Acad. Sci. U.S.A.,* 86, 8034, 1989.
14. **Solari, R.,** Identification and distribution of two forms of the interleukin 1 receptor, *Cytokine,* 2, 21, 1990.
15. **Benjamin, D., Wormsley, S., and Dower, S.K.,** Heterogeneity in interleukin (IL)-1 receptors expressed on human B cell lines. Differences in the molecular properties of IL-1α and IL-1β binding sites, *J. Biol. Chem.,* 265, 9943, 1990.
16. **Horuk, R.,** Differences in internalization and intracellular processing of interleukin-1 associated with the two forms of interleukin-1 receptor found in B-cells and T-cells, *Biochem. J.,* 273, 79, 1991.
17. **Bird, T.A., Gearing, A.J.H., and Saklatvala, J.,** Murine interleukin 1 receptor. Direct identification by ligand blotting and purification to homogeneity of an interleukin 1-binding glycoprotein, *J. Biol. Chem.,* 263, 12063, 1988.
18. **Sims, J.E., March, C.J., Cosman, D., Widmer, M.B., MacDonald, H.R., McMahan, C.J., Grubin, C.E., Wignall, J.M., Jackson, J.L., Call, S.M., Friend, D., Alpert, A.L., Gillis, S., Urdal, D.L., and Dower, S.K.,** cDNA expression cloning of the IL-1 receptor, a member of the immunoglobulin superfamily, *Science,* 241, 585, 1988.

19. **Sims, J.E., Acres, R.B., Grubin, C.E., McMahan, C.J., Wignall, J.M., March, C.J., and Dower, S.K.**, Cloning the interleukin 1 receptor from human T cells, *Proc. Natl. Acad. Sci. U.S.A.*, 86, 8946, 1989.
20. **Horuk, R., Huang, J.J., Covington, M., and Newton, R.C.**, A biochemical and kinetic analysis of the interleukin-1 receptor, *J. Biol. Chem.*, 262, 16275, 1987.
21. **Symons, J.A., Eastgate, J.A., and Duff, G.W.**, A soluble binding protein specific for interleukin 1β is produced by activated mononuclear cells, *Cytokine*, 2, 190, 1990.
22. **McMahan, C.J., Slack, J.L., Mosley, B., Cosman, D., Lupton, S.D., Brunton, L.L., Grubin, C.E., Wignall, J.M., Jenkins, N.A., Brannan, C.I., Copeland, N.G., Huebner, K., Croce, C.M., Cannizzarro, L.A., Benjamin, D., Dower, S.K., Spriggs, M.K., and Sims, J.E.**, A novel IL-1 receptor, cloned from B cells by mammalian expression, is expressed in many cell types, *EMBO J.*, 10, 2821, 1991.
23. **Symons, J.A., Eastgate, J.A., and Duff, G.W.**, Purification and characterization of a novel soluble receptor for interleukin 1, *J. Exp. Med.*, 174, 1251, 1991.
24. **Lowenthal, J.W. and MacDonald, H.R.**, Binding and internalization of interleukin 1 by T cells. Direct evidence from high and low affinity classes of interleukin-1 receptors, *J. Exp. Med.*, 164, 1060, 1986.
25. **Savage, N., Puren, A.J., Orencole, S.F., Ikejima, T., Clark, B.D., and Dinarello, C.A.**, Studies on IL-1 receptors on D10S T-helper cells: demonstration of two molecularly and antigenically distinct IL-1 binding proteins, *Cytokine*, 1, 23, 1989.
26. **Mastushima, K., Yodoi, J., Tagaya, Y., and Oppenheim, J.J.**, Downregulation of interleukin-1 receptor expression by IL-1 and fate of internalized ^{125}I-labeled IL-1β in a human large granular lymphocyte cell line, *J. Immunol.*, 137, 3183, 1986.
27. **Dubois, C.M., Ruscetti, F.W., Palaszynski, E.W., Falk, L.A., Oppenheim, J.J., and Keller, J.R.**, Transforming growth factor β is a potent inhibitor of interleukin 1 (IL-1) receptor expression: proposed mechanism of inhibition of IL-1 action, *J. Exp. Med.*, 172, 737, 1990.
28. **Chiou, W.J., Bonin, P.D., Harris, P.K.W., Carter, D.B., and Singh, J.P.**, Platelet-derived growth factor induces interleukin-1 receptor gene expression in Balb/c 3T3 fibroblasts, *J. Biol. Chem.*, 264, 21442, 1989.
29. **Akahoshi, T., Oppenheim, J.J., and Matsushima, K.**, Interleukin 1 stimulates its own receptor expression on human fibroblasts through the endogenous production of prostaglandin(s), *J. Clin. Invest.*, 82, 1219, 1988.
30. **Dower, S.K., Wignall, J.M., Schooley, K., McMahan, C.J., Jackson, J.L., Prickett, K.S., Lupton, S., Cosman, D., and Sims, J.E.**, Retention of ligand binding activity by the extracellular domain of the IL-1 receptor, *J. Immunol.*, 142, 4314, 1989.
31. **Mancilla, J., Ikejima, I., Clark, B.D., Orencole, S.F., Sirko, S., and Dinarello, C.A.**, Lectin binding suggests different glycosylation patterns of IL-1 receptors on different cells, *Cytokine*, 1, 95, 1989.
32. **Bird, T.A., Gearing, A.J., and Saklatvala, J.**, Murine interleukin-1 receptor: differences in binding properties between fibroblastic and thymoma cells and evidence for a two-chain receptor model, *FEBS Lett.*, 225, 21, 1987.
33. **Ikejima, T., Clark, B.D., Mancilla, J., Sirko, S., Sirko, S.P., Orencole, S.F., Ishii, N., Okuda, K., Wen, H., Zhang, X., and Dinarello, C.A.**, Affinity purified antibodies against a 17 amino acid portion of murine IL-1R recognizes 80 kDa (IL-1RtI) peptide and blocks differentially IL-1α and IL-1β binding on D10S cells, *Lymph. Res.*, 9, 583, 1990.
34. **Scapigliati, G., Ghiara, P., Bartalini, A., Taglibue, A., and Boraschi, D.**, Differential binding of IL-1α and IL-1β to receptors on B and T cells, *FEBS Lett.*, 243, 394, 1989.
35. **Qwarnstrom, E.E., Page, R.C., Gillis, S., and Dower, S.K.**, Binding, internalization and intracellular localization of interleukin-1 beta in human diploid fibroblasts, *J. Biol. Chem.*, 263, 8261, 1988.
36. **Galis, B., Prickett, K.S., Jackson, J., Slack, J., Schooley, K., Sims, J.E., and Dower, S.K.**, IL-1 induces rapid phosphorylation of the IL-1 receptor, *J. Immunol.*, 143, 3235, 1989.
37. **Shimizu, H., Mitomo, K., Watanabe, T., Okamoto, S., and Yamamoto, K.**, Involvement of a NF-kappa B-like transcription factor in the activation of the interleukin-6 gene by inflammatory lymphokines, *Mol. Cell Biol.*, 10, 561, 1990.
38. **O'Neill, L.A., Bird, T.A., Gearing, A.J., and Saklatvala, J.**, Interleukin-1 signal transduction. Increased GTP binding and hydrolysis in membranes of a murine thymoma line (EL4), *J. Biol. Chem.*, 265, 3146, 1990.
39. **Kaur, P., Welch, W.J., and Saklatvala, J.**, Interleukin-1 and tumor necrosis factor increase phosphorylation of the small heat shock protein, *FEBS Lett.*, 258, 269, 1989.
40. **Seckinger, P., Lowenthal, J.W., Williamson, K., Dayer, J.M., and MacDonald, H.R.**, A urine inhibitor of interleukin-1 activity that blocks ligand binding, *J. Immunol.*, 139, 1546, 1987.
41. **Arend, W.P., Joslin, F.G., and Massoni, R.J.**, Effects of immune complexes on production by human monocytes of interleukin 1 or an interleukin 1 inhibitor, *J. Immunol.*, 134, 1985.
42. **Carter, D.B., Deibel, M.R., Jr., Dunn, C.J., Tomich, C.-S.C., Laborde, A.L., Slightom, J.L., Berger, A.E., Bienkowski, M.J., Sun, F.F., McEwan, R.N., Harris, P.K.W., Yem, A.W., Waszak, G.A., Chosay, J.G., Sieu, L.C., Hardee, M.M., Zurcher-Neely, H.A., Reardon, I.M., Heinrikson, R.L., Truesdell, S.E., Shelly, J.A., Eessalu, T.E., Taylor, B.M., and Tracey, D.E.**, Purification, cloning, expression and biological characterization of an interleukin-1 receptor antagonist protein, *Nature*, 344, 633, 1990.

43. **Eisenberg, S.P., Evans, R.J., Arend, W.P., Verderber, E., Brewer, M.T., Hannum, C.H., and Thompson, R.C.,** Primary structure and functional expression from complementary DNA of a human interleukin-1 receptor antagonist, *Nature*, 343, 341, 1990.
44. **Bienkowski, M.J., Eessalu, T.E., Berger, A.E., Truesdell, S.E., Shelly, J.A., Laborde, A.L., Zurcher-Neely, H.A., Reardon, I.M., Heinrikson, R.L., Chosay, J.G., and Tracey, D.E.,** Purification and characterization of interleukin 1 receptor level antagonist proteins from THP-1 cells, *J. Biol. Chem.*, 265, 14505, 1990.
45. **Eisenberg, S.P., Brewer, M.T., Verderber, E., Heimdal, P., Brandhuber, B.J., and Thompson, R.C.,** Interleukin 1 receptor antagonist is a member of the interleukin 1 gene family: evolution of a cytokine control mechanism, *Proc. Natl. Acad. Sci. U.S.A.*, 88, 5232, 1991.
46. **Arend, W.P., Joslin, F.G., and Massoni, R.J.,** Effects of immune complexes on production by human monocytes of interleukin 1 or an interleukin 1 inhibitor, *J. Immunol.*, 134, 3868, 1985.
47. **Roux-Lombard, P., Modoux, C., and Dayer, J.-M.,** Production of interleukin-1 (IL-1) and a specific IL-1 inhibitor during human monocyte-macrophage differentiation: influence of GM-CSF, *Cytokine*, 1, 45, 1989.
48. **Tracey, D.E., Hardee, M.M., Shelly, J.A., Chosay, J.G., Fidler, S.F., Laborde, A.L., and Dunn, C.J.,** IRAP blocks murine type 2 IL-1 receptors and inhibits IL-1 induced neutrophilia at high concentrations, *J. Cell. Biochem. Suppl.*, 15(E), 177, 1991.
49. **McIntyre, K.W., Stepan, G.J., Kolinsky, K.D., Benjamin, W.R., Plocinski, J.M., Kaffka, K.L., Campen, C.A., Chizzonite, R.A., and Kilian, P.A.,** Inhibition of interleukin 1 (IL-1) binding and bioactivity in vitro and modulation of acute inflammation in vivo by IL-1 receptor antagonist and anti-IL-1 receptor monoclonal antibody, *J. Exp. Med.*, 173, 931, 1991.
50. **Arend, W.P. and Dayer, J.M.,** Cytokines and cytokine inhibitors or antagonists in rheumatoid arthritis, *Arthritis Rheum.*, 33, 305, 1990.
51. **Thornberry, N.A., Bull, H.G., Calaycay, J.R., Chapman, K.T., Howard, A.D., Kostura, M.J., Miller, D.K., Molineaux, S.M., Weidner, J.R., Aunins, J., Elliston, K.O., Ayala, J.M., Casano, F.J., Chin, J., Ding, G.J.-F., Egger, L.A., Gaffney, E.P., Limjuco, G., Palyha, O.C., Raju, S.M., Rolando, A.M., Salley, J.P., Yamin, T.-T., Lee, T.D., Shively, J.E., MacCross, M., Mumford, R.A., Schmidt, J.A., and Tocci, M.J.,** A novel heterodimeric cysteine protease is required for interleukin-1β processing in monocytes, *Nature*, 356, 768, 1992.
52. **Carter, D.B., Curry, K.A., Tomich, C.-S.C., Yem, A.W., Deibel, M.R., Tracey, D.E., Paslay, J.W., Carter, J.B., Theriault, N.Y., Harris, P.K.W., Reardon, I.M., Zurcher-Neely, H.A., Heinrikson, R.L., Clancy, L.L., Muchmore, S.W., Watenpaugh, K.D., and Einspahr, H.M.,** Crystallization of purified recombinant human interleukin-1β, *Proteins Struct. Funct. Genet.*, 3, 121, 1988.
53. **Finzel, B.C., Clancy, L.L., Holland, D.R., Muchmore, S.W., Watenpaugh, K.D., and Einspahr, H.M.,** Crystal structure of recombinant human interleukin-1β at 2.0 Å resolution, *J. Mol. Biol.*, 209, 779, 1989.
54. **Priestle, J.P., Schaer, H.-P., and Gruetter, M.G.,** Crystal structure of the cytokine interleukin-1β, *EMBO J.*, 7, 339, 1988.
55. **Priestle, J.P., Schaer, H.-P., and Gruetter, M.G.,** Crystallographic refinement of interleukin 1β at 2.0 Å resolution, *Proc. Natl. Acad. Sci. U.S.A.*, 86, 9667, 1989.
56. **Veerapandian, B., Gilliland, G.L., Raag, R, Svensson, A.L., Masui, Y., Hirai, Y., and Poulos, T.L.,** Functional implications of interleukin-1β based on the three-dimensional structure, *Proteins Struct. Funct. Genet.*, 12, 10, 1992.
57. **Treharne, A.C., Ohlendorf, D.H., Weber, P.C., Wendoloski, J.J., and Salemme, F.R.,** X-ray structural studies of the cytokine interleukin 1-β, in *Cytokines and Lipocortins in Inflammation and Differentiation*, Melli, M. and Parente, L., Eds., Wiley-Liss, New York, 1990, 309.
58. **van Oostrum, J., Priestle, J.P., Gruetter, M.G., and Schmitz, A.,** The structure of murine interleukin-1β at 2.8 Å resolution, *J. Struct. Biol.*, 107, 189, 1991.
59. **Clore, G.M., Wingfield, P.T., and Gronenborn, A.M.,** High-resolution three-dimensional structure of interleukin 1β in solution by three- and four-dimensional nuclear magnetic resonance spectroscopy, *Biochemistry*, 30, 2315, 1991.
60. **Ohlendorf, D.H., Treharne, A., Weber, P.C., Wendoloski, J.J., and Salemme, F.R.,** Accuracy of structures: a comparison of independently refined models of human IL-1β, Abstract G09 in Program and Abstracts of the American Crystallographic Association Meeting, Toledo, Ohio, July 21-26, 1991, Series 2, Vol. 19, 36, 1991.
61. **Clore, G.M. and Gronenborn, A.M.,** Comparison of the solution nuclear magnetic resonance and X-ray crystal structures of human recombinant interleukin-1β, *J. Mol. Biol.*, 221, 47, 1991.
62. **Sweet, R.M., Wright, H.T., Janin, J., Chothia, C.H., and Blow, D.M.,** Crystal structure of the complex of porcine trypsin with soybean trypsin inhibitor (Kunitz) at 2.6-Å resolution, *Biochemistry*, 13, 4212, 1974.
63. **McLachlan, A.D.,** Three-fold structural pattern in the soybean trypsin inhibitor (Kunitz), *J. Mol. Biol.*, 133, 557, 1979.
64. **Onesti, S., Brick, P., and Blow, D.M.,** Crystal structure of a Kunitz-type trypsin inhibitor from *Erythrina caffra* seeds, *J. Mol. Biol.*, 217, 153, 1991.

65. **Einspahr, H.M., Clancy, L.L., Holland, D.R., Muchmore, S.W., Watenpaugh, K.D., and Finzel, B.C.**, The crystal structure of human interleukin-1α, in *Current Research in Protein Chemistry*, Villafranca, J.J., Ed., Academic Press, San Diego, 1990, 35.
66. **Graves, B.J., Hatada, M.H., Hendrickson, W.A., Miller, J.K., Madison, V.S., and Satow, Y.**, Structure of interleukin-1α at 2.7-Å resolution, *Biochemistry*, 29, 2679, 1990.
67. **Zhu, X., Komiya, H., Chirino, A., Faham, S., Fox, G.M., Arakawa, T., Hsu, B.T., and Rees, D.C.**, Three-dimensional structures of acidic and basic fibroblast growth factors, *Science*, 251, 90, 1991.
68. **Zhang, J., Cousens, L.S., Barr, P.J., and Sprang, S.R.**, Three-dimensional structure of human basic fibroblast growth factor, a structural homolog of interleukin 1β, *Proc. Natl. Acad. Sci. U.S.A.*, 88, 3446, 1991.
69. **Eriksson, A.E., Cousens, L.S., Weaver, L.H., and Matthews, B.W.**, Three-dimensional structure of human basic fibroblast growth factor, *Proc. Natl. Acad. Sci. U.S.A.*, 88, 3441, 1991.
70. **Zemke, K.J., Mueller-Fahrnow, A., Jany, K.-D., Pal, G.P., and Saenger, W.**, The three-dimensional structure of the bifunctional proteinase K/α-amylase inhibitor from wheat (PK13) at 2.5 Å resolution, *FEBS Lett.*, 279, 240, 1991.
71. **Habazettl, J., Gondol, D., Wiltscheck, R., Otlewski, J., Schleicher, M., and Holak, T.A.**, Structure of hisactophilin is similar to interleukin-1β and fibroblast growth factor, *Nature*, 359, 855, 1992.
72. **Murzin, A.G., Lesk, A.M., and Chothia, C.**, β-Trefoil fold. Patterns of structure and sequence in the Kunitz inhibitors, interleukins-1β and 1α, and fibroblast growth factors, *J. Mol. Biol.*, 223, 531, 1992.
73. **DeChiara, T.M., Young, D., Semionov, R., Stern, A.S., Batula-Bernardo, C., Fiedler-Nagy, C., Kaffka, K.L., Killian, P.L., Yamazaki, S., Mizel, S.B., and Lomedico, P.T.**, Structure-function analysis of murine interleukin 1: biologically active polypeptides are at least 127 amino acids long and are derived from the carboxyl terminus of a 270-amino acid precursor, *Proc. Natl. Acad. Sci. U.S.A.*, 83, 8303, 1986.
74. **Rosenwasser, L.J., Webb, A.C., Clark, B.D., Irie, S., Chang, L., Dinarello, C.A., Gehrke, L., Wolff, S.M., Rich, A., and Auron, P.E.**, Expression of biologically active human interleukin 1 subpeptides by transfected simian COS cells, *Proc. Natl. Acad. Sci. U.S.A.*, 83, 5243, 1986.
75. **Mosley, B., Dower, S.K., Gillis, S., and Cosman, D.**, Determination of the minimum polypeptide lengths of the functionally active sites of human interleukins 1α and 1β, *Proc. Natl. Acad. Sci. U.S.A.*, 84, 4572, 1987.
76. **Dower, S.K., Mosley, B., Conlon, P.J., Benson, P., Grubin, C., Larsen, A., Gillis, S., and Cosman, D.**, Molecular modification of lymphokines by in vivo mutagenesis, *Ann. N.Y. Acad. Sci.*, 507, 22, 1987.
77. **Lilquist, J.S., Simon, P.L., Summers, M., Jonak, Z., and Young, P.R.**, Structure-activity studies of human IL-1β with mature and truncated proteins expressed in *Escherichia coli*, *J. Immunol.*, 141, 1975, 1988.
78. **Yem, A.W., Richard, K.A., Staite, N.D., and Deibel, M.R., Jr.**, Resolution and biological properties of three N-terminal analogues of recombinant human interleukin-1β, *Lymph. Res.*, 7, 85, 1988.
79. **Daumy, G.O., Merenda, J.M., McColl, A.S., Andrews, G.C., Franke, A.E., Geoghegan, K.F., and Otterness, I.G.**, Isolation and characterization of biologically active murine interleukin-1α derived from expression of a synthetic gene in *Escherichia coli*, *Biochim. Biophys. Acta*, 998, 32, 1989.
80. **Richard, K.A., Yem, A.W., Deibel, M.R., Jr., and Staite, N.D.**, Isolation and bioactivities of three IL-1β N-terminal variants, *Agents Actions*, 27, 268, 1989.
81. **Baird, A., Schubert, D., Ling, N., and Guillemin, R.**, Receptor- and heparin-binding domains of basic fibroblast growth factor, *Proc. Natl. Acad. Sci. U.S.A.*, 85, 2324, 1988.
82. **Antoni, G., Presentini, R., Perin, F., Tagliabue, A., Ghiara, P., Censini, S., Volpini, G., Villa, L., and Boraschi, D.**, A short synthetic peptide fragment of human interleukin 1 with immunostimulatory but not inflammatory activity, *J. Immunol.*, 137, 3201, 1986.
83. **Nencioni, L., Villa, L., Tagliabue, A., Antoni, G., Presentini, R., Perin, F., Silvestri, S., and Boraschi, D.**, In vivo immunostimulatory activity of the 163-171 peptide of human IL-1β, *J. Immunol.*, 139, 800, 1987.
84. **Boraschi, D., Antoni, G., Perin, F., Villa, L., Nencioni, L., Ghiara, P., Presentini, R., and Tagliabue, A.**, Defining the structural requirements of a biologically active domain of human IL-1β, *Eur. Cytokine Net.*, 1, 21, 1990.
85. **Palaszynski, E.**, Synthetic C-terminal peptide of IL-1 functions as a binding domain as well as an antagonist for the IL-1 receptor, *Biochem. Biophys. Res. Commun.*, 147, 204, 1987.
86. **Matsumoto, T., Harada, N., Yamaguchi, K., Komatsu, Y., and Itoh, S.**, Peptides having interleukin-1 activity, European Patent Application 87116824.1, May 18, 1988.
87. **Ferreira, S.H., Lorenzetti, B.B., Bristow, A.F., and Poole, S.**, Interleukin-1β as a potent hyperalgesic agent antagonized by a tripeptide analogue, *Nature*, 334, 698, 1988.
88. **Herzbeck, H., Blum, B., Roenspeck, W., Frenzel, B., Brandt, E., Ulmer, A.J., and Flad, H.-D.**, Functional and molecular characterization of a monoclonal antibody against the 165-186 peptide of human IL-1β, *Scand. J. Immunol.*, 30, 549, 1989.
89. **Obal, F., Opp, M., Cady, A.B., Johannsen, L., Postlethwaite, A.E., Poppleton, H.M., Seyer, J.M., and Krueger, J.M.**, Interleukin 1α and an interleukin 1β fragment are somnogenic, *Am. J. Physiol.*, 259, R439, 1990.

90. **Ogle, J.D., Noel, J.G., Balasurbramanian, A., Sramkoski, R.M., Ogle, C.K., and Alexander, J.W.,** Comparison of abilities of recombinant interleukin-1α and -β and noninflammatory IL-1β fragment 163-171 to upregulate C3b receptors (CR1) on human neutrophils and to enhance their phagocytic capacity, *Inflammation*, 14, 185, 1990.
91. **Joss, U.R., Schmidli, I., and Vosbeck, K.,** Mapping the receptor binding domain of interleukin-1 beta by means of binding studies using overlapping sequence fragments: why did it fail?, *J. Receptor Res.*, 11, 275, 1991.
92. **Staite, N.D., Dortch, K.A., Killar, L.M., Gibbons, A.J., McGee, J.E., Berger, A.E., Maggiora, L.L., Bannow, C.A., Nugent, R.A., Tracey, D.E., Finzel, B.C., and Einspahr, H.M.,** Tests of inhibitory activity of synthesized peptide fragments of human interleukin-1β, unpublished data, 1989.
93. **Gronenborn, A.M., Clore, G.M., Schmeissner, U., and Wingfield, P.,** A ^{1}H-NMR study of human interleukin-1β, *Eur. J. Biochem.*, 161, 37, 1986.
94. **MacDonald, H.R., Wingfield, P., Schmeissner, U., Shaw, A., Clore, G.M., and Gronenborn, A.M.,** Point mutations of human interleukin-1 with decreased receptor binding affinity, *FEBS Lett.*, 209, 295, 1986.
95. **Huang, J.J., Newton, R.C., Horuk, R., Matthew, J.B., Covington, M., Pezzella, K., and Lin, Y.,** Muteins of human interleukin-1 that show enhanced bioactivities, *FEBS Lett.*, 223, 294, 1987.
96. **Kamogashira, T., Masui, Y., Ohmoto, Y., Hirato, T., Nagamura, K., Mizuno, K., Hong, Y.-M., Kikumoto, Y., Nakai, S., and Hirai, Y.,** Site-specific mutagenesis of the human interleukin-1β gene: structure-function analysis of the cysteine residues, *Biochem. Biophys. Res. Commun.*, 150, 1106, 1988.
97. **Gronenborn, A.M., Wingfield, P.T., MacDonald, H.R., Schmeissner, U., and Clore, G.M.,** Site directed mutants of human interleukin-1α: a ^{1}H-NMR and receptor binding study, *FEBS Lett.*, 231, 135, 1988.
98. **Kamogashira, T., Sackaguchi, M., Ohmoto, Y., Mizuno, K., Shimizu, R., Nagamura, K., Nakai, S., Masui, Y., and Hirai, Y.,** Site-specific mutagenesis of the human interleukin-1β gene: the role of arginine residue at the N-terminal region, *J. Biochem.*, 104, 837, 1988.
99. **Wingfield, P., Graber, P., Shaw, A.R., Gronenborn, A.M., Clore, G.M., and MacDonald, H.R.,** Preparation, characterization and application of interleukin-1β mutant proteins with surface-accessible cysteine residues, *Eur. J. Biochem.*, 179, 565, 1989.
100. **Naito, Y., Fukata, J., Masui, Y., Hirai, Y., Murakami, N., Tominaga, T., Nakai, Y., Tamai, S., Mori, K., and Imura, H.,** Interleukin-1β analogues with markedly reduced pyrogenic activity can stimulate secretion of adrenocorticotropic hormone in rats, *Biochem. Biophys. Res. Commun.*, 167, 103, 1990.
101. **Yamayoshi, M., Ohue, M., Kawashima, H., Kotani, H., Iida, M., Kawata, S., and Yamada, M.,** A human IL-1α derivative which lacks prostaglandin E_2 inducing activity and inhibits the activity of IL-1 through receptor competition, *Lymph. Res.*, 9, 405, 1990.
102. **Nakai, S., Kawai, K., Hirai, Y., and Tasaka, K.,** A mutant protein of human interleukin-1β with immunostimulatory but not pyrogenic potency, *Life Sci.*, 47, 1707, 1990.
103. **Yanofsky, S.D. and Zurawski, G.,** Identification of key residues in the amino-terminal third of human interleukin-1α, *J. Biol. Chem.*, 265, 13000, 1990.
104. **Conca, W., Auron, P.E., Aoun-Wathne, M., Bennett, N., Seckinger, P., Welgus, H.G., Goldring, S.R., Eisenberg, S.P., Dayer, J.-M., Krane, S.M., and Gehrke, L.,** An interleukin 1β point mutant demonstrates that *jun/fos* expression is not sufficient for fibroblast metalloproteinase expression, *J. Biol. Chem.*, 266, 16265, 1991.
105. **Tate, S.-I., Kikumoto, Y., Ichikawa, S., Kaneko, M., Masui, Y., Kamogashira, T., Ouchi, M., Takahashi, S., and Inagaki, F.,** Stable isotope aided nuclear magnetic resonance study to investigate the receptor-binding site of human interleukin 1β, *Biochemistry*, 31, 2435, 1992.
106. **Gehrke, L., Jobling, S.A., Paik, L.S., McDonald, B., Rosenwasser, L.J., and Auron, P.E.,** A point mutation uncouples human interleukin-1β biological activity and receptor binding, *J. Biol. Chem.*, 265, 5922, 1990.
107. **Tomich, C.-S.C., Deibel, M.R., Jr., Staite, N.D., Laborde, A.L., Tracey, D.E., Finzel, B.C., and Einspahr, H.M.,** unpublished data, 1990.
108. **Yem, A.W., Zurcher-Neely, H.A., Richard, K.A., Staite, N.D., Heinrikson, R.L., and Deibel, M.R., Jr.,** Biotinylation of reactive amino groups in native recombinant human interleukin-1β, *J. Biol. Chem.*, 264, 17691, 1989.
109. **Chollet, A., Bonnefoy, J.-Y., and Odermatt, N.,** Preparation, application and biological characterization of interleukin-1β mutant protein biotinylated at a single site, *J. Immunol. Methods*, 127, 179, 1990.
110. **Nanduri, V.B., Hulmes, J.D., Pan, Y.-C.E., Kilian, P.L., and Stern, A.S.,** The role of arginine residues in interleukin 1 receptor binding, *Biochim. Biophys. Acta*, 1118, 25, 1991.
111. **Chang, J.-Y., Ngai, P.K., Priestle, J.P., Joss, U., Vosbeck, K.D., and van Oostrum, J.,** Identification of a reactive lysyl residue (Lys^{103}) of recombinant human interleukin-1β. Mechanism of its reactivity and implication of its functional role in receptor binding, *Biochemistry*, 31, 2874, 1992.
112. **Yem, A.W., Epps, D.E., Mathews, W.R., Guido, D.M., Richard, K.A., Staite, N.D., and Deibel, M.R., Jr.,** Site-specific chemical modification of interleukin-1β by acrylodan at cysteine 8 and lysine 103, *J. Biol. Chem.*, 267, 3122, 1992.

113. **Epps, D.E., Yem, A.W., Fisher, J.F., McGee, J.E., Paslay, J.W., and Deibel, M.R., Jr.,** Spectral characterization of environment-sensitive adducts of interleukin-1β, *J. Biol. Chem.*, 267, 3129, 1992.
114. **Gaffney, E.V., Anderson, A.E., Pfanenstiel, Y.T., and Koch, G.A.,** Antibodies and their role in interleukin-1 research, *Immunol. Rev.*, 119, 181, 1991.
115. **van der Loo, A.J., Arntz, O.J., Otterness, I.G., and van den Berg, W.B.,** Protection against cartilage proteoglycan synthesis inhibition by antiinterleukin 1 antibodies in experimental arthritis, *J. Rheumatol.*, 19, 348, 1992.
116. **Labriola-Tomkins, E., Chandran, C., Kaffka, K.L., Biondi, D., Graves, B.J., Hatada, M., Madison, V.S., Karas, J., Kilian, P.L., and Ju, G.,** Identification of the discontinuous binding site in human interleukin 1β for the type I interleukin 1 receptor, *Proc. Natl. Acad. Sci. U.S.A.*, 88, 11182, 1991.
117. **Davies, D.R., Sheriff, S., and Padlan, E.A.,** Antibody-antigen complexes, *J. Biol. Chem.*, 263, 10541, 1988.
118. **Janin, J. and Chothia, C.,** The structure of protein-protein recognition sites, *J. Biol. Chem.*, 265, 16027, 1990.
119. **Granatir, C.A., Reardon, I.M., Finzel, B.C., and Einspahr, H.M.,** unpublished work, 1991.
120. **Veerapandian, B.,** Structure and function of interleukin-1, based on crystallographic and modeling studies, *Biophys. J.*, 62, 112, 1992.
121. **Stockman, B.J., Scahill, T.A., Roy, M., Ulrich, E.L., Strakalaitis, N.A., Brunner, D.P., Yem, A.W., and Deibel, M.R., Jr.,** Secondary structure and topology of interleukin-1 receptor antagonist protein determined by heteronuclear three-dimensional NMR spectroscopy, *Biochemistry*, 31, 5237, 1992.
122. **Stockman, B.J., Scahill, T.A., Strakalaitis, N.A., Brunner, D.P., Yem, A.W., and Deibel, M.R., Jr.,** Proton, carbon, and nitrogen chemical shifts accurately delineate differences and similarities in secondary structure between homologous proteins IRAP and IL-1β, *J. Biomol. NMR*, 2, 591, 1992.
123. **Clancy, L.L., Finzel, B.C., Yem, A.W., Deibel, M.R., Jr., Strakalaitis, N.A., Brunner, D.P., Sweet, R.M., and Einspahr, H.M.,** Preliminary crystallographic analysis of a recombinant human interleukin-1 receptor antagonist protein, *Acta Crystallogr.*, D50, 197, 1994.
124. **Clancy, L.L., Finzel, B.C., Yem, A.W., Deibel, M.R., Jr., Strakalaitis, N.A., Brunner, D.P., Tracey, D.E., and Einspahr, H.M.,** Crystallization of a recombinant human interleukin-1 receptor antagonist protein, Abstract PB41 in Program and Abstracts of the American Crystallographic Association Meeting, Pittsburgh, Pennsylvania, 9-14 August 1992, Series 2, Vol. 20, 118, 1992.
125. **Wang, B.C.,** Resolution of phase ambiguity in macromolecular crystallography, *Methods Enzymol.*, 115, 90, 1985.
126. **Ju, G., Labriola-Tomkins, E., Campen, C.A., Benjamin, W.R., Karas, J., Plocinski, J., Biondi, D., Kaffka, K.L., Kilian, P.L., Eisenberg, S.P., and Evans, R.J.,** Conversion of the interleukin 1 receptor antagonist into an agonist by site-specific mutagenesis, *Proc. Natl. Acad. Sci. U.S.A.*, 88, 2658, 1991.
127. **McGee, J.E., Thomsen, D.R., Carter, D.B., Deibel, M.R., Jr., and Paslay, J.W.,** Purification and characterization of a soluble, truncated form of the interleukin-1 receptor, unpublished work, 1990.
128. **Clancy, L.L., McGee, J.E., Paslay, J.W., and Einspahr, H.M.,** unpublished work, 1991.
129. **Mathias, S., Younes, A., Kan, C.-C., Orlow, I., Joseph, C., and Kolesnick, R.N.,** Activation of the sphingomyelin signaling pathway in intact EL4 cells and in a cell-free system by IL-1β, *Science*, 259, 519, 1993.

Chapter 3

THE HEMATOPOIETIC COLONY-STIMULATING FACTORS

Kenneth Kaushansky

CONTENTS

I. INTRODUCTION

Hematopoiesis, the process of blood cell production, is an enormous undertaking. Each day, the adult human produces 2.5×10^{11} red blood cells (erythrocytes), 1×10^{11} white blood cells (leukocytes), and 2×10^{11} platelets. In addition, in response to infection, inflammation, bleeding, or blood cell breakdown, production must increase many-fold. Thus, the regulation of hematopoiesis becomes a vital process. Central to this response are the hematopoietic colony-stimulating factors (CSFs); acidic glycoproteins essential for the survival, proliferation, and differentiation of blood cell progenitors *in vitro* and *in vivo*. Beginning with the seminal observations and cell culture techniques of Pluznick and Sachs[1] and Bradley and Metcalf[2] 28 years ago, the CSFs have been postulated to exist, biochemically purified, biologically characterized, cloned, expressed in heterologous systems, tested for efficacy, and now routinely used in clinical states of marrow failure.

In 1994, at least 12 biotechnology and pharmaceutical companies have active programs exploring production and modification of these molecules for use as immune modulating agents. This chapter will provide an overview of the biology, biochemistry, and pharmacology of the CSFs in order to better understand their use as therapeutic proteins, and to provide the basis for more recent studies of the structure-function relationships of these clinically valuable

0-8493-9422-8/94/$0.00+$.50

proteins. As the true era of rational drug design often depends upon obtaining the three-dimensional structure of the target of such drugs (in this case each of the CSF receptors), this phase of CSF development awaits us. Despite this caveat, much has been learned of the structural requirements for the biologic function of several CSFs, and will comprise the remainder of this chapter. Although many of these findings are not based on X-ray crystallography or nuclear magnetic resonance (NMR) solution structural determinations, in many respects, these data stand alone, and will become increasingly valuable once additional structural information becomes available. Hopefully, a logical progression from physiology to pharmacology to the rational design of future therapeutics in this important group of proteins will emerge.

II. BACKGROUND

A. PHYSIOLOGY

Colony-stimulating activity was operationally first defined as a substance(s) which supported the clonal growth of blood cells from their progenitors in semisolid cultures.[3] A specific CSF was defined by the cell type(s) in the developing colony. Hence, granulocyte-macrophage (GM)-CSF supported the growth of colonies containing granulocytes (both neutrophils and eosinophils) and monocyte/macrophages, G-CSF supported neutrophilic colony formation, and M-CSF, monocyte and macrophages alone. Multi-CSF, more commonly known as interleukin-3 (IL-3), supported both erythroid and myeloid cell types. Based on a series of refinements in cell culture technique, cell preparation and purification, and the use of defined culture medium, the following biological principles have been discerned. First, one or more CSFs are required for survival of hematopoietic progenitor cells at all stages of development.[3] Second, CSFs are required for each cell division from the most immature progenitor to the final mature blood cell, including the few cell divisions which monocytes may undergo having differentiated into fixed tissue macrophages.[3,4] Third, no single CSF can support the entire developmental progression from stem cell to mature blood cell; at least two CSFs are required and so define the concept of "early-acting" (including SCF [stem cell factor, kit ligand or mast cell growth factor], IL-3, and GM-CSF) and "late-acting" (including G-CSF, M-CSF, and interleukin-5 [IL-5])[5] factors. Fourth, CSFs act by binding to high-affinity cell surface receptors, present on cells of hematopoietic lineage.[6] Recently, the presence of low-affinity receptors for several of the CSFs on nonhematologic cell types, such as placenta,[7] endothelium,[8] and several tumor cell lines,[9] has been described, but with a single exception,[10] the biologic significance of these findings is uncertain. Fifth, in addition to their role in the production of blood cells, the CSFs functionally activate mature leukocytes to participate in the inflammatory response.[11-19] Sixth, the CSFs are produced *in vitro* by cells of the marrow microenvironment or by cells at peripheral sites of inflammation in response to stimulation with inflammatory mediators such as interleukin-1 (IL-1), tumor necrosis factor (TNF), specific antigen, or by bacterial products such as lipopolysaccharide (LPS) or muramidyl dipeptides.[19-31]

In addition to data derived from *in vitro* methods, similar responses have been noted in animal models of inflammation and in human disease. For example, experimental infection of mice with *Listeria monocytogenes* leads to M-CSF, G-CSF, and GM-CSF release into the circulation with subsequent increased leukocyte production and activation.[32] In the human, joint fluid of patients with active rheumatoid arthritis contains substantial levels of GM-CSF; and IL-3 is involved in the histamine release characteristic of asthma[35] and in the eosinophilia associated with a particular type of acute lymphocytic leukemia.[36] In these ways, the CSFs participate in the host response to infectious, inflammatory, and immunologic stimuli.

Based on these observations, the clinical responses to each of the CSFs have been highly predictable. As expected from the spectrum of cell types present in CSF-stimulated cultures, administration of GM-CSF to normal individuals or to patients with marrow suppression has resulted in dose-dependent increases in neutrophil, eosinophil, and monocyte levels. In contrast, G-CSF supports colony growth composed entirely of neutrophils; hence, clinical use results in an exclusive neutrophilia. IL-3 is considered one of the earlier acting CSFs, acting only in concert with other late-acting proteins. Thus, alone, IL-3 leads to a very modest panleukocytosis. In contrast, in combination with other CSFs (such as GM-CSF or G-CSF), IL-3 leads to enhanced responses above that seen with either agent alone.

B. BIOCHEMISTRY

Each of the four well-defined CSFs is the product of a distinct gene.[37-40] The M-CSF, GM-CSF, and IL-3 genes cluster on the long arm of human chromosome 5,[41-43] the G-CSF gene resides on human chromosome 17.[44] G-CSF, GM-CSF, and IL-3 are small (16 to 30 kDa), single-chain polypeptides, each containing one or two disulfide bonds, reduction of which leads to complete loss of biological activity.[45-47] All of the CSFs are modified with N-linked and/or O-linked carbohydrate. Variable degrees of terminal sialation lead to the size and charge heterogeneity characteristic of these proteins. Table 1 lists some of the biochemical features of the CSFs. Despite evidence for their common derivation from a single ancestral gene, and the structural relationship of their receptors,[48,49] G-CSF, GM-CSF, and IL-3 were initially thought to share little or no sequence homology.[45-47] More recently, Sanderson and colleagues described a short stretch of sequence similarity near the carboxyl terminus of IL-5 (an eosinophilic differentiation factor), IL-3, IL-4, IL-6, and GM-CSF.[50] In addition, based on the sites critical for receptor interaction, a second region of primary and secondary structure similarity between GM-CSF and IL-3 has been described.[51] These findings may have important implications for rational drug design and will be discussed in more detail below.

Like the other CSFs, M-CSF displays variable degrees of glycosylation resulting in size and charge heterogeneity.[53] However, in contrast to G-CSF, GM-CSF, and IL-3, M-CSF and the related hemopoietin SCF[53-56] are larger (dimer M_r 45 to 70 kDa and monomer M_r 28 to 35 kDa, respectively) and bind to their receptors as disulfide stabilized (M-CSF) or noncovalently associated (SCF) homodimers. In addition, the genes for M-CSF and SCF encode transmembrane domains.[52-55] Thus, the trafficking of both gene products includes a membrane-bound form. Alternative splicing of the sixth exon of both genes results in the inclusion/exclusion of an additional 298 (M-CSF) or 28 (SCF) amino acids, including a presumptive signal for membrane cleavage.[57] Thus, the shorter form of each protein remains membrane-bound, the longer is cleaved from the membrane to produce the soluble molecule. The relative biologic roles of each form is unclear.

As noted, the CSFs act by binding to high-affinity cell surface receptors which, based on sequence homologies, can be divided into two groups. Receptors for G-CSF (58) GM-CSF,[7,59] and IL-3[60] are members of a growing family of membrane proteins termed the "cytokine receptor superfamily".[48,49] This group additionally includes the IL-2, IL-4, IL-5, IL-6, IL-7, IL-9, IL-11 erythropoietin, prolactin, and growth hormone receptors. Nearly all of these receptors are composed of two or more polypeptides, both being required for high-affinity binding and signal transduction. Of considerable interest to the rationale design of CSF agonists and antagonists is the recent finding that GM-CSF, IL-3, and IL-5 all mutually cross-compete for binding to cells which bear receptors for these cytokines.[61-63] Based on this finding, it was postulated and definitively shown that these receptors share a common subunit, through which such cross-competition is either directly or indirectly manifest. In a search for polypeptides homologous to the IL-3 receptor, Hayashida and colleagues described a cDNA which, when co-expressed with a low-affinity GM-CSF receptor, led to high-affinity GM-CSF binding.[59] Subsequent studies have shown this polypeptide to complex with the previously described IL-5 and recently described low-affinity human IL-3 receptors; moreover, it mediates high-affinity binding and cross-competition among their ligands.[64] This common subunit would seem to present an important target for IL-3-, GM-CSF-, and IL-5-specific therapeutics.

TABLE 1
Biochemistry of the CSFs and Related Hemopoietins

	SCF	IL-3	GM-CSF	G-CSF	IL-5	M-CSF	Epo
				Protein			
M_r(kDa)	28-35	18-30	16-30	18-19	25-60	45-70	39
Quaternary structure	D	M	M	M	D	D	M
N-linked CHO	+	+	+	-	+	+	+
O-linked CHO	+	+	+	+	+	+	+
Disulfide bonds	+	+	+	+	+	+	+
				Nucleic Acid			
Human chromosomal location	12q	5q	5q	17	5	5q	7
No. of exons	10	5	4	5	4	10	5
Alternative splicing	+	-	-	+	-	+	-

SCF, stem cell factor, or kit ligand; IL-3, interleukin-3; IL-5, eosinophil differentiation factor; Epo, erythropoietin; D, dimer; M, monomer.

In contrast to the GM-CSF, G-CSF, and IL-3 receptors, the M-CSF and SCF receptors belong to the tyrosine kinase family of cell surface receptors,[65,66] and like many other members of this group, the M-CSF receptor and the SCF receptors are encoded by protooncogenes, c-*fms* and c-*kit*, respectively. Thus, based on the structural homologies among their receptors and the biochemical properties of the proteins themselves, the CSFs fall into two distinct structural families.

C. PHARMACOKINETICS

Large amounts of purified recombinant CSFs are now available by the methods of recombinant DNA technology. Because of strong clinical interest in these proteins, many pharmacologic preclinical and clinical trials have been reported. A complete discussion of the pharmacology of the CSFs is beyond the scope of this chapter. Rather, general principles will be provided in order to better understand the impetus to rational drug design in the field. First, as the native polypeptides for all the CSFs are at least 15 kDa, parenteral administration is necessary. This, coupled with costly methods of production and purification results in high patient costs. For example, based on the Wholesale Price Listings, the cost in 1994 for a 21-d course of GM-CSF is $3,360.[67] Second, the intravascular clearance of one group of CSFs, that including G-CSF, GM-CSF, and IL-3, is characteristic of many non-carrier bound molecules, i.e. a short α (redistribution) phase and a slightly longer β (predominantly renal elimination) phase.[68,69] Thus, the $t_{1/2}$ of elimination of these CSFs ranges from 7 min (GM-CSF and IL-3) to 2 h (G-CSF). In contrast, the larger M-CSF molecule is cleared primarily by receptor-mediated uptake and destruction resulting in a saturable, prolonged clearance profile.[70] Third, because of the rapid clearance and continuous need for CSF support of progenitor cell proliferation and differentiation, continuous infusions of the CSFs are a more effective hematopoietic stimulus than are intermittent administration schedules.

III. STRUCTURE-FUNCTION ANALYSIS OF THE CSFs

A. CARBOHYDRATES

Several groups have investigated the functional role of carbohydrate modification of the CSFs. Removal of the single site of O-linked carbohydrate leads to slow self-aggregation and inactivation of G-CSF in biological systems.[71] In contrast, removal of the N-linked and O-linked carbohydrate present in M-CSF, GM-CSF, or IL-3 fails to reduce any of the biologic functions of these proteins. In fact, most[68,72,73] but not all[74] groups have found that elimination of the N-linked carbohydrate on GM-CSF leads to enhanced biological activity. This effect is due to enhanced association between non-carbohydrate modified GM-CSF and the GM-CSF receptor.[75] Carbohydrate modification has little or no effect on the blood cell type produced, on the activation of mature blood cells, or on the secretory rate of GM-CSF.[68,69,72] When compared to GM-CSF devoid of N-linked glycosylation, GM-CSF containing its full complement of carbohydrate had a slightly prolonged redistribution phase and an identical β elimination phase.[69] These results are not surprising given the full biologic activity and *in vivo* efficacy characteristic of GM-CSF and IL-3 produced in *Escherichia coli.*

B. POLYPEPTIDE STRUCTURES REQUIRED FOR BIOLOGICAL ACTIVITY

A number of studies suggest that the receptor-binding site of a polypeptide hormone consists of a discrete, highly localized group of amino acids.[76] The majority of the polypeptide appears to be required to generate and maintain the proper conformation of the receptor binding domain. Precise knowledge of the geometry, charge density, potential for hydrogen bonding, and hydrophobic interactions at this site should allow the rationale design of protein mimics and antagonists. With these concepts in mind, a number of approaches have been taken to determine the sites of interaction between the CSFs and their receptors. Clark-Lewis and coworkers have tested a number of synthetic truncated peptides of human GM-CSF in an attempt to identify the receptor-binding domain of the molecule.[77] Based on the biological activities of the peptides, the authors concluded that amino acids Glu14 through Cys96 were critical for biological activity. These results must be interpreted with caution as the truncated polypeptide was three to four orders of magnitude less active than the full-length synthetic polypeptide. However, additional studies using less severely truncated polypeptides suggested that neither the 13 amino-terminal nor the 6 carboxyl-terminal residues were required for activity.

Using a linker-scanning approach to generate a series of internal deletion mutants of murine GM-CSF, two groups have reported disparate results.[78,79] As other work has shown that alterations in protein folding and stability often result from deletional mutagenesis, interpretation of such studies is difficult. Taken together, however, all of the deletions that reduced biological activity in both studies occurred between positions Arg11 and Pro115, results consistent with the synthetic peptide studies of Clark-Lewis.

Using a series of Pro substitution mutants, Altman and colleagues showed that disruption of the first, third, and fourth, but not the second α helix of murine GM-CSF resulted in substantial reductions in biological activity.[80] However, because all of these approaches likely alter the secondary and tertiary conformation of the molecule, conclusions regarding the precise location of receptor interactive residues are, at best, first-order approximations.

On the basis of the lack of cross-species activity of human and murine GM-CSF, we have constructed a series of interspecies hybrids of the growth factor and tested them for species-specific receptor binding and bioactivity. As human and murine GM-CSF share 60% sequence homology,[46] including an identical disulfide structure,[81] and an even greater degree of homology when considering the hydrophobic residues present on the interior surfaces of the four helixes,[51] the two molecules likely share secondary and tertiary structural features. In addition to these theoretical arguments, the overall structural similarity of human and murine GM-CSF has been confirmed experimentally.[82] Thus, the chimeric approach to substitution mutagenesis is much more likely to allow retention of overall structural integrity, allowing more direct interpretation of those sites primarily responsible for species-specific receptor binding. The results of these studies suggested that residues in the first helix of GM-CSF, and residues in the loop between the third and fourth helixes are responsible for receptor binding and biological activity.[83]

Correlation of the binding epitopes of monoclonal antibodies (mAb) with their capacity to block receptor binding or biological activity has been utilized extensively to map domains critical to the biological function of hormones and cytokines. Several groups have reported epitope mapping studies of antibodies which bind GM-CSF. Antibodies to the amino-terminal six residues failed to alter the bioactivity of human GM-CSF.[84] MAb to the first helix,[85] the loop between the third and fourth helix,[84,85] and the fourth helix[85,86] have been described which block GM-CSF receptor binding or neutralize its biological activity. These studies must also be interpreted with some caution, as mAb may neutralize activity by several mechanisms which do not involve direct interaction with the receptor binding sites. The use of Fab fragments can eliminate some of the concern over blocking by steric hindrance from a remote site, but mAbs have also been shown to induce conformational changes in ligands upon binding. The collective experience, however, suggests that GM-CSF binds to its receptor through two nonlinear regions of the polypeptide, which are in close juxtaposition only in the tertiary structure of the molecule. These studies have been supported recently by additional studies of human and murine mutants of GM-CSF and monoclonal antibody mapping studies,[175] which support the role of the amino-terminal α helix in high-affinity GM-CSF receptor-binding interactions, particularly Glu21, while binding to the low-affinity receptor maps to other regions in the molecule.

These data have been used to develop testable models of the tertiary structure of GM-CSF.[87] Based on the primary amino acid sequence, the alignment of its disulfide bonds, and the presence of four predicted α helixes, GM-CSF can be aligned as a four-helix bundle protein similar to that of human growth hormone and interleukin-2, structures which have been determined by X-ray crystallography.[88,89] Based on energy minimization considerations, these models were useful for generating testable hypotheses about amino acid relationships within the GM-CSF structure. The recently determined crystal structure of human GM-CSF confirms the overall orientation as a four-helix bundle but indicates a novel fold which combines a two-stranded anti-parallel β sheet with a relatively open four-helix bundle.[176,177] Based on this crystal structure, a potential binding site is proposed encompassing residues from the first (amino-terminal) and third α helices. These structural data, in combination with mutagenesis and antibody mapping data, identify potential receptor interaction sites that can serve as the basis for future rational design strategies.

A similar range of studies of murine and human IL-3 have been reported. Using a truncated synthetic peptide approach, Clark-Lewis and coworkers demonstrated that the amino-terminal 79 residues of murine IL-3 were partially active, suggesting that this half of the molecule could bind to the IL-3 receptor.[92] However, as the activity of this form of IL-3 was reduced by four orders of magnitude compared to the full-length synthetic peptide, residues in the carboxyl-terminal half were also thought essential for full activity.

Using the interspecies chimeric approach, we have also analyzed the sites of IL-3 which interact with the IL-3 receptor. In this case, residues in the first (Val14 through Asp21) and fourth (Phe107 through Glu119) helixes were required for biological activity.[93] An additional chimeric IL-3 molecule was analyzed which may provide some insights into the IL-3-IL-3 receptor interaction. This chimera, which contained the first 45 human IL-3-specific residues and the 101 carboxyl-terminal murine IL-3-specific residues, bound to the human IL-3 receptor. However, the chimeric protein was nearly devoid of biologic activity. These data suggested that the amino-terminal region binds to the receptor and that the carboxyl-terminal region triggers a biologic response. This concept of distinct "address" and "biologically active" sequences has been reviewed (see Reference 94 and references therein).

Like the studies for GM-CSF, mapping the binding sites of anti-IL-3 mAb has corroborated the findings from structure-activity studies. Neutralizing and receptor blocking mAb have been mapped to sites between Val14 and Glu50, and between Phe107 and Glu133.[93,95,96]

Non-neutralizing mAb, or antipeptide antisera which bind to native murine or human IL-3, bind to the amino-terminal six residues, amino acids between positions 56 and 70, and to residues 130 through 135 near the carboxyl-terminus of the molecule.[93,95,97-99]

Less is known of the structural requirements for action of G-CSF. This molecule contains five Cys residues, reduction of which leads to a complete loss of bioactivity. Circular dichroism (CD) spectral analysis suggests that Cys17 is solvent inaccessible, a result consistent with peptide mapping studies which show that Cys36 is coupled to Cys42, and Cys64 is coupled to Cys74.[100] Further evidence supporting the nonessential character of Cys17 is that mutation at this position to Ser is well tolerated.[101] In contrast, mutation of the other Cys residues or single-amino acid insertions or deletions at positions adjacent to these residues eliminates biological activity.[101]

In addition to the stability induced by the presence of O-linked carbohydrate (see above discussion), residues in the amino-terminus of G-CSF seem to play a role in initiating or stabilizing the proper conformation of G-CSF. These conclusions derive from a study of a series of N-terminal substitution mutants of the molecule.[101] Kuga and co-workers have shown that a four-amino acid substitution within the amino-terminal 17 residues lead to a threefold enhancement in biological activity. As this mutant was more resistant to heat inactivation than the native sequence, and as these polypeptides were produced in an *E. coli* expression system requiring renaturation *in vitro*, it is likely that the amino-terminal substitutions result in higher activity by virtue of their favorable effects on folding. Indeed, other muteins in this same study and the relative lack of homology between human and murine G-CSF in the amino-terminal one third of the molecule strongly suggest that residues in the carboxyl two thirds of G-CSF are essential for interaction with the G-CSF receptor.

Circular dichroism analysis suggests that G-CSF, like GM-CSF and IL-3, is rich in α-helical structure.[100] Parry and coworkers have suggested that G-CSF folds into a four-helix bundle structure, similar to that predicted for GM-CSF and IL-3.[102] However, based on similarities within their genomic organization, disulfide alignment and their similar spectra of biological activities, G-CSF is felt to be structurally most closely related to interleukin-6, a molecule with which it shares sequence homology.[103]

Finally, even less is known about the structure-activity relationships of M-CSF. As noted above, the primary M-CSF transcript undergoes alternative splicing to result in long (555) and short (257) primary translation products, both of which contain an identical 32-amino acid secretory leader and a 24-amino acid transmembrane domain. More recently, a third, intermediate-sized form of M-CSF has also been described.[104] All forms of M-CSF undergo cleavage to release a soluble form of the growth factor, albeit at greatly different rates.[57,105] Despite the uncertainty of the relative roles of each form of M-CSF, it is clear that the released polypeptides share only the 149 N-terminal amino acids. As the biologic activity of the various forms of soluble M-CSF are identical, it is clear that all of the determinants of receptor binding and activation reside in these residues. Further characterization of the receptor-binding domain has been hampered by the complex disulfide structure of the molecule and the requirement for an intact homodimeric structure.

Efforts are currently underway to determine the physical structure the CSFs.[90,91] These efforts, when coupled with studies based on analysis of peptides, muteins, mcAb epitope mapping, and computer-assisted modeling, will provide important insights into the structure-activity relationships of the CSFs. These comparisons will begin the truc cra of rational drug design of the CSFs.

IV. THE USE OF NATIVE SEQUENCE CSFs AS THERAPEUTIC PROTEINS

Therapeutic or pharmaceutical proteins have been defined as "proteins or polypeptides which by reason of their native functions in the human body are suitable as therapeutic substances."[106] In the greater sense, the CSFs have fulfilled this definition. As expected from their physiology, the CSFs were predicted to be useful for states of marrow failure. Recombinant GM-CSF produced in CHO cells was first tested in patients with the acquired immune deficiency syndrome (AIDS) in whom a concomitant fall in neutrophil count had occurred.[107] GM-CSF produced a dose-dependent rise in peripheral blood neutrophil levels which began within 3 d of the start of therapy and which returned to baseline within a few days of discontinuation. Bone marrow morphology in these patients suggested that the rise was due to substantial increases in cell production, rather than simply due to premature release of a marrow storage pool of cells. This finding was later confirmed for both GM-CSF and G-CSF by careful quantitative analysis.[108,109] A follow-up study demonstrated sustained effects of subcutaneous administration of GM-CSF to patients with AIDS for up to 6 months.[110] Dose-dependent neutrophilia was again noted, without the development of tachyphylaxis. These studies suggested the feasibility of long-term use.

Reports of *in vitro* enhancement of human immunodeficiency virus (HIV) production from HIV-infected cell lines grown in the presence of GM-CSF[111] have tempered enthusiasm for the use of GM-CSF in patients with AIDS. This, coupled with the mild nature of neutropenia in many patients with AIDS (as opposed to the severe infectious complications of lymphopenia) has urged caution in this clinical setting. However, more recent reports have called into question the significance of these *in vitro* findings, especially since the concurrent use of GM-CSF and the anti-HIV agent Zidovudine (AZT) leads to a decrease in HIV production *in vitro*.[112] Furthermore, the occurrence of significant neutropenia and anemia related to the treatment of AIDS with Zidovudine and dideoxyinosine (DDI) has renewed interest in the use of CSFs to permit ongoing therapy with these drugs in the setting of marrow toxicity.

Recent reports suggest that this combined approach is feasible; severely leukopenic patients with AIDS given GM-CSF along with Zidovudine had reduced treatment-induced hematologic toxicity compared to patients given comparable Zidovudine therapy alone.[113] Similar studies have been reported using G-CSF along with erythropoietin in patients in whom the dose of Zidovudine had to be lowered because of neutropenia.[114] In this study, not only was Zidovudine-associated neutropenia abrogated, but anemia was partially to completely corrected in all 20 patients. Further study of the optimal dose, timing, and combination of agents is presently underway.

In patients undergoing bone marrow transplantation for lymphoid malignancies, Nemunaitis and coworkers showed that the use of GM-CSF hastened the recovery of neutrophils compared to a closely matched group of historical controls.[115] The GM-CSF-treated patients had fewer febrile days and were discharged from hospital earlier. In a study of patients undergoing autologous marrow transplantation following high-dose chemotherapy for refractory solid tumors, GM-CSF was shown to elevate the neutrophil count by day 14 of transplantation and was associated with a reduced incidence of bacteremia.[116] Similar studies using G-CSF in marrow transplantation have been reported. Again, patients treated with G-CSF had a more rapid return of neutrophil counts following autologous marrow transplantation for Hodgkin's disease.[117] These agents have also been used, with some success, for marrow graft failure following conventional protocols of bone marrow transplantation.[118,119]

The potential usefulness of the CSFs in myeloid leukemias and in some solid malignancies has been restricted by the occurrence of receptors for these growth factors on a number of cell lines and clinical samples.[9,120,121] In addition, leukemic blasts from fresh marrow samples from many of these patients are stimulated to proliferate *in vitro* by IL-3, GM-CSF, or G-CSF.[122] Thus, caution in these clinical settings has been the general rule. However, more recent proposals have included the use of CSFs in patients with CSF receptor-bearing leukemias undergoing chemotherapy or marrow transplantation, both to speed hematologic recovery, and potentially as a way to enhance tumor cell kill induced by the conventional therapy. In this latter way CSFs may be envisaged as acting as chemotherapy-sensitizing agents. One recent report of the use of G-CSF for patients with acute myeloid leukemias (AML) found the drug to be effective (a more rapid neutrophil recovery following high-dose chemotherapy) and showed no evidence of enhanced leukemic relapse.[123] In another study of eight patients with AML, GM-CSF did not appear to accelerate leukemic recurrence following conventional chemotherapy.[124] Further studies are clearly required to assess the relative merits and risks of CSF therapy in patients with CSF receptor-bearing malignancies.

A number of trials have been reported using CSFs to reduce the myelotoxicity associated with conventional high-dose chemotherapy for malignancy. Gabrilove and co-workers administered G-CSF to 27 patients undergoing intensive chemotherapy for transitional cell carcinoma of the bladder.[131] The study design incorporated each patient as his/her own control; G-CSF was administered during the first cycle of chemotherapy and not during the second, or vice versa. Treatment cycles with G-CSF had a 91% reduction in days with neutrophil count below 1000, substantially reduced mucositis, and a reduced number of days on which antibiotics were required to treat febrile infections. In addition, G-CSF therapy significantly increased the proportion of patients hematologically capable of undergoing their subsequent course of chemotherapy on schedule. Similar favorable results have been reported for G-CSF therapy in support of patients given Melphelan for a variety of malignancies,[132] for patients given G-CSF following therapy with cyclophosphamide, doxorubicin, and etoposide for small cell carcinoma of the lung,[133] for GM-CSF therapy following doxorubicin, dacarbazine, ifosfamide, and mesna therapy for metastatic carcinoma,[134] and for treatment with IL-3 during high-dose 5-fluorouracil therapy in a preclinical study in cynomologous primates.[135] It is clear that comparative trials of the CSFs are required to determine whether one therapy is superior to the others for a given clinical setting. Such trials are currently underway.

Myelodysplasia (MDS) is the term given to a variety of entities all characterized by dysplastic features of marrow development, one or more cytopenias and often functional failure of neutrophils or platelets. The most clinically devastating syndromes are usually those associated with neutropenia, as red cell and platelet transfusions can often forestall life-threatening symptoms from anemia and thrombocytopenia.

Therapy with hematopoietic growth factors for patients with myelodysplasia is difficult due to the chronic nature of the disease (requiring continuous therapy), the often poor response of myelodysplastic progenitor cells to growth factors *in vitro,* and the potential for leukemic cells (which may become part of the dysplastic process) to proliferate in response to growth factors.[122,125] Despite these considerations, the lack of alternative therapies and the potential for leukemic or preleukemic cells to differentiate rather than proliferate in response to hematopoietic growth factors has led to a number of clinical trials. Two endpoints for these studies have been considered; elevation of the white blood cell count and functional activation of neutrophils. The first reported trial utilized continuous-infusion GM-CSF therapy in eight patients with MDS.[126] Overall, treatment was associated with a marked leukocytosis and a moderate increase in red cell and platelet production. Analysis of the circulating cells in these patients demonstrated their derivation from the abnormal clone. These results suggested that therapy lead to increased production and differentiation of the dysplastic cells, rather than production from residual normal progenitor cells. However, subsequent studies have been far less optimistic. When patients with marrow blast cell counts above 14% were included in treatment arms containing GM-CSF (approximately 15% of MDS patients), an alarmingly high proportion developed frank leukemia. In one study, four such patients progressed within 4 weeks of the beginning of treatment.[127] A similar result was reported by Ganser and coworkers, who treated nine MDS patients with IL-3.[128] Although neutrophil and platelet counts responded in several patients, another patient developed increased numbers of leukemic blast cells during therapy. A number of similar results have been reported; in some patients reversal of the high blast counts has not occurred upon discontinuation of therapy. Clearly, this group of patients must be excluded from therapy with GM-CSF or IL-3.

The results with G-CSF in patients with MDS are more promising. This may be explained, at least in part, by the propensity of G-CSF to preferentially stimulate MDS progenitor cell *differentiation*. In contrast, progenitor cell *proliferation* predominates in the presence of GM-CSF.[129] In most clinical studies reporting the use of G-CSF for patients with MDS, a dose-dependent elevation of neutrophil count and neutrophil function was noted. Prolonged periods of response were noted in many studies, even in patients with high initial blast counts.[129] These results have translated into a reduction in infectious complications for responding patients. As a result of these studies, most patients with MDS are presently treated with G-CSF, especially if marrow blast cell counts are elevated prior to therapy.

The success of single agent CSF therapy of aplastic anemia is uncertain regardless of the type of CSF utilized. In most studies, a variable increase in leukocytes has occurred, with less impressive platelet and reticulocyte responses.[136-139] Unfortunately, most studies have found the response proportionate to the level of pretherapy hematopoiesis; patients with the least severe aplasia respond most favorably. Furthermore, all responses have been transient. In addition, even in those patients with a favorable leukocyte response, the level of marrow progenitor cells has not been altered,[136] suggesting that CSF therapy alone had not altered the basic defect in most patients with marrow aplasia, reduced stem cell numbers. Based on the necessity of both early-acting and late-acting factors for the complete program of blood cell development, combinations of factors are envisaged as being superior to single-agent therapy in the setting of stem cell failure. In this regard, IL-3 and GM-CSF, administered sequentially, was associated with an enhanced hematopoietic response in normal macaques.[140] Similar results have been reported for IL-3 and G-CSF.[141] The clinical utility of this approach is presently under study. However, at present, CSF therapy of aplastic anemia should be reserved for those patients who have failed conventional therapy, who are not eligible for bone marrow transplantation, and who manifest complications from one or more cytopenias.

In addition to conventional aplastic anemia, a number of isolated neutropenic states have been treated with the CSFs. In children with severe congenital neutropenia (Kostmann Syndrome), G-CSF therapy has been overwhelmingly successful. In two studies, the administration of G-CSF lead to substantial neutrophilic responses, clearing of infectious complications, and resumption of a near-normal lifestyle.[142,143] The use of GM-CSF has been far less promising in this setting.[143] In cyclic neutropenia, G-CSF therapy has nearly eliminated the infectious complications of neutropenic periods.[144] In addition, an occasional adult patient with acquired agranulocytosis has been successfully treated with G-CSF.[145]

One of the predictable effects of all of the CSFs is to mobilize hematopoietic progenitor cells from the marrow to the peripheral blood. For example, IL-3 lead to a 9- to 12-fold rise in peripheral blood granulocyte-macrophage colony-forming units, erythroid burst-forming units, and megakaryocytic colony-forming cells.[146] GM-CSF and G-CSF have similar effects. Together, multiple CSFs act in synergy, resulting in a substantial rise in these cells.[146] Further studies have now suggested that stem cells capable of repopulating the marrow following ablative chemotherapy are mobilized following CSF therapy. A recent study has shown that murine peripheral blood stem cells following G-CSF therapy are a rich source of marrow and lymphoid repopulating cells.[147] This technique could eventually replace the need for marrow harvest in the rescue of patients treated with very high doses of chemotherapy and radiation for malignancy.

Finally, therapy with M-CSF has taken a different clinical direction. *In vitro*, the predominant activity of human M-CSF has been macrophage activation. In fact, unless special culture conditions are used,[148] it is difficult to demonstrate any proliferative effects of human M-CSF using human progenitor cells. In contrast, M-CSF is a potent stimulus of macrophage inflammatory mediator release (IL-1 and TNF), antibody-dependent cellular cytotoxicity, and non-specific tumor cell killing.[14,15] Thus, M-CSF has been applied as adjuvant therapy in the treatment of malignancy. In this setting, combination with specific antitumor antibody therapy seems especially attractive. Clinical trials to assess the efficacy and toxicity in this setting are currently underway.

Pharmacokinetic studies have shown that IL-3, GM-CSF, and G-CSF have short intravascular transit times.[68,69] Thus, when given as an intravenous bolus, GM-CSF is without hematologic effect.[149] Therapy with all of the CSFs was initially administered by continuous intravenous infusion.[107,131] Subsequent studies have shown that although somewhat less effective, 2-h daily infusions of GM-CSF are effective,[15] and subcutaneous administration, especially of G-CSF, has also gained acceptance.[130,133,134]

In general, therapy with the CSFs has been well tolerated. Initial phase I studies of GM-CSF revealed dose-limiting toxicities of capillary leak and large vessel thrombosis at doses above 15 μg/kg,[67,110] doses which are clearly in excess of those needed in most clinical settings. Lower doses have been complicated by bone pain, myalgia, fever, anorexia, and an occasional erythematous rash at the injection site. These effects have been reversible upon dose reduction or discontinuation of the drug. For G-CSF, bone pain and fever have also complicated therapy, but higher doses have not been associated with the capillary leak syndrome. Bolus administration of both drugs is associated with an immediate *neutropenia,* which revolves within 1 to 6 h despite continuation of drug. It is likely that these complications of CSF therapy are directly related to their effects on mature leukocytes.[150] GM-CSF and M-CSF activate monocytes and neutrophils to release a number of inflammatory mediators, including TNF and IL-1.[151-153] In addition, both GM- and G-CSF activate neutrophil prostaglandin synthesis, cause the release of proteases and toxic oxygen radicals, and trigger homotypic aggregation.[12,18] Thus, nearly all of the listed side effects of the two drugs can be predicted by their effects on mature leukocytes.

It is unclear whether the source of production of CSF has any effect on its clinical utility or on the development of side effects. Materials produced by *E. coli,* yeast, and mammalian tissue culture cells have been utilized in the clinical trials noted above. With the exception of a shorter redistribution phase (but not steady-state elimination kinetics) for GM-CSF devoid of carbohydrate, all of the products appear to be clinically equivalent. Only a single report of an immunologic reaction to a CSF has appeared in the literature; 4 of a group of 13 patients given GM-CSF produced in yeast developed anti-GM-CSF antibodies.[153] In only one patient was the response associated with GM-CSF failure. Until further reports appear, the incidence of this complication is difficult to determine; it is likely to be a rare event. Finally, very few long-term effects of administration of the CSFs have appeared. Initially, theoretical concerns were raised that the CSFs might act to deplete hematopoietic stem cells. Thus far no evidence of marrow exhaustion has been presented, despite continuous administration of up to 6 years in animals and 5 years in humans. The only long-term complications that have appeared are mild splenomegaly, more common with G-CSF than with GM-CSF.[110]

V. RATIONAL DRUG DESIGN — THE SECOND GENERATION

As should be obvious from the previous discussion, although the clinical responses to the CSFs as therapeutic proteins have been gratifying, many problems remain. Costs are high. The agents have short circulatory survivals, and must be administered parenterally. In addition, as the CSFs may be involved in the pathogenesis of leukemia, asthma, and chronic inflammation, CSF antagonists may potentially provide important therapeutics for these disorders.

Several goals for improved CSF therapeutics might be set. First, agents with prolonged circulatory survival might allow less frequent dosing. Second, the development of superagonists, agents of increased potency or effects, might also reduce costs or side effects. Third, the development of peptide or small organic mimics would allow alternate routes of administration and reduced costs. Fourth, selective agonists (agents which dissociate the multiple functions of the CSFs) would likely reduce toxicity. And fifth, CSF antagonists might prove useful in pathologic states wholly or in part dependent on the CSFs. In this section a discussion of potential routes to realize these goals will be presented to illustrate some of the directions presently being pursued towards the rational drug design of the CSFs.

A. PROLONGED CSF SURVIVAL

Polyethylene glycol (PEG) modification of proteins has long been known to increase the residence time of proteins in the vascular compartment.[155] One of the three mechanisms may account for this finding. First, for small proteins which may pass through the glomerulus, PEG modification may increase the molecular weight sufficiently to preclude rapid renal clearance. Second, the metabolism of larger proteins can be altered due to PEG interference in the recognition and degradation process. And third, PEG modification can reduce the immunogenicity of foreign proteins and thus reduce immune clearance mechanisms.[156] A number of therapeutic proteins, including L-asparaginase, adenosine deaminase, superoxide dismutase, IL-2, streptokinase, and blood clotting factor VIII have been PEG-modified and are in various stages of drug development.

PEG is added to free amino groups of the polypeptide. In addition to the amino-terminal residue, free Lys groups may be modified if surface accessible. Thus, if inadequate Lys residues are available in the native amino acid sequence, additional sites may be added by recombinant DNA techniques. Usually, site-directed mutagenesis of Arg to Lys accomplishes this goal. Conversely, modification at biologically critical Lys sites can lead to protein inactivation; this problem can usually be overcome by Lys → Arg mutation.

Delgado and colleagues have applied this technology to human GM-CSF.[157] Using a new method to link PEG under physiologic conditions, PEG-GM-CSF proteins were generated which retained full *in vitro* biological activity. Furthermore, certain levels of PEG modification resulted in enhanced neutrophil activation.[158] The *in vivo* characteristics of these PEG-modified GM-CSF proteins are undergoing evaluation. More recently, Shaw and colleagues at Genetics Institute have begun to modify IL-3 with PEG.[178] These products are also scheduled to begin testing shortly. The rat SCF used in preclinical trials has been PEG modified. Preliminary studies comparing the natural protein to PEG-modified rat SCF indicate that modification leads to a twofold enhancement in circulatory survival.[179]

B. SUPERAGONISTS

More potent CSFs could reduce costs of administration and possibly reduce the side effects of therapy if related to total dose of foreign protein administered. Two approaches have been taken, mutation of the native polypeptide sequence, and the linking together of different growth factors.

A number of groups have shown that removal of the N-linked carbohydrate from human GM-CSF enhances the *in vitro* specific activity of the resultant polypeptide.[68,72,73] This occurs whether the GM-CSF is synthesized by bacteria (which are incapable of N-linked carbohydrate modification) or if the critical Asn residues have been replaced. Similar results have been noted for human IL-3.[180] As the role of N-linked carbohydrate in the secretion, processing, or biological activities of GM-CSF or IL-3 is uncertain, deglycosylated GM-CSF might provide a more potent CSF for clinical use. Preliminary pharmacokinetic studies have not borne out this promise.[68,69] The enhanced activity of these forms of GM-CSF appears to be at least partially offset by a reduced circulatory survival.[69] Further studies will be necessary to determine if deglycosylated CSFs offer any advantage over unmodified recombinant proteins.

Using cassette mutagenesis. Kuga and coworkers have screened a number of mutants of the N-terminal region of human G-CSF and found one with enhanced granulopoietic activity both *in vitro* and *in vivo*.[101] Based on receptor-binding studies, the enhanced activity appears to be due to higher receptor-binding affinity. However, as the mutein also displayed enhanced thermal stability, a greater proportion of the *E. coli*-produced mutant may refold or remain in the active conformation compared to the native polypeptide, and thus explain the enhanced biological activity and receptor affinity. This explanation is also consistent with a number of independent studies which suggest that the receptor-binding domain of G-CSF, and the highly related cytokine IL-6, resides in the carboxyl-, not the amino-terminal region of each molecule.[101,159-161]

A second approach to enhance CSF potency has been to combine growth factors which exhibit synergistic effects. This was recently accomplished by Williams and coworkers at Immunex.[162] Using a polyglycine linker, a GM-CSF/IL-3 fusion protein was produced. The fusion protein was 10-fold more potent that either GM-CSF or IL-3 alone at stimulating colony formation and proliferation *in vitro*. The reason for the enhanced activity was likely due to enhanced receptor-binding kinetics. *In vivo* studies will be required to confirm that the increase in activity in cell culture assays will be reproduced in the clinical setting. Enhanced clearance by immune and nonimmune mechanisms likely pose the greatest challenge to this approach.

C. CSF MIMICS

In addition to a better understanding of the atomic basis for protein-protein interactions, an ultimate goal of structure-function analysis of physiologically important molecules lies in their application to the design of altered therapeutics; smaller molecules whose structure is designed from a knowledge of the protein-protein interaction. The development of peptides which mimic the structure and function of a parent protein is an intermediate in this process. Success at this stage has been reported for many hormones, such as parathormone.[163] The ultimate expression of this process is the rational design of small organic molecules which bind to receptor in the same fashion as the native protein. This exciting step has now been accomplished for a mAb (termed 87.92.6) which binds to the cell surface receptor for reovirus type 3.[164] Given the cost and likely ongoing utility of CSF therapy, application of this technology seems inevitable.

In the two cited examples, PTH and mAb 87.92.6, the receptor-binding domain consists of a linear array of amino acids. The technologic feat was to design mimics which conform to the spatial characteristics of the parent molecules. In the case of GM-CSF and IL-3, for which the greatest CSF structure-function data base presently exists, the receptor-binding domain appears to be comprised of two nonlinear regions of the polypeptide. Thus, simple peptide subsets are unlikely to be sufficient for biologic activity.

Although a detailed discussion of present theories of polypeptide folding is beyond the scope of this chapter, they predict that individual units of secondary structure (e.g., an α-helical segment) assemble independently (the "molten globule" state).[165] The spatial relationships between secondary structural units is thought to be dependent on folding signals derived from additional sequence elements. For example IL-3 is predicted to resemble a four-helix bundles, the active site being comprised of one helix and a loop[83] or of two of the four helixes.[51] As noted above, these predictions need structural (crystallography or NMR) verification. Thus, a possible route to synthesize a CSF mimic would be the template-assisted synthetic protein approach (TASP).[166] In this methodology critical elements for receptor interaction are sequentially added to a preformed synthetic template. Knowledge of the structural constraints of the protein-receptor interaction allows optimal juxtaposition of each receptor interactive element. In this way, the majority of the polypeptide required for folding can be eliminated. Thus far, model systems have had limited success.[166] Given the complexity of the CSF-receptor interaction, much work remains to realize these goals.

D. CSF ANTAGONISTS

Finally, the CSFs appear to play an important role in a number of neoplastic, immunologic, and inflammatory processes. Interventions in CSF pathophysiology may be of therapeutic benefit. For example, antisera to GM-CSF and IL-3, when simultaneously administered to mice with an experimental form of cerebral malaria, lead to a significant amelioration of invasive disease.[167] CSF antagonists could play a similar role in acute leukemia, asthma, and chronic inflammatory joint disease. The rational development of a CSF antagonist will depend upon developing mimics which bind to receptor but fail to trigger receptor signal transduction. This has been recently described for IL-1,[168] glucagon,[169] and parathyroid hormones.[163] Our recent description of an interspecies chimeric IL-3 polypeptide which binds to the human IL-3 receptor but which fails to elicit a proliferative response,[51] and Landgraf and coworkers' description of a conformational mutant of human IL-2 with similar properties[170] point to the feasibility of this approach for cytokine therapeutics. Like most of the other goals of rational CSF drug design, the development of antagonists is far from complete.

VI. SUMMARY

The CSFs are a family of acidic glycoproteins which are critical for the host response to infectious, inflammatory, and immunologic stimuli. Within 30 years, this family has been postulated to exist, cloned, expressed, and tested as clinical therapeutics. Overall, the application of these physiologic regulators to clinical medicine has been an unqualified success. Nearly all of the physiologic responses predicted from their behavior *in vitro* have been realized *in vivo*. GM-CSF and G-CSF are useful to enhance the recovery of marrow function following cytotoxic radiation and chemotherapy. Their use has reduced the toxicity of these therapies. However, whether this can be translated into improved survival or cure rates has yet to be determined. The CSFs have also improved the care of patients with congenital neutropenias and many patients with myelodysplastic syndromes. And the CSFs offer a method to increase the hematologic tolerance of therapies for the acquired immunodeficiency syndrome, toxicities which often limit the effectiveness of these agents. The era of rational drug design is upon us; therapeutic CSFs are but the beginning. The techniques of recombinant DNA research, physical structure determination, molecular modeling, and medicinal chemistry promise to improve upon this expanding area of science.

REFERENCES

1. **Pluznick, D.H. and Sachs, L.**, The cloning of normal "mast" cells in tissue culture, *J. Cell Comp. Physiol.*, 66, 319, 1965.
2. **Bradley, T.R. and Metcalf, D.**, The growth of mouse bone marrow cells in vitro, *Aust. J. Exp. Biol. Med. Sci.*, 44, 287, 1966.
3. **Burgess, A.W. and Metcalf, D.**, The nature and action of granulocyte-macrophage colony-stimulating factors, *Blood*, 56, 947, 1980.
4. **Metcalf, D.**, The molecular biology and functions of the granulocyte-macrophage colony-stimulating factors, *Blood*, 67, 257, 1986.
5. **Migliaccio, G., Migliaccio, A.R., Kaushansky, K., and Adamson, J.W.**, Regulation of differentiation of murine progenitor cells derived from blast cell colonies under serum-deprived conditions, *Exp. Hematol.*, 17, 110, 1989.
6. **Nicola, N.A.**, Hemopoietic growth factors and their interactions with specific receptors, *J. Cell. Physiol.*, 5 (Suppl.), 9, 1987.
7. **Gearing, D., King, J., Gough, N., and Nicola, N.**, Expression cloning of a receptor for human granulocyte-macrophage colony-stimulating factor, *EMBO J.*, 8, 3667, 1989.
8. **Bussolino, F., Wang, J.M., and Defilippi, P.**, Granulocyte- and granulocyte-macrophage colony-stimulating factors induce human endothelial cells to migrate and proliferate, *Nature*, 337, 471, 1989.
9. **Baldwin, G.C., Golde, D.W., Widhopf, G.F., Economou, J., and Gasson, J.C.**, Identification and characterization of a low-affinity granulocyte-macrophage colony-stimulating factor receptor on primary and cultured human melanoma cells, *Blood*, 78, 609, 1991.
10. **Pollard, J.W., Bartocci, A., Arceci, R., Orlofsky, A., Ladner, M.B., and Stanley, E.R.**, Apparent role of the macrophage growth factor, CSF-1, in placental development, *Nature*, 330, 484, 1987.

11. **Grabstein, K.H., Urdal, D.L., Tushinski, R.J., Mochizuki, D.Y., Price, V.L., Cantrell, M.A., Gillis, S., and Conlon, P.J.,** Induction of macrophage tumoricidal activity by granulocyte-macrophage colony-stimulating factor, *Science*, 232, 506, 1986.
12. **Silberstein, D.S., Owen, W.F., Gasson, J.C., DiPersio, J.F., Golde, D.W., Bina, J.C., Soberman, R., Austen, K.F., and David, J.R.,** Enhancement of human eosinophil cytotoxicity and leukotriene synthesis by biosynthetic (recombinant) granulocyte-macrophage colony-stimulating factor, *J. Immunol.*, 137, 3290, 1986.
13. **Weisbart, R.H., Golde, D.W., Clark, S.C., Wong, G.G., and Gasson, J.C.,** Human granulocyte-macrophage colony stimulating factor is a neutrophil activator, *Nature*, 314, 361, 1985.
14. **Wing, E.J., Waheed, A., Shadduck, R.K., Nagle, L.S., and Stephenson, K.,** Effect of colony stimulating factor on murine macrophages, *J. Clin. Invest.*, 69, 270, 1982.
15. **Ralph, P., Nacy, C.A., Meltzer, M.S., Williams, N., Nakoinz, I., and Leonard, E.J.,** Colony-stimulating factors and regulation of macrophage tumoricidal and microbicidal activities, *Cell. Immunol.*, 76, 10, 1983.
16. **Rothenberg, M.E., Owen, W.F., Silberstein, D.S., Woods, J., Soberman, R.J., Austen, K.F., and Stevens, R.L.,** Human eosinophils have prolonged survival, enhanced functional properties, and become hypodense when exposed to human interleukin 3, *J. Clin. Invest.*, 81, 1986, 1988.
17. **Lopez, A.F., To, L.B., Yang, Y.-C., Gamble, J.R., Shannon, M.F., Burns, G.F., Dyson, P.G., Juttner, C.A., Clark, S.C., and Vadas, M.A.,** Stimulation of proliferation, differentiation, and function of human cells by primate interleukin 3, *Proc. Natl. Acad. Sci. U.S.A.*, 84, 2761, 1987.
18. **Souza, L., Boone, T.C., Gabrilove, J., Lai, P.H., Zsebo, K.M., Murdoch, D.C., Chazin, V.R., Bruszewski, J., Lu, H., Chen, K.K., Barendt, J., Platzer, E., Moore, M.A.S., Mertlesmann, R., and Welte, K.,** Recombinant human granulocyte colony-stimulating factor: effects on normal and leukemic myeloid cells, *Science*, 232, 61, 1986.
19. **Golde, D.W., Finley, T.N., and Cline, M.J.,** Production of colony-stimulating factor by human macrophages, *Lancet*, 1397, 1972.
20. **Bagby, G.C., Dinarello, C.A., Wallace, P., Wagner, C., Hefeneider, S., and McCall, E.,** Interleukin 1 stimulates granulocyte macrophage colony-stimulating activity release by vascular endothelial cells, *J. Clin. Invest.*, 78, 1316, 1986.
21. **Bagby, G.C., Rigas, V.D., Bennett, R.M., Vandenbark, A.A., and Garewal, H.S.,** Interaction of lactoferrin, monocytes, and T lymphocyte subsets in the regulation of steady-state granulopoiesis *in vitro*, *J. Clin. Invest.*, 68, 56, 1981.
22. **Quesenberry, P.J. and Gimbrone, M.A.,** Vascular endothelium as a regulator of granulopoiesis: production of colony-stimulating activity by cultured human endothelial cells, *Blood*, 56, 1060, 1980.
23. **Zucali, J.R., Dinarello, C.A., Oblon, D.J., Gross, M.A., Anderson, L., and Weiner, R.S.,** Interleukin 1 stimulates fibroblasts to produce granulocyte-macrophage colony-stimulating activity and prostaglandin E_2, *J. Clin. Invest.*, 77, 1857, 1986.
24. **Broudy, V.C., Kaushansky, K., Harlan, J.M., and Adamson, J.W.,** Interleukin 1 stimulates human endothelial cells to produce granulocyte-macrophage colony-stimulating factor and granulocyte colony-stimulating factor, *J. Immunol.*, 139, 464, 1987.
25. **Kaushansky, K., Miller, J.E., Morris, D.R., Wilson, C.B., and Hammond, W.P.,** The role of lymphocytes and monocytes in hematopoietic growth factor production by peripheral blood mononuclear cells, *Cell. Immunol.*, 122, 62, 1989.
26. **Munker, R., Gasson, J., Ogawa, M., and Koeffler, H.P.,** Recombinant human TNF induces production of granulocyte-macrophage colony-stimulating factor, *Nature*, 323, 79, 1986.
27. **Kaushansky, K., Lin, N., and Adamson, J.W.,** IL-1 stimulates fibroblasts to synthesize granulocyte/macrophage (GM) and granulocyte (G) colony-stimulating factors: a mechanism for the hematopoietic response to inflammation, *J. Clin. Invest.*, 81, 92, 1988.
28. **Koeffler, H.P., Gasson, J.C., Ranyard, J., Souza, L., Shepard, M., and Munker, R.,** Recombinant human TNF alpha stimulates production of granulocyte colony-stimulating factor, *Blood*, 70, 55, 1987.
29. **Niemeyer, C.M., Sieff, C.A., Mathey-Prevot, B., Wimperis, J.Z., Bierer, B.E., Clark, S.C., and Nathan, D.G.,** Expression of human interleukin-3 (multi-CSF) is restricted to human lymphocytes and T-cell lines, *Blood*, 73, 945, 1989.
30. **Wimperis, J.Z., Niemeyer, C.M., Sieff, C.A., Mathey-Prevot, B., Nathan, D.G., and Arceci, R.J.,** Granulocyte-macrophage colony-stimulating factor and interleukin-3 mRNAs are produced by a small fraction of blood mononuclear cells, *Blood*, 74, 1525, 1989.
31. **Broudy, V.C., Kaushansky, K., Shoemaker, S.G., Aagarwal, B., and Adamson, J.W.,** Muramyl dipeptide and lipopolysaccharide induce production of hematopoietic growth factors in vivo by different mechanisms, *J. Immunol.*, 144, 3789, 1990.
32. **Cheers, C., Haigh, A.M., Kelso, A., Metcalf, D., Stanley, E.R., and Young, A.M.,** Production of colony-stimulating factors during infection: separate determinations of macrophage, granulocyte, granulocyte-macrophage and multi-CSFs, *Infect. Immun.*, 56, 247, 1988.

33. **Xu, W.D., Firestein, G.S., Taetle, R., Kaushansky, K., and Zvaifler, N.J.,** Cytokines in chronic inflammatory arthritis: granulocyte-macrophage colony-stimulating factor in rheumatoid synovial effusions, *J. Clin. Invest.*, 83, 876, 1989.
34. **Alvaro-Gracia, J.M., Zvaifler, N.J., Brown, C.B., Kaushansky, K., and Firestein, G.S.,** Cytokines in chronic inflammatory arthritis. VI. Analysis of the synovial cells involved in granulocyte-macrophage colony-stimulating factor production and gene expression in rheumatoid arthritis and its regulation by IL-1 and tumor necrosis factor-α, *J. Immunol.*, 146, 3365, 1991.
35. **Valent, P., Besemer, J., Muhm, M., Majdic, O., Lechner, K., and Bettelheim, P.,** Interleukin 3 activates human blood basophils via high-affinity binding sites, *Proc. Natl. Acad. Sci. U.S.A.*, 86, 5542, 1989.
36. **Meeker, T.C., Hardy, D., Willman, C., Hogan, T., and Abrams, J.,** Activation of the interleukin-3 gene by chromosome translocation in acute lymphocytic leukemia with eosinophilia, *Blood*, 72, 285, 1990.
37. **Kaushansky, K., O'Hara, P.J., Berkner, K., Segal, G.M., Hagen, F.S., and Adamson, J.W.,** Genomic cloning, characterization, and multilineage expression of human granulocyte-macrophage colony-stimulating factor, *Proc. Natl. Acad. Sci. U.S.A.*, 83, 3101, 1986.
38. **Nagata, S., Tsuchiya, M., Asano, S., Yamamoto, O., Hirata, Y., Kubota, N., Oheda, M., Nomura, H., and Yamazaki, T.,** The chromosomal gene structure and two mRNAs for human granulocyte colony-stimulating factor, *EMBO J.*, 5, 575, 1986.
39. **Kawasaki, E.S., Ladner, M.B., Wang, A.M., Van Arsdell, J., Warren, M.K., Coyne, M.Y., Schweickart, V.L., Lee, M.-T., Wilson, K.J., Boosman, A., Stanley, E.R., Ralph, P., and Mark, D.F.,** Molecular cloning of a complementary DNA encoding human macrophage-specific colony stimulating factor (CSF-1), *Science*, 230, 291, 1985.
40. **Yang, Y.-C. and Clark, S.C.,** Molecular cloning and characterization of the human gene for interleukin-3 (IL-3), in *Molecular Basis of Lymphokine Action*, Webb, D.R., Pierce, C.W., and Cohen, S., Eds., Humana Press, Totowa, NJ, 1987, 325.
41. **Pettenati, M.J., Le Beau, M.M., Lemons, R.S., Shima, E.A., Kawasaki, E.S., Larson, R.A., Sherr, C.J., Diaz, M.O., and Rowley, J.D.,** Assignment of CSF-1 to 5q33.1: evidence for clustering of genes regulating hematopoiesis and for their involvement in the deletion of the long arm of chromosome 5 in myeloid disorders, *Proc. Natl. Acad. Sci. U.S.A.*, 84, 2970, 1987.
42. **Hueber, K., Isobe, M., Croce, C.M., Golde, D.W., Kaufman, S.E., and Gasson, J.C.,** The human gene encoding GM-CSF is at 5q21-q32, the chromosome region deleted in the 5q-anomaly, *Science*, 230, 1282, 1985.
43. **Le Beau, M.M., Epstein, N.D., O'Brien, S.J., Nienhuis, A.W., Yang, Y.-C., Clark, S.C., and Rowley, J.D.,** The interleukin 3 gene is located on human chromosome 5 and is deleted in myeloid leukemias with a deletion of 5q, *Proc. Natl. Acad. Sci. U.S.A.*, 84, 5913, 1987.
44. **Le Beau, M.M., Lemons, R.S., Carrino, J.J., Pettenati, M.J., Souza, L.M., Diaz, M.O., and Rowley, J.D.,** *Leukemia*, 1, 795, 1987.
45. **Yang, Y.-C., Ciarletta, A.B., Temple, P.A., Chung, M.P., Kovacic, S., Witek-Giannotti, J.S., Leary, A.C., Kriz, R., Donahue, R.E., Wong, G.G., and Clark, S.C.,** Human IL-3 (multi-CSF): identification by expression cloning of a novel hematopoietic growth factor related to murine IL-3, *Cell*, 47, 3, 1986.
46. **Wong, G.G., Witek, J.S., Temple, P.A., Wilkens, K.M., Leary, A.C., Luxenberg, D.P., Jones, S.S., Brown, E.L., Kay, R.M., Orr, E.C., Shoemaker, C., Golde, D.W., Kaufman, R.J., Hewick, R.M., Wang, E.A., and Clark, S.C.,** Human GM-CSF: molecular cloning of the complementary DNA and purification of the natural and recombinant proteins, *Science*, 228, 810, 1985.
47. **Nagata, S., Tsuchiya, M., Asano, S., Kaziro, Y., Yamazaki, T., Yamamoto, O., Hirata, Y., Kubota, N., Oheda, M., Nomura, H., and Ono, M.,** Molecular cloning and expression of cDNA for human granulocyte colony-stimulating factor, *Nature*, 319, 415, 1986.
48. **Bazan, J.F.,** Structural design and molecular evolution of a cytokine receptor superfamily, *Proc. Natl. Acad. Sci. U.S.A.*, 87, 6934, 1990.
49. **Cosman, D., Lyman, S.D., Idzerda, R.L., Beckmann, M.P., Park, L.S., Goodwin, R.G., and March, C.J.,** A new cytokine receptor superfamily, *TIBS*, 265, 1990.
50. **Sanderson, C.J., Campbell, H.D., and Young, I.G.,** Molecular and cellular basis of eosinophil differentiation factor (IL-5) and its effects on human and mouse B-cells, *Immunol. Rev.*, 102, 29, 1988.
51. **Kaushansky, K.,** Structure-function relationships of the hematopoietic colony-stimulating factors, *Proteins Struct. Funct. Genet.*, 12, 1, 1992.
52. **Kawasaki, E.S., Ladner, M.B., Wang, A.M., Van Arsdell, J., Warren, M.K., Coyne, M.Y., Schweikart, V.L., Lee, M.-Y., Wilson, K.J., Boosman, A., Stanley, E.R., Ralph, P., and Mark, D.F.,** Molecular cloning of a complementary DNA encoding human macrophage-specific colony-stimulating factor (CSF-1), *Science*, 230, 291, 1985.
53. **Zsebo, K.M., Wypych, J., McNiece, I.K., Lu, H.S., Smith, K.A., Karkare, S.B., Sachdev, R.K., Yuschenkoff, V.N., Birkett, N.C., Williams, L.R., Satyagal, V.N., Tung, W., Bosselman, R.A., Mendiaz, E.A., and Langley, K.E.,** Identification, purification, and biological characterization of hematopoietic stem cell factor from buffalo rat liver-conditioned medium, *Cell*, 63, 195, 1990.

54. **Anderson, D.M., Lyman, S.D., Baird, A., Wignall, J.M., Eisenman, J., Rauch, C., March, C.J., Bosewell, H.S., Gimpel, S.D., Cosman, D., and Williams, D.E.**, Molecular cloning of mast cell growth factor, a hematopoietin that is active in both membrane bound and soluble forms, *Cell*, 63, 235, 1990.
55. **Huang, E., Nocka, K., Beier, D.R., Chu, T.Y., Buck, J., Lahm, H.W., Wellner, D., Leder, P., and Besmer, P.**, The hematopoietic growth factor KL is encoded by the SI locus and is the ligand of the c-kit receptor, the gene product of the W locus, *Cell*, 63, 225, 1990.
56. **Bazan, J.F.**, Genetic and structural homology of stem cell factor and macrophage colony-stimulating factor (letter), *Cell*, 65, 9, 1991.
57. **Rettenmier, C.W. and Roussel, M.F.**, Differential processing of colony-stimulating factor 1 precursors encoded by two human cDNAs, *Mol. Cell. Biol.*, 8, 5026, 1988.
58. **Larsen, A., Davis, T., Curtis, B.M., Gimpel, S., Sims, J.E., Cosman, D., Park, L., Sorensen, E., March, C.J., and Smith, C.A.**, Expression cloning of a human granulocyte colony-stimulating factor receptor: a structural mosaic of hematopoietin receptor, immunoglobulin, and fibronectin domains, *J. Exp. Med.*, 172, 1559, 1990.
59. **Hayashida, K., Kitamura, T., Gorman, D.M., Aria, K.I., Yokota, T., and Miyajima A.**, Molecular cloning of a second subunit of the receptor for human granulocyte-macrophage colony-stimulating factor (GM-CSF): reconstitution of a high-affinity GM-CSF receptor, *Proc. Natl. Acad. Sci. U.S.A.*, 87, 9655, 1990.
60. **Itoh, N., Yonehara, S., Schreurs, J., Gorman, D.M., Maruyama, K., Ishii, A., and Yahara, I.**, Cloning of an interleukin-3 receptor gene: a member of a distinct receptor gene family, *Science*, 247, 324, 1990.
61. **Park, L.S., Friend, D., Price, V., Anderson, D., Singer, J., Prickett, K.S., and Urdal, D.L.**, Heterogeneity in human interleukin-3 receptors, *J. Biol. Chem.*, 264, 5420, 1989.
62. **Lopez, A.F., Eglinton, J.M., Gillis, D., Park, L.S., Clark, S., and Vadas, M.A.**, Reciprocal inhibition of binding between interleukin 3 and granulocyte-macrophage colony-stimulating factor to human eosinophils, *Proc. Natl. Acad. Sci. U.S.A.*, 86, 7022, 1989.
63. **Lopez, A.F., Eglinton, J.M., Lyons, A.B., Tapley, P.M., To, L.B., Park, L.S., Clark, S.C., and Vadas, M.A.**, Human interleukin-3 inhibits the binding of granulocyte-macrophage colony-stimulating factor and interleukin-5 to basophils and strongly enhances their functional activity, *J. Cell. Physiol.*, 145, 69, 1990.
64. **Kitamura, T., Sato, N., Arai, K.-I., and Miyajima, A.**, Expression cloning of the human IL-3 receptor cDNA reveals a shared β subunit for the human IL-3 and GM-CSF receptors, *Cell*, 66, 1165, 1991.
65. **Sherr, C.J., Rettenmier, C.W., Sacca, R., Roussel, M.F., Look, A.T., and Stanley, E.R.**, The *c-fms* proto-oncogene product is related to the receptor for the mononuclear phagocyte growth factor, CSF-1, *Cell*, 41, 665, 1985.
66. **Williams, D.E., Eisenman, J., Baird, A., Rauch, C., Van Ness, K., March, C.J., Park, L.S., Martin, U., Mochinzuki, D.Y., Boswell, H.S., Burgess, G.S., Cosman, D., and Lyman, S.D.**, Identification of a ligand for the *c-kit* proto-oncogene, *Cell*, 63, 167, 1990.
67. Granulocyte colony-stimulating factors, in *The Medical Letter*, Vol 33, Issue 847, Abramowicz, M., Ed., 1991.
68. **Donahue, R.E., Wang, E.A., Kaufman, R.J., Foutch, L., Leary, A.C., Witek-Giannetti, J.S., Metzker, M., Hewick, R.M., Steinbrink, D.R., Shaw, G., Kamen, R., and Clark, S.C.**, Effects of N-linked carbohydrate on the in vivo properties of human GM-CSF, *Cold Spring Harbor Symp. Quant. Biol.*, 51, 685, 1986.
69. **Kaushansky, K.**, Structure-function relationship of granulocyte-macrophage colony-stimulating factor, *UCLA Symp. Mol. Cell. Biol.*, 120, 1, 1989.
70. **Bartocci, A., Mastrogiannis, D.S., Migliorati, G., Stockert, R.J., Wolkoff, A.W., and Stanley, E.R.**, Macrophages specifically regulate the concentration of their own growth factor in the circulation, *Proc. Natl. Acad. Sci. U.S.A.*, 84, 6179, 1987.
71. **Oh-eda, M., Hasegawa, M., Hattori, K., Kuboniwa, H., Kojima, T., Orita, T., Tomonou, K., Yamazaki, T., and Ochi, N.**, O-Linked sugar chain of human granulocyte colony-stimulating factor protects it against polymerization and denaturation allowing it to retain its biological activity, *J. Biol. Chem.*, 265, 11432, 1990.
72. **Kaushansky, K., O'Hara, P.J., Hart, C.E., Forstrom, J.W., and Hagen, F.S.**, Role of carbohydrate in the function of human granulocyte-macrophage colony-stimulating factor, *Biochemistry*, 26, 4861, 1987.
73. **Moonen, P., Mermod, J.J., Ernst, J.F., Hirschi, M., and DeLamarter, J.F.**, Increased biological activity of deglycosylated recombinant human granulocyte macrophage colony-stimulating factor produced by yeast or animal cells, *Proc. Natl. Acad. Sci. U.S.A.*, 84, 4428, 1987.
74. **Cosman, D., Deeley, M.C., Price, V., Klinke, R., Clevenger, T.H., Anderson, D., Sassenfeld, H., and Urdal, D.L.**, Human interleukin-3 and granulocyte-macrophage colony stimulating factor: site-specific mutangenesis and expression in yeast. 20th IABS Congress on Cytokines: Laboratory and Clinical Evaluation, London, UK, 1987, Devel. Biol. Standard., S. Karger, Basel, 1988, vol. 69, 9.
75. **Cebon, J., Nicola, N., Ward, M., Gardner, I., Dempsey, P., Layton, J., Duhrsen, U., Burgess, A.W., Nice, E., and Morstyn, G.**, Granulocyte-macrophage colony stimulating factor from human lymphocytes, *J. Biol. Chem.*, 265, 4483, 1990.
76. **Janin, J. and Clothia, C.**, The structure of protein-protein recognition sites, *J. Biol. Chem.*, 265, 16027, 1990.
77. **Clark-Lewis, I., Lopez, A., To, L.B., Vadas, M.A., Schrader, J.W., Hood, L.E., and Kent, S.B.H.**, Structure-function studies of human granulocyte-macrophage colony-stimulating factor, identification of residues required for activity, *J. Immunol.*, 141, 881, 1988.

78. **Gough, N.M., Grail, D., Gearing, D.P., and Metcalf, D.,** Mutagenesis of murine GM-CSF reveals critical residues near the N-terminus, *Eur. J. Biochem.*, 169, 353, 1987.
79. **Shanafelt, A.B. and Kastelein, R.A.,** Identification of critical regions in mouse granulocyte-macrophage colony-stimulating factor by scanning deletion analysis, *Proc. Natl. Acad. Sci. U.S.A.*, 86, 4872, 1989.
80. **Altmann, S.W., Johnson, G.D., and Prystowsky, M.B.,** Single proline substitutions in predicted alpha helices of murine granulocyte-macrophage colony-stimulating factor result in a loss in bioactivity and altered glycosylation, *J. Biol. Chem.*, 266, 5333, 1991.
81. **Schrimsher, J.L., Rose, K., Simona M.G., and Wingfield, P.,** Characterization of human and mouse granulocyte-macrophage colony-stimulating factors derived from Escherichia coli, *Biochem. J.*, 247, 195, 1987.
82. **Wingfield, P., Graber, P., Moonen, P., Craig, S., and Pain, R.H.,** The conformation and stability of recombinant granulocyte-macrophage colony stimulating factors, *Eur. J. Biochem.*, 173, 65, 1988.
83. **Kaushansky, K., Shoemaker, S.G., Alfaro, S., and Brown, C.,** The hematopoietic activity of granulocyte-macrophage colony-stimulating factor is dependent upon two distinct regions of the molecule: a functional analysis based upon the activities of hybrid growth factors, *Proc. Natl. Acad. Sci. U.S.A.*, 86, 1213, 1989.
84. **Kanakura, T., Cannsitra, S.A., Brown, C.B., Nakamura, M., Seelig, G.F., Prosise, W.W., Hakins, J.C., Kaushansky, K., and Griffen, J.D.,** Identification of functionally distinct domains of human granulocyte-macrophage colony-stimulating factor using monoclonal antibodies, *Blood*, 77, 1033, 1991.
85. **Brown, C.B., Hart, C.E., Curtis, D.M., Baily, M.C., and Kaushansky, K.,** Two neutralizing monoclonal antibodies against human granulocyte-macrophage colony-stimulating factor recognize the receptor binding domain of the molecule, *J. Immunol.*, 144, 2184, 1990.
86. **Seelig, G.F., Prosise, W.W., Scheffler, J.E., Nagabhushan, T.L., and Trotta, P.P.,** Evidence for a direct involvement of the carboxyl terminus of human granulocyte-macrophage colony-stimulating factor in receptor binding, *J. Cell. Biochem. Suppl.*, 14c, 246, 1990.
87. **Kaushansky, K., Brown, C.B., and O'Hara, P.J.,** Molecular modeling of human granulocyte-macrophage colony-stimulating factor, *Int. J. Cell Cloning*, 8 (Suppl. 1), 26, 1990.
88. **Abdel-Meguid, S.S., Shieh, H.-S., Smith, W.W., Dayringer, H.E., Violand, B.N., and Bentle, L.A.,** Three-dimensional structure of a genetically engineered variant of porcine growth hormone, *Proc. Natl. Acad. U.S.A.*, 84, 6434, 1987.
89. **Brandhuber, B.J., Boone, T., Kenney, W.C., and McKay, D.B.,** Three-dimensional structure of interleukin-2, *Science*, 238, 1707, 1987.
90. **La Londe, J.M., Hanna, L.S., Rattoballi, R., Berman, H.M., and Voet, D.,** Crystallization and preliminary X-ray studies of recombinant human granulocyte-macrophage colony stimulating factor, *J. Mol. Biol.*, 205, 783, 1989.
91. **Reichert, P., Cook, W.J., Ealick, S.E., Hammond, G.S., Le, H.V., Nagabhushan, T.L., Trotta, P.P., and Bugg, C.E.,** Crystallization and preliminary X-ray investigation of recombinant human granulocyte-macrophage colony-stimulating factor, *J. Biol. Chem.*, 265, 452, 1990.
92. **Clark-Lewis, I., Aebersold, R., Ziltener, H., Schrader, J.W., Hood, L.E., and Kent, S.B.H.,** Automated chemical synthesis of a protein growth factor for hemopoietic cells, interleukin-3, *Science*, 231, 134, 1986.
93. **Kaushansky, K., Shoemaker, S.G., and Broudy, V.C.,** Structure-function relationships of IL-3, *J. Clin. Invest.*, 90, 1879, 1992.
94. **Hruby, V.J., Al-Obeidi, F., and Kazmierski, W.,** Emerging approaches in the molecular design of receptor-selective peptide ligands: conformational, topographical and dynamic considerations. A Review Article, *J. Biochem.*, 268, 249, 1990.
95. **Abrams, J.S. and Pearce, M.K.,** Development of rat anti-mouse interleukin 3 monoclonal antibodies which neutralize bioactivity in vitro, *J. Immunol.*, 140, 131, 1988.
96. **Lokker, N.A., Strittmatter, U., Steiner, C., Fagg, B., Graff, P., Kocher, H.P., and Zenke, G.,** Mapping the epitopes of neutralizing anti-human IL-3 monoclonal antibodies, *J. Immunol.*, 146, 893, 1991.
97. **Conlon, P.J., Luk, K.H., Park, L.S., March, C.J., Hopp, T.P., and Urdal, D.L.,** Generation of anti-peptide monoclonal antibodies which recognize mature CSF-*2α*(IL3) protein, *J. Immunol.*, 135, 328, 1985.
98. **Ziltener, H., Clark-Lewis, I., de St. Groth, B., Hood, L., Kent, S., and Schrader, J.,** Antipeptide antibodies define the NH_2-terminal structure of the panspecific hemopoietin interleukin 3, *J. Immunol.*, 138, 1105, 1987.
99. **Ziltener, H., Clark-Lewis, I., de St. Groth, B., Orban, P., Hood, L., Kent, S., and Schrader, J.,** Monoclonal antipeptide antibodies recognize IL-3 and neutralize its bioactivity *in vivo*, *J. Immunol.*, 140, 1182, 1988.
100. **Lu, H.S., Boone, T.C., Souza, L.M., and Lai, P.H.,** Disulfide and secondary structures of recombinant human granulocyte colony stimulating factor, *Arch. Biochem. Biophys.*, 68, 81, 1989.
101. **Kuga, T., Komatsu, Y., Yamasaki, M., Sekine, S., Miyaji, H., Nishi, T., Sato, M., Yokoo, Y., Asano, M., Okabe, M., Morimoto, M., and Itoh, S.,** Mutagenesis of human granulocyte colony stimulating factor, *Biochem. Biophys. Res. Commun.*, 159, 103, 1989.
102. **Parry, D.A.D., Minasian, E., and Leach, S.J.,** Conformational homologies among the cytokines: interleukins and colony-stimulating factors, *Mol. Recognition*, 1, 107, 1988.

103. **Yasukawa, K., Hirano, T., Watanabe, Y., Muratani, K., Matsuda, T., Nakai, S., and Kishimoto, T.,** Structure and expression of human B cell stimulatory factor-2 (BSF-2/IL-6) gene, *EMBO J.*, 6, 2939, 1987.
104. **Cerretti, D.P., Wignall, J., Anderson, D., Tushinski, R.J., Gallis, B.M., Stya, M., Gillis, S., Urdal, D.L., and Cosman, D.,** Human macrophage-colony stimulating factor: alternative RNA and protein processing from a single gene, *Mol. Immunol.*, 25, 761, 1988.
105. **Manos, M.M.,** Notes: Expression and processing of recombinant human macrophage colony-stimulating factor in mouse cells, *Mol. Cell. Biol.*, 8, 5035, 1988.
106. **Blohm, D., Bollschweiler, C., and Hillen, H.,** Pharmaceutical proteins, *Angew. Chem. Int. Ed. Engl.*, 27, 207, 1988.
107. **Groopman, J.E., Mitsuyasu, R.T., DeLeo, M.J., Oette, D.H., and Golde, D.W.,** Effect of recombinant human granulocyte-macrophage colony-stimulating factor on myelopoiesis in the acquired immunodeficiency syndrome, *N. Engl. J. Med.*, 317, 593, 1987.
108. **Aglietta, M., Piacibello, W., Sanavio, F., Stacchini, A., Apra, F., Schena, M., Mossetti, C., Carnino, F., Caligaris-Cappio, C., and Gabosto, F.,** Kinetics of human hemopoietic cells after *in vivo* administration of granulocyte-macrophage colony-stimulating factor, *J. Clin. Invest.*, 83, 551, 1989.
109. **Lord, B.I., Bronchud, M.H., Ownens, S., Chang, J., Howell, A., Souza, L., and Dexter, T.M.,** The kinetics of human granulopoiesis following treatment with granulocyte colony-stimulating factor *in vivo*, *Proc. Natl. Acad. Sci. U.S.A.*, 86, 9499, 1989.
110. **Groopman, J.E., Molina, J.M., and Scadden, D.T.,** Medical progress: hematopoietic growth factors, *N. Engl. J. Med.*, 321, 1449, 1989.
111. **Koyanagi, Y., O'Brien, W.A., Zhao, J.Q., Golde, D.W., Gasson, J.C., and Chen, I.S.Y.,** Cytokines alter production of HIV-1 from primary mononuclear phagocytes, *Science*, 241, 1673, 1988.
112. **Hammer, S.M. and Gillis, J.M.,** Synergistic activity of granulocyte-macrophage colony-stimulating factor and 3′-azido-3′dideoxythymidine against human immunodeficiency virus in vitro, *Antimicrob. Agents Chemother.*, 31, 1046, 1987.
113. **Pluda, J.M., Yarchoan, R., Smith, P.D., McAtee, N., Shay, L.E., Oette, D., Maha, M., Wahl, S.M., Myers, C.E., and Broder, S.,** Subcutaneous recombinant granulocyte-macrophage colony-stimulating factor used as a single agent and in an alternating regimen with azidothymidine in leukopenic patients with severe human immunodeficiency virus infection, *Blood*, 76, 463, 1990.
114. **Miles, S.A., Mitsuyasu, R.T., Moreno, J., Baldwin, G., Alton, N.K., Souza, L., and Glaspy, J.A.,** Combined therapy with recombinant granulocyte colony-stimulating factor and erythropoietin decreases hematologic toxicity from Zidovudine, *Blood*, 77, 2109, 1991.
115. **Nemunaitis, J., Singer, J.W., and Buckner, C.D.,** Use of recombinant human granulocyte-macrophage colony-stimulating factors in autologous marrow transplantation for lymphoid malignancies, *Blood*, 72, 834, 1988.
116. **Brandt, S.J., Peters, W.P., Atwater, S.K., Kurtzberg, J., Borowitz, M.J., Jones, R.B., Shpall, E.J., Bast, R., Gilbert, C.J., and Oette, D.H.,** Effect of recombinant human granulocyte-macrophage colony-stimulating factor on hematopoietic reconstitution after high-dose chemotherapy and autologous bone marrow transplantation, *N. Engl. J. Med.*, 318, 869, 1988.
117. **Taylor, K.McD., Jagannath, S., Spitzer, G., Spinolo, J.A., Tucker, S.L., Fogel, B., Cabanillas, F.F., Hagemeister, F.B., and Souza, L.M.,** Recombinant human granulocyte colony-stimulating factor hastens granulocyte recovery after high-dose chemotherapy and autologous bone marrow transplantation in Hodgkin's disease, *J. Clin. Oncol.*, 7, 1791, 1989.
118. **Brandwein, J.M., Nayar, R., Baker, M.A., Sutton, D.M.C., Scott, J.G., Sutcliffe, S.B., and Keating, A.,** GM-CSF therapy for delayed engraftment after autologous bone marrow transplantation, *Exp. Hematol.*, 19, 191, 1991.
119. **Nemunaitis, J., Singer, J.W., Buckner, C.D., Durnam, D., Epstein, C., Hill, R., Storb, R., Thomas, E.D., and Appelbaum, F.R.,** Use of recombinant human granulocyte-macrophage colony-stimulating factor in graft failure after bone marrow transplantation, *Blood*, 76, 245, 1990.
120. **Park, L.S., Waldron, P.E., Friend, D., Sassenfeld, H.M., Price, V., Anderson, D., Cosman, D., Andrews, R.G., Bernstein, I.D., and Urdal, D.L.,** Interleukin-3, GM-CSF, and G-CSF receptor expression on cell lines and primary leukemia cells: receptor heterogeneity and relationship to growth factor responsiveness, *Blood*, 74, 56, 1989.
121. **Griffin, J.D. and Young, D.C.,** The role of colony stimulating factors in leukaemogenesis, *Clin. Hematol.*, 15, 995, 1986.
122. **Demetri, G.D., and Griffin, J.D.,** Hemopoietins and leukemia, *Hematol. Oncol. Clin. North Am.*, 3, 535, 1989.
123. **Ohno, R., Tomonaga, M., Kobayashi, T., Kanamaru, A., Shirakawa, S., Masaoka, T., and Omine, M.,** Effect of granulocyte colony-stimulating factor after intensive induction therapy in relapsed or refractory acute leukemia, *N. Engl. J. Med.*, 323, 871, 1990.
124. **Estey, E.H., Dixon, D., Kantarjian, H.M., Keating, M.J., McCredie, K., and Bodey, G.P.,** Treatment of poor-prognosis, newly diagnosed acute myeloid leukemia with ara-C and recombinant human granulocyte-macrophage colony-stimulating factor, *Blood*, 75, 1766, 1990.

125. **Delwel, R., van Buitenen, C., Salem, M., Bot, F., Gillis, S., Kaushansky, K., Altrock, B., and Lowenberg, B.**, Interleukin 1 stimulates proliferation of acute myeloblastic leukemia cells by induction of granulocyte-macrophage colony-stimulating factor (GM-CSF) release, *Blood*, 74, 586, 1989.
126. **Vadhan-Raj, S., Keating, M., LeMaistre, A., Hittelman, W.N., McCredie, K., and Trujillo, J.M.**, Effects of recombinant human granulocyte-macrophage colony-stimulating factor in patients with myelodysplastic syndromes, *N. Engl. J. Med.*, 317, 1545, 1987.
127. **Ganser, A., Volkers, B., Greher, J., Ottmann, O.G., Becher, W.R., Bergmann, L., Schulz, G., and Hoelzer, D.**, Recombinant human granulocyte-macrophage colony-stimulating factor in patients with myelodysplastic syndromes — A phase I/II trial, *Blood*, 73, 31, 1989.
128. **Ganser, A., Seipelt, G., Lindemann, A., Ottman, O.G., Falk, S., Eder, M., and Herrmann, F.**, Effects of recombinant human interleukin-3 in patients with myelodysplastic syndromes, *Blood*, 76, 455, 1990.
129. **Nagler, A., Binet, C., Mackichan, M.L., Negrin, R., Bangs, C., Donlon, T., and Greenberg, P.**, Impact of marrow cytogenetics and morphology on in vitro hematopoiesis in the myelodysplastic syndromes: comparison between recombinant human granulocyte colony-stimulating factor (CSF) and granulocyte-monocyte CSF, *Blood*, 76, 1299, 1990.
130. **Negrin, R.S., Haeuber, D.H., Nagler, A., Kobayashe, Y., Sklar, J., Donlon, T., Vincent, M., and Greenberg, P.L.**, Maintenance treatment of patients with myelodysplastic syndromes using recombinant human granulocyte colony-stimulating factor, *Blood*, 76, 36, 1990.
131. **Gabrilove, J.L., Jakubowski, A., Scher, H., Sternberg, C., Wong, G., Grous, J., and Yagoda, A.**, Effect of granulocyte colony-stimulating factor on neutropenia and associated morbidity due to chemotherapy for transitional-cell carcinoma of the urothelium, *N. Engl. J. Med.*, 318, 141, 1988.
132. **Morstyn, G., Souza, L.M., Keech, J., Seridan, W., Campbell, L., Alton, N.K., Green, M., and Metcalf, D.**, Effect of granulocyte colony-stimulating factor on neutropenia induced by cytotoxic chemotherapy, *Lancet*, 667, 671, 1988.
133. **Crawford, J., Ozer, H., Stoller, R., Johnson, D., Lyman, G., Tabbara, I., Kris, M., Grous, J., and Picozzi, V.**, Reduction by granulocyte colony-stimulating factor of fever and neutropenia induced by chemotherapy in patients with small-cell lung cancer, *N. Engl. J. Med.*, 325, 164, 1991.
134. **Antman, K.S., Griffin, J.D., Ellias, A., Socinski, M.A., Ryan, L., Cannistra, S.A., Oette, D., and Whitley, M.**, Effect of recombinant human granulocyte-macrophage colony-stimulating factor on chemotherapy-induced myelosuppression, *N. Engl. J. Med.*, 319, 593, 1988.
135. **Gillio, A.P., Gasparetto, C., Laver, J., Abboud, M., Bonilla, M.A., Garnick, M.B., and O'Reilly, R.J.**, Effects of interleukin-3 on hematopoietic recovery after 5-fluorouracil or cyclophosphamide treatment of cynomolgus primates, *J. Clin. Invest.*, 85, 1560, 1990.
136. **Vadhan-Raj, S., Buescher, S., Broxmeyer, H.E., LeMaistre, A., and Lepe-Zuniga, J.L.**, Stimulation of myelopoiesis in patients with aplastic anemia by recombinant human granulocyte-macrophage colony-stimulating factor, *N. Engl. J. Med.*, 319, 1628, 1988.
137. **Champlin, R.E., Nimer, S.D., Ireland, P., Oette, D.H., and Golde, W.D.**, Treatment of refractory aplastic anemia with recombinant human granulocyte-macrophage colony stimulating factor, *Blood*, 73, 694, 1989.
138. **Kojima, S., Fukuda, M., Miyajima, Y., Matsuyama, T., and Horibe, K.**, Treatment of aplastic anemia in children with recombinant human granulocyte colony-stimulating factor, *Blood*, 77, 937, 1991.
139. **Ganser, A., Lindemann, A., Seipelt, G., Ottmann, O.G., Hermann, F., and Eder, M.**, Effects of recombinant human interleukin-3 in patients with normal hematopoiesis and in patients with bone marrow failure, *Blood*, 76, 666, 1990.
140. **Donahue, R.E., Seehra, J., Metzger, M., Lefebvre, D., Rock, B., Carbone, S., Nathan, D.G., and Garnick, M.**, Human IL-3 and GM-CSF act synergistically in stimulating hematopoiesis in primates, *Science*, 241, 1820, 1988.
141. **Ulich, T.R., del Castillo, J., McNiece, I.K., Yin, S., Irwin, B., Busser, K., and Guo, K.**, Acute and subacute hematologic effects of multi-colony stimulating factor in combination with granulocyte colony-stimulating factor *in vivo*, *Blood*, 75 48, 1990.
142. **Bonilla, M.A., Gillio, A.P., Ruggeiro, M., Kernan, N., and Brochstein, J.A.**, Effects of recombinant human granulocyte colony-stimulating factor on neutropenia in patients with congenital agranulocytosis, *N. Engl. J. Med.*, 320, 1574, 1989.
143. **Welte, K., Zeidler, C., Reiter, A., Muller, W., Odenwald, E., Souza, L., and Riehm, H.**, Differential effects of granulocyte-macrophage colony-stimulating factor and granulocyte colony-stimulating factor in children with severe congenital neutropenia, *Blood*, 75, 1056, 1990.
144. **Hammond, W., Price, T., Souza, L.M., and Dale, D.C.**, Treatment of cyclic neutropenia with granulocyte colony-stimulating factor, *N. Engl. J. Med.*, 320, 1306, 1989.
145. **Jakubowski, A.A., Souza, L., Kelly, F., Fain, K., Budman, D., Clarkson, B., Bonill, M.A., Moore, M.A.S., and Gabrilove, J.**, Effects of human granulocyte colony-stimulating factor in a patient with idiopathic neutropenia, *N. Engl. J. Med.*, 320, 38, 1989.

146. **Geissler, K., Valent, P., Mayer, P., Liehl, E., Hinterberger, W., Lechner, K., and Bettelheim, P.,** Recombinant human interleukin-3 expands the pool of circulating hematopoietic progenitor cells in primates — synergism with recombinant human granulocyte/macrophage colony-stimulating factor, *Blood*, 75, 2305, 1990.
147. **Molineau, G., Pojda, Z., Hampson, I.N., Lord, B.I., and Dexter, T.M.,** Transplantation potential of peripheral blood stem cells induced by granulocyte colony-stimulating factor, *Blood*, 76, 2153, 1990.
148. **Broxmeyer, H.E., Cooper, S., Lu, L., Miller, M.E., Langefeld, C.D., and Ralph, P.,** Enhanced stimulation of human bone marrow macrophage colony formation in vitro by recombinant human macrophage colony-stimulating factor in agaros medium and at low oxygen tension, *Blood*, 76, 323, 1990.
149. **Lieschke, G.J., Maher, D., O'Connor, M., Green, M., Sheridan, W., Rallings, M., Bonnem, E., Burgess, A.W., McGrath, K., Fox, R.M., and Morstyn, G.,** Phase I study of intravenously administered bacterially synthesized granulocyte-macrophage colony-stimulating factor and comparison with subcutaneous administration, *Cancer Res.*, 50, 606, 1990.
150. **Klausmann, M., Pfluger, K.H., Krumwieh, D., Seiller, F.R., and Havemann, K.,** Modulation of functions of granulocytes by recombinant human GM-CSF and possible complications of GM-CSF therapy, *Leukemia*, 2 (Suppl.), 63S, 1988.
151. **Cannistra, S.A., Rambaldi, A., Spriggs, D.R., Hermann, F., Kufe, D., and Griffin, J.D.,** Human granulocyte-macrophage colony-stimulating factor induces expression of the tumor necrosis factor gene by the U937 cell line and by normal human monocytes, *J. Clin. Invest.*, 79, 1720, 1987.
152. **Lindemann, A., Riedel, D., Oster, W., Meuer, S.C., Blohm, D., Mertelsmann, R.H., and Herrmann, F.,** Granulocyte/macrophage colony-stimulating factor induces interleukin 1 production by human polymorphonuclear neutrophils, *J. Immunol.*, 140, 837, 1988.
153. **Evans, R., Duffy, T.M., Blake, S.S., and Lin, H.S.,** Regulation of systemic macrophage *IL-1* gene transcription: the involvement of tumor-derived macrophage growth factor, CSF-1, *J. Leuk. Biol.*, 46, 428, 1989.
154. **Gribben, J.G., Devereux, S., Thomas, N.S.B., Keim, M., Jones, H.M., Goldstone, A.H., and Linch, D.C.,** Development of antibodies to unprotected glycosylation sites on recombinant human GM-CSF, *Lancet*, 335, 434, 1990.
155. **Abuchowski, A., McCoy, J.R., Palczuk, N.C., Van, E.T., and Davis, F.F.,** Effect of covalent attachment of polyethylene glycol on immunogenic and circulating life of bovine liver catalase, *J. Biol. Chem.*, 252, 3582, 1977.
156. **Goddard, P.,** Therapeutic proteins — a pharmaceutical perspective, *Adv. Drug Deliv. Rev.*, 6, 103, 1991.
157. **Delgado, C., Malik, F., Knusli, C., Fisher, D., and Francis, G.E.,** New preparative and analytical procedures for polyethylene glycol (PEG) modified cytokines, *Exp. Hematol.*, 18, 617, 1990.
158. **Knusli, C., Delgado, C., Malik, F., Irvine, S.A., Smith, O.P., Fisher, D., and Francis, G.E.,** Dissociation of two biological activities of granulocyte-macrophage colony stimulating factor (GM-CSF) by polyethylene glycol (PEG), *Exp. Hematol*, 18, 608, 1990.
159. **Brakenhoff, J.P.J., Hart, M., and Aarden, L.A.,** Analysis of human IL-6 mutants expressed in *Escherichia coli* biologic activities are not affected by deletion of amino acids 1-18, *J. Immunol.*, 143, 1175, 1989.
160. **Ida, N., Sakurai, S., Hosaka, T., Hosoi, K., Kunitomo, T., Shimazu, T., Maruyama, T., Matsuura, Y., and Kohase, M.,** Establishment of strongly neutralizing monoclonal antibody to human interleukin-6 and its epitope analysis, *Biochem. Biophys. Res. Commun.*, 165, 728, 1989.
161. **Kruttgen, A., Rose-John, S., Moller, C., Wroblowski, B., Wollmer, A., Mullberg, J., Hirano, T., Kishimoto, T., and Heinrich, P.C.,** Structure-function analysis of human interleukin-6, evidence for the involvement of the carboxy-terminus in function, *FEBS Lett.*, 262, 323, 1990.
162. **Williams, D.E., Broxmeyer, H.E., Curtis, B.M., Dunn, J., Price, V., Craig, V., March, C.J., Cosman, D., and Park, L.S.,** Enhanced biological activity of a human GM-CSF/IL-3 fusion protein, *Exp. Hematol.*, 18, 615, 1990.
163. **Chorev, M., Goldman, M.E., McKee, R.L., Roubini, E., Levy, J.J., Gay, T., Reagan, J.E., Fisher, J.E., Caporale, L.H., Golub, E.E., Caulfield, M.P., Nutt, R.F., and Rosenblatt, M.,** Modifications of position 12 in parathyroid hormone and parathyroid hormone related protein: toward the design of highly potent antagonists, *Biochemistry*, 29, 1580, 1990.
164. **Saragovi, H.U., Fitzpatrick, D., Raktabutr, A., Nakanishi, H., Kahn, M., and Greene, M.I.,** Design and synthesis of a mimetic from an antibody complementarity-determining region, *Science*, 253, 792, 1991.
165. **Fischer, G. and Schmid, F.X.,** The mechanism of protein folding. Implications of in vitro refolding models for *de novo* protein folding and translocation in the cell, *Biochemistry*, 29, 2205, 1990.
166. **Altmann, K.H. and Mutter, M.,** A general strategy for the *de novo* design of proteins — template assembled synthetic proteins, *Int. J. Biochem.*, 22, 947, 1990.
167. **Grau, G., Kindler, V., Piguet, P.-F., Lambert, P.-H., and Vassalli, P.,** Prevention of experimental cerebral malaria by anticytokine antibodies, *J. Exp. Med.*, 168, 1499, 1988.
168. **Yamayoshi, M., Ohue, M., Kawashima, H., Kotani, H., Iida, M., Kawata, S., and Yamada, M.,** A human IL-1*a* derivative which lacks prostaglandin E_2 inducing activity and inhibits the activity of IL-1 through receptor competition, *Lymphokine Res.*, 9, 405, 1990.

169. **Unson, C.G., MacDonald, D., Ray, K., Durrah, T.L., and Merrifield, R.B.,** Position 9 replacement analogs of glucagon uncouple biological activity and receptor binding, *J. Biol. Chem.*, 266, 2763, 1991.
170. **Ladgraf, B.E., Williams, D.P., Murphy, J.R., Smith, K.A., and Ciardelli, T.L.,** Conformational perturbation of interleukin-2: a strategy for the design of cytokine analogs, *Proteins Struct. Funct. Genet.*, 9, 207, 1991.
171. **Meropol, N.J., Altmann, S.W., Shanafelt, A.B., Kastelein, R.A., Johnson, G.D., and Prystowsky, M.B.,** Requirement of hydrophilic amino-terminal residues for granulocyte-macrophage colony-stimulating factor bioactivity and receptor binding, *J. Biol. Chem.*, 267, 14266, 1992.
172. **Shanafelt, A.B., Miyajima, A., Kitamura, T., and Kastelein, R.A.,** The amino-terminal helix of GM-CSF and IL-5 governs high affinity binding to their receptors, *EMBO J.*, 10, 4105, 1991.
173. **Shanafelt, A.B. and Kastelein, R.A.,** High affinity ligand binding is not essential for granulocyte-macrophage colony-stimulating factor receptor activation, *J. Biol. Chem.*, 267, 25466, 1992.
174. **Lopez, A.F., Shannon, M.F., Hercus, T., Nicola, N.A., Cambareri, B., Dottore, M., Layton, M.J., Eglinton, L., and Vadas, M.A.,** Residue 21 of human granulocyte-macrophage colony-stimulating factor is critical for biological activity and for high but not low affinity binding, *EMBO J.*, 11, 909, 1992.
175. **Meropol, N.J., Kreider, B.L., Lee, V.M., Kaushansky, K., and Prystowsky, M.B.,** A neutralizing monoclonal antibody binds to an epitope near the amino terminus of murine granulocyte-macrophage colony-stimulating factor, *Hybridoma*, 10, 433, 1991.
176. **Diederichs, K., Jacques, S., Boone, T., and Karplus, P.A.,** Low-resolution structure of recombinant human granulocyte-macrophage colony stimulating factor, *J. Mol. Biol.*, 221, 55, 1991.
177. **Diederichs, K., Boone, T., and Karplus, P.A.,** Novel fold and putative receptor binding site of granulocyte-macrophage colony-stimulating factor, *Science*, 254, 1779, 1991.
178. **Shaw, G. and colleagues,** personal communication.
179. **Martin, F.,** personal communication.
180. **Clark, S.,** personal communication.

Chapter 4

MONOCLONAL ANTIBODIES: TECHNICAL DEVELOPMENT AND THERAPEUTIC INDICATIONS

Margaret R. Dalesandro, Martin E. Sanders, and John A. Lipani

CONTENTS

I. INTRODUCTION

The year 1975 witnessed the quiet birth of a new technology in the field of immunology. A graduate student named Georges Kohler[1] working in the London laboratories of Cesar Milstein created a myeloma cell hybridoma, an immortal cell line producing antibody. This cell line was capable of growing in tissue culture and secreting unlimited quantities of antibody of single specificity. The development of the hybridoma, originally intended to study the genetics of antibody formation, revolutionized the field and allowed the production of an unlimited supply of monoclonal antibody.[2] Hybridomas produced from antigen-stimulated B cells secrete a single species of antibody (monoclonal antibody) which can be selected for the desired antigen specificity. A vast number of monoclonal antibodies (mAbs) have been made

0-8493-9422-8/94/$0.00+$.50

which specifically bind proteins, carbohydrates, nucleic acids, and haptens. Some antibodies bind to transition-state analogs of enzymatic reactions and act as enzymelike catalysts.[3] Such catalytic antibodies increase by several hundred to 200,000-fold the reaction rates of ester and carbonate hydrolysis,[4,5] as well as hydrolysis of alkyl esters[6] and amide bonds.[7] The important potential of this technology in both diagnostics and in therapy has been exploited over the subsequent 19 years. Today's widespread experimental use of monoclonals gives testimony to this fact. By 1985, over 500 million dollars had been spent on diagnostic kits using monoclonal antibodies. In recent years many more millions have been spent on the development of monoclonal antibodies as therapies for human disease.

This chapter will deal with an overview of the monoclonal antibody, a description of the laboratory techniques used in their development and close with a discussion of their uses in disease intervention.

Tapping the vast human repertoire for the appropriate therapeutic specificity sounds like the ideal way to produce antibodies, but the reality is that most monoclonal antibodies available today are of rodent origin.[8] This is due both to the ethical problems involved in immunizing humans to generate high-affinity antibodies produced by "memory" B cells[9] and also to the instability of many human hybridomas in culture.[10]

The usefulness of monoclonal antibodies is based on their specificity and homogeneity. They could not be developed as therapeutic entities, however, until a method was found for extending the *in vitro* viability of antibody-producing B cells. Kohler and Milstein[1] solved this problem by successfully fusing antibody-secreting cells from immunized mice with myeloma cells. The hybridoma resulting from this fusion is an immortal somatic cell hybrid which continuously secretes monoclonal antibody. The myeloma cells provide the genes which allow continued cell division in culture and the antibody-producing cell provides the functionally rearranged immunoglobulin genes.[11]

Myelomas can be induced in certain strains of mice by injecting mineral oil into the peritoneum. The first examples of these cells were isolated from BALB/c mice by Potter.[12] Myeloma cells have the ability to make antibodies themselves. To avoid the generation of hybridomas that produce two antibodies, myelomas that lack the genetic machinery to make antibodies are chosen as fusion partners in the making of hybridomas.[13] Theoretically, any fusogen can be used to effect the fusion between myeloma and antibody-secreting cells. However, soon after its introduction, the use of polyethylene glycol (PEG) became the standard method for hybridoma production.[14] PEG fuses the plasma membranes of adjacent myeloma and antibody-secreting cells forming a heterokaryon. During subsequent mitotic divisions, the chromosomes from the discrete nuclei resegregate into daughter cells. The newly formed hybridomas are then cloned and the supernatant produced by growing cells is screened for antibody titer.

In very efficient hybridoma fusions, 1% of the starting cells are fused and 1 in 10^5 form viable hybrids. This leaves a large number of unfused cells in the culture. Unfused antibody-secreting cells pose no problem since they die in culture, but unfused myeloma cells are adapted to tissue culture and must be killed to avoid confusing them with antibody-producing hybridomas. Usually the myeloma partner has an enzyme mutation which blocks use of the salvage pathway of purine nucleotide biosynthesis. A common example of this is a mutated hypoxanthine-guanine phosphoribosyl transferase gene (HPRT). The addition of any compound that blocks the *de novo* synthesis of nucleotide, thereby forcing use of the salvage pathway, will be lethal to unfused myeloma cells with this mutation. Hybrids between myelomas with a nonfunctional HPRT and antibody-secreting cells with a functional HPRT will be able to grow.[15]

The frequency of obtaining viable hybridomas is increased when both fusion partners are of the same species. Most of the myelomas available are of mouse origin and immunized mice are the most common source of antibody-secreting cells. Finding a suitable fusion partner for human cells proved difficult so the first mAbs used therapeutically were murine.

The therapeutic use of rodent mAbs, however, presents several problems. As foreign immunoglobulins, the rodent antibodies may elicit anti-immunoglobulin responses which interfere with therapy or may result in anaphylactic or immune complex hypersensitivity.[16] Additionally, the half-life of rodent antibodies is considerably shorter in humans than that of human antibodies and rodent antibodies interact less efficiently with human effector cells than do human antibodies.

Antibodies are composed of disulfide-linked heavy and light chains, each of which is comprised of a constant region that defines isotype and a variable region that confers antigen specificity. The variable region itself is composed of hypervariable loops called complementarity-determining regions (CDRs), which are held together by a beta-pleated sheet of framework residues to form an antigen-binding groove.

Chimerization of a murine antibody, wherein the constant region is made human by recombinant techniques and the entire variable region is of murine origin, results in a decreased immune response when it is administered to humans. This is expected since 90% of the human immune response to xenogeneic antibodies is directed against constant domains and 10% against the variable domain.[17] Chimerization also produces up to a sixfold increase of the *in vivo* half-life of the antibody in humans.[18] Another advantage of human antibodies, or at the very least, antibodies with a human Fc portion, is their enhanced ability to bind to Fc receptors on the surface of human effector cells such as phagocytes or natural killers and initiate phagocytosis or antibody-dependent cell-mediated cytolysis (ADCC).[17] Finally, they interact optimally with human complement components to lyse target cells. Studies with various chimeric antibodies have substantiated their ability to lyse human cells via ADCC at 100-fold lower concentrations than the parental murine antibodies from which they were developed.[19] Other researchers have shown the increased effectiveness of chimeric antibodies relative to murine antibodies in mediating complement-dependent cytolysis of human cancer cells.[20]

II. PRODUCTION OF MONOCLONAL ANTIBODIES WITH HUMAN CHARACTERISTICS

The widespread use of the monoclonal antibody as a diagnostic and therapeutic was predicated on the development of hybridoma technology. The goal of this hybridoma technology was to produce a hybrid combining only the desirable characteristics of two cells. The resulting hybrid cell would have the capacity to produce antibody indefinitely like a B lymphocyte and the ability to grow like the myeloma cell. In the Kohler and Milstein experiments, mice were immunized with sheep red blood cells. Then spleen lymphocytes were added to mouse myeloma cells in culture, in the presence of a fusing agent. The resulting hybrid cells produced antibody against sheep red cells and could reproduce in tissue culture, as their parent B cell and myeloma cell, respectively. The hybrids so produced were a mixture of cells producing a variety of antibodies. As the hybrids had the capacity to grow in tissue culture, a dilute solution of these cells was spread over the surface of a dish. The individual cells were spaced sufficiently far apart to form separate and distinct clones. All of the cells of an individual clone have the antibody-producing characteristics of a single progenitor cell. The antibody so produced was named a "monoclonal" antibody (mAb).

The technique of antigen-focused fusion has been used with mixed results to generate human hybridomas with high antigen affinity.[21,22] In one variation on this technique, immune B cells are coated with a limited amount of an antigen-biotin conjugate to encourage binding to B cells with the highest affinity antibodies bound to their surface. The B cells are then mixed with biotin-coated myeloma cells. Avidin is added to bring the B cells and myelomas together and they are then electrofused. Several other methods have been used to immortalize B cells. Calcium phosphate-precipitated DNA is commonly used to introduce genes into nonlymphoid cells but this method works poorly with myeloma lines.[23] Both DNA electroporation[24] and bacterial protoplast fusion[25] are reasonable methods for the introduction of DNA into human cells. Both have transfection frequencies between 1×10^{-4} and 1×10^{-5}.

Currently, however, the two most common ways to immortalize human B cells are by conventional PEG fusion or by initial infection using the B lymphotropic Epstein-Barr herpesvirus (EBV) followed by a PEG fusion, according to the method of Kozbor et al.[26] Compared with PEG fusion alone, EBV infection has been reported to increase the fusion frequency by several orders of magnitude. Furthermore, human B lymphocytes are subject to suppression from other cell populations in peripheral blood which prevents them from being antigen-specifically activated. This suppression is mediated by lysosome-rich natural killer cells, monocytes, and $CD8^+$ cytotoxic T cells. Elimination of suppressor cells by treating peripheral blood cells with the lysosomotropic agent leucyl-leucyl methyl ester after *in vitro* immunization and before EBV infection significantly increased the outgrowth of antigen-specific B cell clones.[27] The EBV activated cells are generally fused with a heteromyeloma (mouse × human) to insure a more stable phenotype and better antibody production than with the EBV line itself.

Although the aforementioned techniques have proven successful to a degree, the frequency of obtaining high-affinity, antigen-specific human antibodies even after labor-intensive fusion and screening procedures has been disappointing. These problems stem in part from the fact that the most accessible source of human B cells is peripheral blood, since spleen and lymph nodes must be obtained by surgery. Peripheral blood B cells are poor sources of antibody production, apparently because they are subject to suppression mechanisms which are not encountered by B cells that populate lymphoid organs.[28] In fact, *in vitro* antigen activation of B lymphocytes can be accomplished by providing the required lymphokines. In contrast, peripheral blood B cells cannot be antigen-activated *in vitro* by the addition of lymphokines alone. Activation does not occur unless T, B, and accessory cell components are reconstituted in a specific ratio, a fact which is taken as proof that cell-mediated suppression mechanisms function in the blood.[29] This is reasonable since the blood is primarily a transport organ while spleen and lymph nodes are activation sites.

A. RECONSTITUTION OF IMMUNODEFICIENT MICE

Production of human antibodies is faced with the double problem of inaccessibility of those B cells most easily activated to antibody production and also by the ethical problems encountered in immunizing humans with potentially hazardous antigens. Yet, without this immunization, the memory compartment producing high-affinity human antibody responses remains untapped. One way of circumventing both of these problems is through the use of severe combined immunodeficiency (SCID) mice reconstituted with human lymphocytes.[30,31] These mice can be repopulated with lymphocytes from a donor recently boosted for an antigen or, where that is not feasible, the cells can be removed from the donor and immunized *in vitro*. After the SCID mouse is repopulated, it is immunized to promote the selective proliferation of human lymphocytes producing antibodies specific for the immunogen.[32] Human reconstituted SCID mice (SCID-hu) are useful for the direct generation of human mAbs using the conventional hybridoma methods previously discussed, or for the isolation of mRNA from immune human B cells, which will allow cloning via polymerase chain reaction (PCR) of an entire library of heavy and/or light chain variable regions. The latter method bypasses completely the generation of hybridomas and will be discussed in detail in a subsequent section.

In recent studies, Duchosal et al.[33] populated SCID mice with blood from human donors who had been exposed to tetanus toxoid (TT) antigen at widely varying times ranging from immediately before the study to a donor who had not had contact with antigen for 20 years. This last donor had no significant serum anti-TT IgG. Likewise, nonimmunized SCID mice reconstituted with blood from this donor had no detectable serum anti-TT IgG. However, SCID mice reconstituted with the blood from this donor and immunized with TT showed high anti-TT antibody levels. In several donors who had not been boosted for 4 years prior to the study, a mouse reconstituted and then immunized with TT showed an average 55-fold increase in serum IgG anti-TT relative to both the donors and to mice reconstituted with the same donor's cells but not immunized. The reconstituted SCID anti-TT response was skewed to IgG1 as is the case in humans.[34] This technique can be employed to amplify the yield of antigen-specific human B cells.

B. TRANSGENIC MICE

A second way in which mice can produce human antibodies is to make them transgenic with human antibody genes. For example, the genes encoding for a given human mAb could be introduced into a mouse. After immunization with the appropriate antigen, the responsive murine B cells would rearrange the human immunoglobulin transgenes and produce human antibody. Bruggemann et al.[35] created a mouse that carried an unrearranged human heavy chain locus comprising variable, diversity, and joining regions linked to a human mu chain gene. A large portion of the thymus and spleen cells rearranged the human gene segments and 4% of the total B lymphocyte population synthesized human mu chains. Stable hybridomas secreting several micrograms per milliliter of antibody containing human mu chains were established from these transgenic mice. These preliminary results and the continued advances in techniques to clone large pieces of DNA make feasible in the near future the insertion of a complete human immunoglobulin gene region into a mouse germline.[36]

III. CHIMERIC ANTIBODIES

Although hybridoma technology enabled the research scientist to produce an unlimited supply of a large repertoire of antibodies, only the rat and mouse myeloma lines appear to be reliably stable in long-term tissue culture. Rodent monoclonals, however, have serious drawbacks when used as therapeutic agents, especially in diseases requiring repetitive treatments. They induce an immune response to themselves that may neutralize their effect, and lead to rapid clearance. In addition, murine monoclonals have a short serum half-life in humans. In view of the persistent difficulties in making human monoclonals by conventional fusion techniques, recombinant DNA technology has become an important mode of human antibody production.

In order to circumvent these problems, i.e., decrease immunogenicity and increase half-life, the chimeric monoclonal was engineered. In Greek mythology the Chimera was a fire-breathing monster with a lion's head, a goat's body, and the tail of a dragon. In antibody terminology chimeras are antibodies constructed of disparate parts. They can be constructed in various ways. Immunoglobulin gene segments not normally associated can be assembled within or between species. For example, murine-derived variable regions can be conjoined with constant regions of human origin. Chimeric antibodies have properties that naturally occurring antibodies lack. With the appropriate manipulations, antigen-binding specificity and affinity can be optimized; and constant-region effector functions can be increased, decreased, or eliminated altogether. Finally, functions not present in antibodies can be introduced.[37]

In 1984 Morrison et al. published a description of chimeric antibody molecules containing murine antigen-binding variable regions with human constant regions.[38,39] For example, a chimeric anti-colorectal cancer mAb was constructed by combining the gene that encodes the variable heavy chain region (V_H) of the murine anti-tumor antibody with the human constant region, and the murine variable light chain region (V_L) was joined to the human kappa light chain constant region. The genes encoding the chimeric light and heavy chains were transfected simultaneously into mouse Sp 2/0 myeloma cells. The resulting antibodies produced by the myeloma cell line had the ability to inhibit tumor growth and to lyse tumor cell targets in assays measuring ADCC and were less antigenic themselves.[40,41]

Current techniques employ PCR primers to amplify rearranged human immunoglobulin genes from hybridomas or individual antigen-reactive B cells.[42] Fragments can then be directly sequenced or cloned into expression vectors. To make mouse/human chimeric antibodies where the entire antibody-binding variable region is murine and the constant region is human, the heavy and light chain murine variable regions are cloned from a murine hybridoma by screening with J_H and J_K probes, respectively. The murine V region fragments are then cloned into separate expression vectors containing the light chain or heavy chain human constant region of the desired isotype. Heavy and light chain plasmids are then cotransfected into a nonsecreting murine myeloma such as Sp 2/0 and the antibodies produced are screened for high affinity, antigen specificity, and a human Fc portion.[38]

An alternate method of producing chimeric antibodies is through homologous recombination, which refers to the ability of cells to join together pieces of DNA that have regions of similar or identical sequence. Fell et al.[43] have demonstrated the ability of murine hybridoma cells (J558L) to mediate homologous recombination. They used this method to produce a fusion protein that is a chimeric mAb with a human IgG1 heavy chain constant region and specificity for a human tumor-associated antigen. This was accomplished by cotransfecting the J558L cells with phage DNA encoding the murine IgA heavy chain gene and a plasmid vector bearing the heavy chain constant region exons of the human IgG1 isotype. Analysis of the resulting heavy chain producing cell lines demonstrated that homologous recombination between the two molecules occurred at a frequency of 30% and the frequency of productive genomic recombinations was ~1 in 200 transfectants, with accumulation of the chimeric protein reaching >20 μg/ml in culture supernatants.

IV. HUMANIZED ANTIBODIES

To further reduce the immunogenicity of the rodent variable region, humanized monoclonal antibodies have been constructed. Jones et al.[39] produced a rat/human antibody in which only the hypervariable regions were of rat origin, i.e., only the antigen-binding site rather than the entire variable domain was from the rodent. Two years later, Reichman et al.[44] published the use of humanized CAMPATH-1, a rat monoclonal antibody capable of recognizing an antigen on human lymphocytes that could be applied to the therapy of leukemia and graft-vs.-host disease. The humanized monoclonal bound antigen, fixed complement, performed cell-mediated lysis, and was effective in complement-mediated lysis of human B cell lymphocytic leukemia cells *in vitro*.[45]

In an early clinical trial in non-Hodgkin's lymphoma, two patients studied showed tumor regression without an antibody response against the humanized molecule.[45] Larger studies will be required to determine the immunogenicity of this antibody in comparison with its chimeric form. Humanized antibodies retain foreign idiotypic and human allotypic markers that are potentially immunogenic. Response to an immunogenic allotype could require matching the allotype of the therapeutic antibody with that of the recipient. In humanized antibodies where only the antigen-binding sites are foreign, anti-immunoglobulin responses could be focused on these sites and might have an undesirable effect on antibody therapy. Alternatively, restriction of the anti-immunoglobulin response to the antigen-binding site could be advantageous in the development of anti-idiotypic vaccines.

The variable regions of the heavy and light chains of antibodies are each comprised of three hypervariable loops, the CDRs, which actually make contact with antigen. The rest of the V domain is a framework of beta-pleated sheets which supports the loops in a manner permitting them to make high-affinity contact with the antigen. Current humanization technology has resulted in the ability to graft rodent antigen-binding loops onto human framework regions which support the loops in a way that results in high-affinity functional antibody. Grafting of human CDRs onto human framework regions does not guarantee a humanized antibody with the binding affinity of the murine. Riechman et al.[44] found that their first attempt to humanize CAMPATH-1 antibody resulted in an antibody that bound with 40-fold less affinity to CAMPATH-1 antigen than did the murine antibody, suggesting an error in the packing of the reshaped antigen-binding domains in the human framework regions. Site-directed mutagenesis restored the affinity of the reshaped antibody, possibly by altering the packing between the hypervariable regions and the framework. This shows that CDR contacts with framework residues as well as antigen are critical to affinity, and indicates one major difficulty that can be encountered in the humanization process. CDRs can be cycled through a series of framework architectures until the combination resulting in the best antibody is identified. However, this is an extremely labor-intensive process.

Grafting of CDRs onto human framework regions involves the synthesis of cDNA from the mRNA extracted from the hybridoma producing the antibody of interest. Several grafting techniques have been used. In one, the rodent hypervariable regions were excised using three large mutagenic oligonucleotides for each variable domain. These were grafted onto human heavy or light chain framework regions.[44] Others accomplished CDR grafting by reconstructing the whole V region using overlapping oligonucleotide incorporating the rodent CDRs on a human framework.[39,46]

Recently, recombinant PCR techniques have been used to graft rodent CDRs onto human immunoglobulin frameworks. This process decreased the time and effort required for humanization. No nucleotide errors were found in the 1463-bp sequence of a grafted anti-digoxin antibody even after sequential rounds of PCR.[47] A humanized antibody directed against the CD18 component of human leukocyte integrins was also generated by the use of overlapping PCR fragments.[48] The expression vectors used by Daugherty et al.[48] in this work enabled them to combine various human framework regions (FRs) with identical murine CDRs to explore the effects of FR on antibody affinity. They also developed a transient expression system for recombinant humanized antibodies driven by an adenovirus major late promoter in nonlymphoid mammalian cells. The applications of these approaches allows the functional evaluation of recombinant humanized antibody just 6 weeks after the cDNA cloning of the murine mAb.

V. SINGLE-CHAIN ANTIGEN-BINDING PROTEINS

A new development in antibody technology is the single-chain antigen-binding protein. These are novel recombinant polypeptides, composed of an antibody variable light chain amino acid sequence linked to a variable heavy chain sequence.[49] The linkage connects the carboxyl-terminus of the light chain to the amino-terminus of the heavy chain by means of a designed peptide. These proteins have the same specificities and affinities as the parent monoclonal antibodies whose V_L and V_H sequences were used to construct the recombinant genes that were expressed.

These antigen-binding proteins are expected to have advantages in clinical application because of their small size. They should be cleared faster than their larger parent antibodies and parent Fab fragments. Because they lack the Fc portion of an antibody, which is recognized by cell receptors, they should have a lower background in imaging applications. They should also be less immunogenic. Clinical applications are anticipated in the areas of cardiovascular and oncologic imaging and therapeutics.[50-52]

A. COMBINATORIAL PHAGE EXPRESSION LIBRARIES

In classical antibody engineering, antigen-specific hybridomas provide the rearranged V_H and V_L genes for cloning. The use of hybridomas, especially for human antibodies, is problematic. This has been bypassed by the development of PCR techniques using universal primers to rescue V region genes from terminally differentiated B lymphocytes which are rich in V region mRNA, but are unable to fuse. By building restriction sites into these primers, the amplified DNA can be cloned directly for expression in mammalian cells,[53] bacteria,[51] or even directly on the surface of phage.[54] In this process, the V_H and V_L genes expressed through λ phage libraries combine randomly, and the chance of recovering the original pairs of V_H and V_L that produced high-affinity antibodies is small. The likelihood of recovery of V region gene pairs encoding for Fab fragments with high antigen affinity is increased by making combinatorial libraries from antigen-selected B cells rather than from heterogeneous cell populations. Critical to the usefulness of the combinatorial approach, however, are the size of the library and the power of the screening methods. The larger the library, the greater the opportunity to recover original or even novel high-affinity V region gene pairs.

Motivated by their desire to identify catalytic antibodies, Huse et al.[55] searched for a way to generate mAbs in vast numbers to provide for an adequate survey of the possible antibody V region gene repertoire. They devised a method for expressing the antibody repertoire in *Escherichia coli* by creating a large combinatorial library in λ phage. In fact a plasmid expression library of V_H fragments with specificity for keyhole limpet hemocyanin (KLH) and lysozyme was constructed in *E. coli*.[48,53] X-ray crystallography, however, showed considerable contact between the V_L domain and the antigen, making it unlikely that V_H fragments would have the affinity of intact antibodies.[56] Huse et al.[55] devised a novel system that was a breakthrough in allowing them to construct bacteriophage λ libraries for the expression of Fab antibody fragments. They succeeded in cloning into separate λ vectors the PCR-amplified products of mRNA that code for either heavy or light chain variable regions. Combinatorial constructs expressing Fab fragments were then generated by cutting DNA isolated from light and heavy chain libraries at the asymmetric *Eco* R1 site of each vector and religating the resulting arms. The constructs generated contained random combinations of heavy and light chains, including combinations which are not necessarily present in the B cell population of the parent animal. Using this method, mRNA isolated from a mouse that had been immunized with *p*-nitrophenyl phosphonamidate (NPN) coupled to KLH was isolated from spleen cells and amplified with various oligonucleotide primers. After ligation and packaging, 2.5×10^7 clones were obtained and screened for affinity for the binding of ^{125}I-NPN.

Both negative and positive effects accompany the use of combinatorial phage library technology. On the negative side, the mAbs generated have not undergone the affinity maturation that occurs with *in vivo* selection of the appropriately rearranged V_H-V_L pair. Attempts to mimic affinity maturation involve the creation of point mutations through use of error-prone polymerases or multiple rounds of PCR.[17] One positive aspect of building random phage libraries, particularly from unimmunized or naive individuals, is that it might allow for the recovery of combinations which physiological tolerance would eliminate *in vivo*.

Mullinax et al.[57] have applied this technology to the building of a relevant human antibody. They immunized volunteers with TT and harvested mRNA from lymphocytes 6 d later. They used PCR primers to amplify H or L chain sequences creating a mAb fragment of the IgG1 isotype with conservation of the H-L disulfide bond. In the library that was screened with radiolabeled TT, approximately 0.2% of the clones were positive with affinities of 9×10^8 M^{-1}. In principle, it should be possible to immortalize the entire antigen-combining repertoire as well as many novel V_H-V_L combinations not normally associated *in vivo*. However, the ability to recover antibody of a given specificity will rely on the efficiency of the screening protocol. In the Mullinax system, the frequency of B cells producing anti-TT mAb was <1/500,000 for unimmunized individuals and as high as 1/3000 after immunization.

B. PHAGE ANTIBODIES

Libraries made from unimmunized individuals can bypass the need for an immune human or reconstituted system, but the frequency of antigen-specific recombinations is very low and therefore the relative importance of screening methods is increased. Phage combinatorial library expression of Ig V region genes in bacteria is currently screened by enzyme-linked immunosorbent assay (ELISA) techniques. Screening of V region genes, however, has been revolutionized by the expression of antigen-binding antibody variable domain directly on the surface of bacteriophage. Phages expressing V region genes which produce antibody fragments with the correct configuration to bind antigen can be isolated from millions of nonspecific phages by affinity chromatography. McCafferty et al.[54] showed that the heavy and light chain variable domains of the anti-lysozyme antibody D1.3 associate tightly as a single chain

Fv (scFv) fragment whose affinity is similar to that of the intact antibody. To allow expression of both domains on the same polypeptide, they were joined by a flexible linker and a single-chain fragment was cloned into a filamentous phage (fd) vector at the N-terminal region of the gene III protein. This protein is expressed at the tip of fd phage and is responsible for attachment of phage to the bacterial F. pilus. Phages displaying the scFv-gene III fusion protein on their surface were then purified from parental phages by passage over a Sepharose-lysozyme column. Each passage over the column enriched the eluted phages 1000-fold for the presence of antibody Fv, giving evidence of the usefulness of this technique in selecting rare phages from large populations.

Whereas McCafferty et al. preselected the antigen-specific V genes which they expressed on filamentous phage, Clackson et al.[58] challenged this system further and displayed a random combinatorial library of the rearranged heavy and light chains from mice immunized with the hapten 2-phenyloxazol-5-one (phOx) on the surface of phage. Passage of the phage over a hapten affinity column detected several high-affinity binders ($K_d = 10^8$ M^{-1}). Interestingly, they were encoded by V region genes found in the anti-phOx hybridomas but in promiscuous combinations (i.e., the same V_H gene was found combined with several different partners). To exploit this finding, Clackson et al. generated "hierarchical" libraries by assembling the frequently found V_H genes with an entire repertoire of V_K genes from the same immunized mice. They then did the same for a frequently used V_K, pairing it with an entire V_H repertoire. The resulting hierarchical libraries were subjected to several rounds of antigen selection. The high-affinity combinations of V region genes were identified using this technique. Random combinatorial libraries (2×10^6 members) from unimmunized mice produced no phOx-binding clones after two rounds of selection. With libraries of this size ($\sim 10^6$), immunization seems to be necessary for V_H or V_K domains with the features required for hapten binding to be represented at high enough frequency to reconstitute a binding site. With the use of larger libraries ($>10^7$), which are now manageable through affinity column selection, immunization may become unnecessary for the generation of antibody fragments. We will then have bypassed the need not only for hybridomas but for immunization. In the case of human antibodies, this is an attractive prospect.

One disadvantage in the scFv fragments which have been expressed on phage is that they often have lower affinities than do their parent antibodies. Hoogenboom et al.[59] have taken phage technology another step further by demonstrating the display of heterodimeric Fab fragments on the surface of phage. They accomplished this by cloning libraries of heavy and light chains into the same or different vectors and by linking one chain to the phage gene III coat protein and co-expressing the complementary chain in the bacterial periplasm. The antibody heavy and light chains then reassociate into a functional Fab fragment. The libraries of heavy and light chains can be encoded by the same vector, giving a potential diversity of displayed Fab fragments of 10^7 light and 10^7 heavy (10^{14} members). Alternatively, two vectors can be used with the light chain encoded on one and the heavy on the other. This latter approach facilitates the construction of "hierarchical" libraries in which a fixed heavy or light chain is paired with a library of partners expressed on the second vector.

VI. CATALYTIC ANTIBODIES

Work by Lerner and Tramantano at the Research Institute of the Scripps Clinic has provided details of the interaction between antibody and its target molecule.[60] They have been able to utilize the energy with which antibodies bind to their target for catalysis. The catalytic antibody can potentially produce a limitless variety of molecules for use in biotechnology, in clinical medicine and in the investigation of protein structure and function.

Antigen-antibody and enzyme-substrate reactions have several similar characteristics. They are highly specific, interact with high affinity, and are usually reversible. Antibodies recognize a substrate with specificity and enzymes accelerate a reaction without being used up themselves. The catalytic antibodies combine these characteristics into a molecule that couples the diversity of the antibody with catalytic power. Monoclonal antibodies have been designed to increase the reaction rates of ester and carbonate hydrolysis by several hundred to 10,000 times, catalyze the hydrolysis of alkyl esters and enhance by 250,000-fold the hydrolysis of an amide bond.

A catalytic antibody for a reaction, e.g., an ester hydrolysis, is made by coupling a transition state analog, a stable substance mimicking a labile transition state molecule in the reaction, to a carrier protein and injecting the combination into an experimental animal. Antibody-secreting spleen cells are taken from the animal and fused with myeloma cells. A clone making antibody specific for the analog is then selected. The antibody may also be capable of binding to the transition state itself and thereby catalyze the reaction.[61,62]

VII. CLINICAL APPLICATION OF MONOCLONAL ANTIBODIES

Because of the rapid advances in recombinant technology, hybridoma technology, and in the understanding of disease pathogenesis, the monoclonal antibody has emerged as a potent therapeutic approach. Monoclonals, murine as well as chimeric, have been used in the clinic to interfere with the inflammatory cascade, abrogate endotoxic shock, restrict the coagulation process, and interfere with tumor growth. The first attempts to utilize monoclonals to modulate immune functions in humans involved treatment of acute renal allograft rejection with a monoclonal to the pan-T-cell antigen CD3(T3).[63-65] Cosimi and coworkers in Massachusetts used monoclonals to define the functional subsets of T lymphocytes, describing the helper/inducer cell-surface antigen (OKT4) and the suppressor/cytotoxic cell-surface antigen (OKT8). Carrying these studies into the clinic and monitoring these subpopulations in renal allograft recipients, it was seen that the OKT4 subset was associated with rejection. A major goal of the transplantation process is to suppress the immune response to the allograft. As CD4 molecules are expressed on T cells that react with class II major histocompatibility complex (MHC) restricted antigens, a key interaction in the rejection process, anti-CD4 monoclonals, have proven extremely effective in inhibiting rejection in renal, liver, and heart transplantation. Studies both in the nonhuman renal allograft model and in human transplantation demonstrated an efficacious role for these monoclonals.

A. ANTI-THROMBOSIS MONOCLONAL ANTIBODIES

Platelets are implicated in a variety of serious vaso-occlusive and thromboembolic disorders that together constitute the most common cause of death in the U.S. Antibodies directed to three components of the thrombus: fibrin, the platelet GPIIb/IIIa receptor, and α2-anti-plasmin have been used in the targeting of plasminogen activators by conjugating plasminogen activators to mAbs.[66] By targeting fibrin or platelet glycoprotein (GP)IIb/IIIa, concentration of plasminogen activation at the thrombus is increased and more rapid clot lysis is achieved.[67] Using an α2-anti-plasmin mAb, Haber at Bristol-Myers Squibb selectively inactivated a component of thrombus and produced clot lysis.[68]

A chimeric monoclonal, a genetically constructed mouse/human IgG antibody against the GPIIb/IIIa receptor on human platelets, has been developed. The papain cleavage fragment, Fab, is currently in clinical trials. The high affinity of the Fab fragment to the GPIIb/IIIa receptor prevents the adhesion of platelets to natural ligands for GPIIb/IIIa, e.g., fibrinogen and von Willebrand factor, and interferes with platelet aggregation and thrombosis.

B. ANTI-TUMOR MONOCLONAL ANTIBODIES

The development of intensive combination chemotherapeutic regimens has been accompanied by the appearance of significant toxicity. The resulting poor therapeutic index has spurred the development of novel approaches, such as targeted therapies using monoclonal antibodies and fusion-toxin molecules, which will be discussed in a later section. The oncologic applications of monoclonal antibody therapy are as diverse as the variety of tumor cell types presenting in the clinic. Monoclonal antibodies can detect a number of antigens which are specifically expressed by cancer cells. The mAb can be used both as a therapeutic as well as a diagnostic tool, especially when combined with a radioisotope. Radioimmunotherapy with a labeled, tumor-specific mAb is an approach being widely tested with a variety of radionuclides[69] (see also Chapter 5). Such radionuclides are theoretically able to deliver high-energy particulate radiation capable of penetrating numerous cell layers, resulting in tumor destruction. This method caused excessive nonspecific tissue toxicity. As an alternative approach to killing individual tumor cells, a low-energy electron emitter such as iodine-125(^{125}I) was used. The low-energy electrons have been shown to cause specific subcellular damage to the chromosomes of dividing cells. This method has resulted in clinical efficacy with acceptable nonspecific tissue toxicity.

Radiolabeled monoclonal antibodies may be able to deliver an additional increment of radiotherapy to sites of leukemic involvement in hematopoietic and lymphoid tissue while sparing the normal organs, particularly liver and lung, which are usually the site of dose-limiting toxicity.

Chimeric mAbs for oncologic indications have been developed to decrease the immunogenicity incurred with repeated administration. These have found clinical application. For example, the mouse/human chimeric monoclonal antibody, 17-1A,[70] produced and initially characterized at the Wistar Institute, has a relative specificity for cells of human gastrointestinal malignancies, such as colon, pancreas, and stomach adenocarcinoma. It has been used successfully in radioimmune imaging studies in man,[71] as well as in phase I and phase II therapeutic trials in patients with pancreas and colon cancer.[72,73]

Radiolabeled antibodies may be used alone to remit cancer or to cycle cells making them more susceptible to conventional chemotherapy or radiation. The therapeutic potential of a ^{131}I labeled anti-B-cell monoclonal was evaluated by Press et al.[74] in 26 patients with advanced non-Hodgkin's lymphoma who had failed conventional therapy. Twelve of these patients had favorable biodistributions of the monoclonal and were treated with therapeutic doses. Of those treated, eight had complete remissions, and one had a partial remission.

C. ANTI-INFLAMMATORY MONOCLONALS

CD4 T cells have been implicated in the pathogenesis of inflammatory diseases such as rheumatoid arthritis, systemic lupus erythematosus, multiple sclerosis, and Crohn's disease.[75-80] After antigen has been processed and presented on the antigen-presenting cell surface in the context of a class II MHC, it is recognized by T cell receptors on CD4 expressing helper T cells. This interaction between the class II MHC complex, the T cell receptor, and the CD4 surface molecule has become the target for intervention in the autoimmune diseases. Monoclonal antibodies have been developed to inhibit MHC recognition using anti-MHC mAbs or by the inhibition of T cell activation with anti-TCR mAbs or anti-CD4 mAbs. Chimeric mouse/human monoclonal antibodies directed against the CD4 epitope of T lymphocytes have been developed to treat these T cell-mediated entities.[81]

Animal models of autoimmune diseases have shown resolution of inflammatory processes when treated with an anti-CD4 monoclonal antibody. This efficacy has been shown in murine models of collagen arthritis,[82] systemic lupus erythematosus,[83] myasthenia gravis,[84] experimental allergic encephalitis,[85] diabetes mellitus,[86] thyroiditis,[87] and uveitis.[88]

In clinical trials, anti-CD4 chimeric monoclonal antibody has shown promising results in patients with rheumatoid arthritis and multiple sclerosis. Anecdotal data of its use in other T cell-mediated diseases, such as Crohn's disease, systemic lupus erythematosus, relapsing polychondritis, and uveitis, suggest application in these diseases.

The mechanism of action of anti-CD4 chimeric antibody has not been fully explained. Potential mechanisms of action include: depletion of CD4 T cells by ADCC; depletion through complement-mediated cytotoxicity (CDC); modulating the CD4 antigen from the T cell surface; and blocking of early and late events in T cell activation, i.e., calcium mobilization and IL-2 receptor expression, respectively.[89]

A chimeric anti-human tumor necrosis factor (TNF-α) monoclonal antibody has been developed. This antibody has high affinity and the ability to neutralize the cytotoxic effects of human TNF. TNF-α has been shown to play a prominent role in the inflammatory cascade.[92] Along with interleukin (IL)-1α it is produced by macrophages and monocytes and stimulates systemic responses, including fever, release of acute-phase proteins from the liver, increased superoxide production, and decreased chemotaxis.[91] mRNA for TNF is increased in rheumatoid arthritis synovial tissue. Clinical trials using anti-TNF mAbs to treat patients with rheumatoid arthritis have recently been initiated.

D. ANTI-ADHESION MONOCLONAL ANTIBODIES

Several monoclonal antibodies specific for molecules involved in leukocyte adhesion to endothelial cells are under development as therapies for a variety of autoimmune and anti-inflammatory diseases. Extensive animal model experimentation with anti-adhesion molecule monoclonal antibodies has indicated promise for this approach in a diverse set of clinical indications, including arthritis,[92] asthma,[93] myocardial reperfusion injury,[94] stroke,[95] and transplant rejection.[96] Humanized monoclonal antibodies specific for CD18, ICAM-1, ELAM-1, and GMP-140 will soon enter clinical trials for some of these indications.

E. ANTI-INFECTIVE MONOCLONAL ANTIBODIES

The application of monoclonal antibody technology to the therapy of infective processes has demonstrated clinical efficacy in the treatment of Gram-negative sepsis, with and without endotoxic shock. The mAb has either been used as an adjunctive therapy or as a new modality for intervention in some viremias.

1. Preventing the Biological Effects of Endotoxin

Gram-negative bacteremia is a leading cause of death in hospitalized patients. These infections most often stem from urinary tract infections, the postoperative complications of bowel surgery, postpartum sepsis, and from open, traumatic wounds. Mortality is increased in the presence of endotoxic shock.

Endotoxins exist in most microorganisms as complexes of lipid, polysaccharide, and protein. The biological activity appears to be a property of the lipid portion. It was demonstrated a decade ago that therapy with human antiserum against core lipopolysaccharide (LPS) of Gram-negative enteric bacilli greatly reduced mortality in Gram-negative bacteremia.[97] It was hypothesized that antibodies that recognize conserved epitopes in the core region of LPS may cross react with a wide variety of endotoxins and therefore might be able to counter their lethal effects. An important clinical trial supported the hypothesis that passive immunization of patients with human antisera against the heat-activated rough J5 mutant of *E. coli* is an efficacious adjunct to antibiotics resulting in reduced mortality. However, human polyclonal J5 antiserum was not suitable for widespread clinical use. The titer of hemagglutinating antibody to J5 LPS was highly variable, prepared units could be stored for only a short period of time, and the use of pooled sera carried the risk of transmitting blood-borne pathogens.

These limitations were circumvented with the development of mAb technology. An appropriate monoclonal would bind to the lipid A moiety of endotoxin. It would demonstrate the ability of the antibody to activate complement when complexed with endotoxin, thereby clearing the complexes more rapidly and conferring greater protection. Finally, a human mAb would be less immunogenic than a mAb derived from a nonhuman species. Teng and colleagues[98] developed a cell line that produced a human monoclonal IgM antibody that bound to the lipid A portion of Gram-negative bacterial endotoxin. The cell line was developed by fusing the splenocytes from a patient who had been immunized using a J5 vaccine with a mouse-human heteromyeloma cell line.[98]

2. Human Immunodeficiency Virus Type I (HIV I)

HIV is transmitted most commonly through an exchange of body fluids, sexual activity, or blood transfusion. The virus invades cells by attachment of the virus envelope protein gp120 to the cell-associated CD4 molecule, which is expressed on the surface of a number of cell populations, including T cells, macrophages, megakaryocytes, and glial cells. After attachment to the CD4 binding site for gp120, the virus enters the cell through a combination of activities mediated by gp120 and gp41.

Attempts have been made to utilize the CD4 protein as a method of blocking the viral entry into target cells. A human IgG1 kappa monoclonal antibody was produced by a hybridoma constructed from an EBV transformant fused with a human myeloma analog. The antibody reacts with the CD4 binding region of gp120. This mAb neutralized the IIIB and MN strains of HIV at concentrations which are readily achievable *in vivo*. The design of the mAb in this case offers a potential advantage as a biologic treatment for HIV infection because it reacts with an epitope on gp120, and thus avoids the problems related to interference with the normal functions of CD4.[99]

Several other viral entities have been addressed as potential targets for monoclonal therapy. Cytomegalovirus (CMV), Herpes zoster, and murine picornaviruses have been studied. Human IgG1 monoclonal antibodies have been generated against Hepatitis B virus, CMV, Herpes simplex, and Varicella zoster virus. CMV infection causes most interstitial pneumonia in bone marrow transplant recipients. Two neutralizing human IgG1 monoclonal antibodies to CMV have been developed. In a 1991 trial in Germany 13 patients, 8 seropositive and 5 seronegative for CMV, were treated with bone marrow transplantation. The antibodies were administered over a 3-month period showing both a satisfactory safety profile and significant neutralizing activity against CMV.[100]

F. IMMUNOCONJUGATES

Due to the inability of some mouse anti-human mAbs to fix complement or to activate human cytolytic cells, treatment with these antibodies may not adequately deplete or inactivate the desired target cells. For this reason, cell-specific antibodies linked to a toxin have been constructed (see also Chapter 5). The German scientist Paul Ehrlich first suggested that hybrid molecules (*Zauberkugln*, the magic bullet) consisting of cell-specific antibodies linked to a toxin be constructed for therapeutic purposes.[101] He envisioned that immunotoxins, the magic bullets, could be used to destroy a highly selective population of target cells.

The genetic replacement of either the native diphtheria toxin or *Pseudomonas* exotoxin A receptor-binding domain with cell receptor-specific polypeptide hormones or growth factor sequences has resulted in the development of a new class of biological response modifiers, the fusion-toxin. One such construct was made by Chaudhary et al.,[102] who expressed in *E. coli* a fusion protein consisting of the *Pseudomonas* exotoxin and the single-chain Fv portion of an anti-IL-2 receptor antibody. This reagent selectively binds to and kills activated T cells. This same group used PCR to clone antibody-toxin conjugates, including a single-chain immunotoxin with specificity for the OVB3 antigen present on ovarian cancer cells.[103] Once again the advantage is the specificity of killing afforded by this reagent.

In another study, antibody specificity and effector function were combined to make a fusion protein by joining the variable region from the heavy chain of an anti-fibrin antibody (59D8) with a mouse constant region, most of whose exons were replaced by the DNA sequences encoding the catalytic β chain of tissue plasminogen activator (t-PA).[104] This heavy chain fusion gene was transfected into a heavy chain loss variant of the original antifibrin hybridoma. The cells produced a 65-kDa heavy chain t-PA fusion protein that was secreted in association with the 59D8 antifibrin light chain to form a 170-kDa disulfide-linked dimer. The fusion protein had 70% of the peptidolytic activity of the native t-PA but the affinity for fibrin was diminished 100-fold compared with the native antibody. This underscores the lesson that the effective use of recombinant DNA techniques for creating therapeutic antibodies requires copying binding site sequences and maintaining the proper folding to preserve active domains.

In the therapy of rheumatoid arthritis (RA) a recently described immunotoxin molecule is the DAB_{486} IL-2, which consists of a portion of IL-2 sufficient in size to recognize the high-affinity IL-2 receptor, fixed to a potent fragment of diphtheria toxin.[105] DAB_{486} IL-2 was observed to be efficient in killing cells expressing IL-2 receptor.[106] In rats, this molecule markedly downregulates the induction of adjuvant arthritis. When administered to patients with advanced RA, 5 of 13 patients responded to a 7-d administration of the immunotoxin. A cytokine release syndrome, including fever, chills, myalgias, and transient hypotension may accompany the administration. Some transient liver enzyme abnormalities were also seen.[107]

Another immunoconjugate combining an anti-CD5 monoclonal with the A chain of the ricin molecule has also been used in the clinic to treat refractory RA. Ricin, a 33-kDa glycoprotein purified from castor beans, inhibits ribosomal protein synthesis resulting in cell death. The CD5 antibody is a murine IgG1 which binds to the CD5 molecule expressed on 95% of mature T lymphocytes and a subpopulation of B lymphocytes. Treatment resulted in significant improvement in over 50% of patients in the early trials. The magnitude of acute improvement was comparable to methotrexate.[108] This toxin conjugate has also been used to treat patients with lupus nephritis refractory to 1 year of treatment with prednisone and cyclophosphamide.[109] Preliminary results to date demonstrated that the therapy was well tolerated and several patients had an improvement in renal function for 5 or more months after treatment. Interfering with the pathogenesis of inflammatory diseases by receptor-targeted toxins and blocking monoclonal antibodies requires more thorough *in vitro* and clinical testing.

G. DIAGNOSTIC ASSAYS

The use of monoclonals to increase diagnostic sensitivity and specificity in immunocytoassays has become widespread. Tumor detection can be enhanced by using a monoclonal antibody specific for tumor antigen. The site of disease can also be more accurately localized and the follow-up of the patient facilitated. For example, radiolabeling of monoclonal anti-tumor antibodies has been utilized in such entities as melanoma with ^{131}I-labeled mAb,[110] against carcinoembryonic antigen,[111] in colon cancer,[112] as well as improving conventional cytodiagnosis in disseminated ovarian cancer.[113] These are described more fully in Chapter 5.

REFERENCES

1. **Kohler, G. and Milstein, C.,** Continuous cultures of fused cells secreting antibody of predefined specificity, *Nature*, 256, 495, 1975.
2. **Milstein C.,** Monoclonal antibodies, *Sci. Am.*, 243, 66, 1980.
3. **Jencks, W.P.,** *Catalysis in Chemistry and Enzymology*, McGraw-Hill, New York, 1969, 288.
4. **Tramontano, A., Janda, K.D., and Lerner, R.A.,** Catalytic antibodies, *Science*, 234, 1566, 1986.
5. **Pollack, S.J., Jacobs, J.W., and Schultz, P.G.,** Selective chemical catalysis by an antibody, *Science*, 234, 1570, 1986.
6. **Janda, K.D., Benkovic, S.J., and Lerner, R.A.,** Catalytic antibodies with lipase activity and R or S substrate selectivity, *Science*, 244, 437, 1989.
7. **Janda, K.D., Schloeder, D., Benkovic, S.J., and Lerner, R.A.,** Induction of an antibody that catalyzes the hydrolysis of an amide bond, *Science*, 241, 1188, 1988.

8. **Morrison, S.L., Canfield, S., Porter S. et al.,** Production and characterization of genetically engineered antibody molecules, *Clin. Chem.*, 34, 1668, 1988.
9. **Pirofski, L., Casadevall, A., Rodriguez, L. et al.,** Current state of hybridoma technology, *J. Clin. Immunol.*, 10 (6 Suppl.) 5S, 1990.
10. **Borrebaeck, C.A.,** Strategy for the production of human monoclonal antibodies using in vitro activated B-cells, *J. Immunol. Methods*, 123, 157, 1989.
11. **Dreyer, W.J. and Bennett, J.C.,** The molecular basis of antibody formation: A paradox, *Proc. Natl. Acad. Sci. USA*, 54, 864, 1964.
12. **Potter, M.,** Immunoglobulin-producing tumors and myeloma proteins of mice, *Physiol. Rev.*, 52, 631, 1972.
13. **Kearney, J.F., Radbruch, A., Liesegang, B. et al.,** A new mouse myeloma line that has lost immunoglobulin expression but permits the construction of antibody-secreted hybrid cell lines, *J. Immunol.*, 123, 1548, 1979.
14. **Pontecorvo, G.,** Production of mammalian somatic cell hybrids by means of polyethylene glycol treatment, *Somatic Cell Genet.*, 1, 397, 1975.
15. **Harlow, E. and Lane, D., Eds.,** *Antibodies: A Laboratory Manual*, Cold Spring Harbor Laboratory, Cold Spring Harbor, NY, 1988, 146.
16. **Bruggemann, M., Winter, G., Waldmann, H., and Neuberger, M.S.,** The immunogenicity of chimeric antibodies, *J. Exp. Med.*, 170, 2153, 1989.
17. **Winter, G. and Milstein, C.,** Man-made antibodies, *Nature*, 349, 293, 1991.
18. **LoBuglio, A.F., Wheeler, R.H., Trang, J., Haynes, A., Rogers, K., Harvey, E.B., Sun L., Ghrayeb, J., and Khazaeli, M.B.,** Mouse/human chimeric monoclonal antibody in man: kinetics and immune response, *Proc. Natl. Acad. Sci. U.S.A.*, 86, 4220, 1989.
19. **Koga, H., Kanda, H., Nakashima, M., Watanabe, Y., Endo, K., and Watanabe, T.,** Mouse-human chimeric monoclonal antibody to carcinoembryonic antigen (CEA): in vitro and in vivo activities, *Hybridoma*, 9, 43, 1990.
20. **Liu, A.Y., Robinson, R.R., Hellstrom, K.E., Murray, E.D., Chang, C.P., and Hellstrom, I.,** Chimeric mouse-human IgG1 antibody that can mediate lysis of cancer cells, *Proc. Natl. Acad. Sci. U.S.A.*, 84, 3439, 1987.
21. **Bankert, R., DesSoye, U., and Powers, L.,** Antigen promoted cell fusion: antigen coated myeloma cells fuse with antigen reactive spleen cells, *Transplant. Proc.*, 12, 443, 1980.
22. **Lo, M., Tsong, T., Conrad, U., Stillmatter, S., Hester, L., and Snyder, S.,** Monoclonal antibody production by receptor mediated electronically induced cell fusion, *Nature*, 310, 792, 1984.
23. **Oi, V.T., Morrison, S.L., Herzenberg, L.A., and Berg, P.,** Immunoglobulin gene expression in transformed lymphoid cells, *Proc. Natl. Acad. Sci. U.S.A.*, 80, 825, 1983.
24. **Jonak, Z.L., Owen, J.A., and Machy, P.,** Strategies for the immortalization of B lymphocytes, in vitro immunization in hybridoma technology, in *Progress in Biotechnology*, Vol. 5, Borrebaeck, C.A.K., Ed., Elsevier, Amsterdam, 1988, 163.
25. **Oi, V.T. and Morrison, S.L.,** Chimeric antibodies, *Biotechniques*, 4, 214, 1986.
26. **Kozbor, D., Lagarde, A.E., and Roder, J.C.,** Human hybridomas constructed with antigen-specific Epstein-Barr virus transformed cell lines, *Proc. Natl. Acad. Sci. U.S.A.*, 79, 6651, 1982.
27. **Ohlin, M., Danielsson, L., Carlsson, R., and Borrebaeck, C.A.K.,** The effect of leucyl-leucylmethyl ester on proliferation and Ig-secretion of EBV-transformed human B lymphocytes, *Immunology*, 66, 485, 1989.
28. **Lagace, J. and Brodeur, B.R.,** Parameters affecting in vitro immunization of human lymphocytes, *J. Immunol. Methods*, 85, 127, 1985.
29. **Danielsson, L., Moller, S.A., and Borrebaeck, C.A.K.,** Effect of cytokines on specific in vitro immunization of human peripheral B lymphocytes against T-cell dependent antigens, *Immunology*, 61, 51, 1987.
30. **Mosier, D.E., Gulizin, R.J., Baird, S.M., and Wilson, D.B.,** Transfer of a functional human immune system to mice with severe combined immunodeficiency, *Nature*, 335, 256, 1988.
31. **McCune, J.M., Nawikama, A., Kaeshima, H., Shultz, D., Lieberman, M., and Weissman, I.,** The SCID-hu mouse: a murine model for the analysis of human hematolymphoid differentiation and function, *Science*, 241, 1632, 1988.
32. **Cavacini, L.A., Kennel, M., Lally, E.V., Posner, M.R., and Quinn, A.,** Human immunoglobulin production in immunodeficient mice: enhancement by immunosuppression of host and preactivation of human PBMC, *Clin. and Exp. Immunol.*, 90, 135, 1992.
33. **Duchosal, M.A., Eming, S.A., Fischer, P., Leturcq, D., Barbas, C.F., McConahey, P.J., Caothien, R.H., Thornton, G.B., Dixon, F.J., and Burton, D.R.,** Immunization of hu-PBL-SCID mice and the rescue of human monoclonal Fab fragments through combinatorial libraries, *Nature*, 355, 258, 1992.
34. **Seppala, I., Routonen, N., Sarnesto, A., Mattila, P., and Makela, O.,** The percentage of six immunoglobulin isotypes in human antibodies to tetanus toxoid: standardization of isotype-specific second antibodies in solid-phase assay, *Eur. J. Immunol.*, 14, 868, 1984.
35. **Bruggemann, M., Caskey, H.M., Teal, C., Waldmann, H., Williams, G.T., Sunani, H.A., and Neuberger, M.S.,** A repertoire of monoclonal antibodies with human heavy chains, *Proc. Natl. Acad. Sci. U.S.A.*, 86, 6709, 1989.

36. **Burke, D., Carle, G.F., and Olson, M.V.,** Cloning of large segments of exogenous DNA into yeast by means of artificial chromosome vectors, *Science*, 236, 806, 1987.
37. **Morrison, S.L.,** Genetically engineered (chimeric) antibodies, *Hosp. Prac.*, 24, 65, 1989.
38. **Morrison, S.L., Johnson, M.J., Herzenberg, L.A., and Oi, V.T.,** Chimeric human antibody molecules: mouse antigen-binding domains with human constant region domains, *Proc. Natl. Acad. Sci. (USA)*, 81, 6851, 1984.
39. **Jones, P.T., Dear, P.H., Foote, J. et al.,** Replacing the complementarity-determining regions in human antibody with those from a mouse, *Nature*, 321, 522, 1986.
40. **Steplewski, Z., Sun, L.K., Shearman, C.W. et al.,** Biological activity of human-mouse IgG1, IgG2, IgG3 and IgG4 chimeric monoclonal antibodies with anti-tumor specificity, *Proc. Natl. Acad. Sci. (USA)*, 85, 4852, 1988.
41. **Alters, S.E., Steinman, L., and Oi, V.T.,** Comparison of rat and rat-mouse chimeric anti-murine CD4 antibodies *in vitro*; chimeric antibodies lyse low-density $CD4^+$ cells, *J. Immunol.*, 142, 2018, 1989.
42. **Looney, J., Knight, D., Arevalo-Moore, M., Trinh, H., Pak, K.-Y., Dalesandro, M., Rieber, E.P., Riethmüller, G., Daddona, P., and Ghrayeb, J.,** High level expression and characterization of a mouse/human chimeric CD4 antibody with therapeutic potential, *Human Hybridomas and Antibodies*, 3, 191, 1992.
43. **Fell, H.P., Yarnold, S., Hellstrom, I. et al.,** Homologous recombination in hybridoma cells: heavy chain chimeric antibody produced by gene targeting, *Proc. Natl. Acad. Sci. U.S.A.*, 86, 8507, 1989.
44. **Riechman, L. et al.,** Reshaping human antibodies for therapy, *Nature*, 332, 323, 1988.
45. **Hale, G., Clark, R., Marcus, R., Winter, G., Dyer, M., Phillips, J., Reichmann, L., and Waldmann, H.,** Remission induction in non-Hodgkins lymphoma with reshaped human monoclonal antibody CAMPATH-1H, *Lancet*, 2, 1394, 1988.
46. **Queen, C., Schneider, W.P., Selick, H., Payne, P.W., Landolfi, N.F., Duncan, J.F., Avdalovic, N.M., Levitt, M., Junghans, R.P., and Waldmann, T.A.,** A humanized antibody that binds to the interleukin 2 receptor, *Proc. Natl. Acad. Sci. U.S.A.*, 86, 10029, 1989.
47. **Lewis, A.P. and Crowe, J.S.,** Immunoglobulin complementarity-determining region grafting by recombinant polymerase chain reaction to generate humanized monoclonal antibodies, *Gene*, 101, 297, 1991.
48. **Daugherty, B.L., DeMartino, J.A., Law, M.-F., Kawka, D.W., Singer, I.I., and Mark, G.E.,** Polymerase chain reaction facilitates the cloning, CDR-grafting, and rapid expression of a murine monoclonal antibody directed against the CD18 component of leukocyte integrins, *Nucleic Acids Res.*, 19, 2471, 1991.
49. **Mayforth, R.D. and Quintans, J.,** Designer and catalytic antibodies, *N. Engl. J. Med.*, 323, 173, 1990.
50. **Bird, R.E., Hardman, K.D., Jacobson, J.W. et al.,** Single-chain antigen-binding proteins, *Science*, 242, 423, 1988.
51. **Ward, E.S., Güssow, D., Griffiths, A.D. et al.,** Binding activities of a repertoire of single immunoglobulin variable domains secreted from Escherichia coli, *Nature*, 341, 544, 1989.
52. **Williams, W., Moss, D.A., Kieber-Emmons, T.A. et al.,** Development of biologically active peptides based on antibody structure, *Proc. Natl. Acad. Sci. U.S.A.*, 86, 5537, 1989.
53. **Orlandi, R., Gussow, D.H., Jones, P.T., and Winter, G.,** Cloning immunoglobulin variable domains for expression by the polymerase chain reaction, *Proc. Natl. Acad. Sci. U.S.A.*, 86, 3833, 1989.
54. **McCafferty, J., Griffith, A.D., Winter, G., and Chiswell, D.J.,** Phage antibodies: filamentous phage displaying antibody variable domains, *Nature*, 348, 552, 1990.
55. **Huse, W., Sastry, L., Iverson, S.A. et al.,** Generation of a large combinatorial library of the immunoglobulin repertoire in phage lambda, *Science*, 246, 1275, 1989.
56. **Davies, D.P. and Padlan, E.A.,** Antibody-antigen complexes, *Annu. Rev. Biochem.*, 59, 439, 1990.
57. **Mullinax, R.L., Gross, E.A., Amberg, J.R., Jr. et al.,** Identification of human antibody fragment clones specific for tetanus toxoid in a bacteriophage lambda expression library, *Proc. Natl. Acad. Sci. U.S.A.*, 87, 8095, 1990.
58. **Clackson, T., Hoogenboom, H.R., Griffiths, A.D., and Winter, G.,** Making antibody fragments using phage display libraries, *Nature*, 352, 624, 1991.
59. **Hoogenboom, H.R., Griffiths, A.D., Johnson, K.S. et al.,** Multi-subunit protein on the surface of filamentous phage: methodologies for displaying antibody (Fab) heavy and light chains, *Nucleic Acids Res.*, 19, 4133, 1991.
60. **Lerner, R.A. and Tramontano, A.,** Catalytic antibodies, *Sci. Am.*, 258, 58, 1988.
61. **Green, B.S.,** Monoclonal antibodies as catalysts and templates for organic chemical reactions, *Adv. Biotechnol. Processes*, 11, 359, 1989.
62. **Schultz, P.G.,** The interplay between chemistry and biology in the design of enzymatic catalysts, *Science*, 240, 426, 1988.
63. **Burton, R.C., Cosimi, A.B., Colvin, R.B. et al.,** Monoclonal antibodies to human T-cell subsets: use for immunological monitoring and immunosuppression in renal transplantation, *J. Clin. Immunol.*, 2, 142S, 1982.
64. **Cosimi, A.B., Colvin, R.B., Burton, R.C. et al.,** Use of monoclonal antibodies to T-cell subsets for immunologic monitoring and treatment in recipients of renal allografts, *N. Engl. J. Med.*, 305, 308, 1981.

65. **Cosimi, A.B., Burton, R.C., Kung, P.C. et al.,** Evaluation in primate renal allograft recipients of monoclonal antibody to human T-cell subclasses, *Transplant. Proc.*, 13, 499, 1981.
66. **Coller, B.S., Folts, J.D., Scudder, L.E. et al.,** Anti-thrombotic effect of a monoclonal antibody to the platelet glycoprotein IIb/IIIa receptor in an experimental animal model, *Blood*, 68, 783, 1986.
67. **Coller, B.S., Folts, J.D., Smith, S.R. et al.,** Abolition of in vivo platelet thrombus formation in primates with monoclonal antibodies to the platelet GP IIb/IIIa receptor, *Circulation*, 80, 1766, 1989.
68. **Haber, E.,** Antibody targeting in cardiovascular diseases, *J. Cell Biochem.*, Suppl. 15E, 112, 1991.
69. **Brady, L.W. et al.,** The present and future role of monoclonal antibodies in the management of cancer, Vaeth, J.M., Meger, S.L., Ed., Vol. 24, *Front Radiat. Ther. Oncol.*, S. Karger, Basel, 1990, 247.
70. **Shaw, D.R., Khazaeli, M.B., Sun, L.K. et al.,** Characterization of a mouse/human chimeric monoclonal antibody (17-1A) to a colon cancer tumor-associated antigen, *J. Immunol.*, 138, 4535, 1987.
71. **Moldofsky, P.J., Powe, J., Mulhern, C.B. et al.,** Metastatic colon cancer detected with radiolabeled monoclonal antibody fragments, *Radiology*, 149, 549, 1983.
72. **Sears, H.F., Herlyn, D., Steplewski, Z. et al.,** Effect of monoclonal antibody immune therapy in patients with gastrointestinal adenocarcinoma, *J. Biol. Response Mod.*, 3, 138, 1984.
73. **LoBuglio, A.F., Saleh, M., Peterson, L. et al.,** Phase I clinical trial of C012-1A monoclonal antibody, *Hybridoma*, 5 (Suppl. 1), S117, 1986.
74. **Press, O.W., Eary, J., Badger, C. et al.,** Treatment of refractory non-Hodgkin's lymphoma with radiolabeled MB-1 (anti-CD37) antibody, *J. Clin. Oncol.*, 7, 1027, 1989.
75. **Paulus, N.E., Machleder, N.I. et al.,** Lymphocyte involvement in rheumatoid arthritis: studies during thoracic duct drainage, *Arthritis Rheum.*, 20, 1249, 1977.
76. **Duke, O., Panayi, G.S. et al.,** An immunohistological analysis of lymphocyte subpopulations and their microenvironment in the synovial membranes of patients with rheumatoid arthritis using monoclonal antibodies, *Clin. Exp. Immunol.*, 49, 22, 1982.
77. **Carteron, N.L., Wofsy, D., Schimenti, C. et. al.,** F $(ab')_2$ anti-CD4 and intact anti-CD4 monoclonal antibodies inhibit the accumulation of CD4+ T cells, CD8+ T cells and B cells in the kidneys of lupus-prone NZB/NZW mice, *Clin. Immunol. Immunopathol.*, 56, 373, 1990.
78. **Acha-Orbea, H., Mitchell, D.J., Timmerman, L. et al.,** Limited heterogeneity of T-cell receptors from lymphocytes mediating autoimmune encephalomyelitis allows specific immune intervention, *Cell*, 54, 263, 1988.
79. **Hafler, D.A., Duby, A., Lee, S.J. et al.,** Oligoclonal T-lymphocytes in the cerebrospinal fluid of patients with multiple sclerosis, *J. Exp. Med.*, 167, 1313, 1988.
80. **Selby, W.S., Janossy, G. et al.,** Intestinal lymphocyte subpopulations in inflammatory bowel disease: an analysis by immunohistologic and cell isolation techniques, *Gut*, 25, 32, 1984.
81. **Herzog, C., Walker, C., Muller, W. et al.,** Anti-CD4 antibody treatment in patients with rheumatoid arthritis: effect on clinical course and circulating T-cells, *J. Autoimmun.*, 2, 627, 1989.
82. **Ranges, G.E., Sriram, S., and Cooper, S.M.,** Prevention of type II collagen-induced arthritis by in vivo treatment with anti-L3T4, *J. Exp. Med.*, 162, 1105, 1985.
83. **Wofsy, D. and Seaman, W.E.,** Reversal of advanced murine lupus in NZB/NZW F1 mice by treatment with monoclonal antibody to L3T4, *J. Immunol.*, 138, 3247, 1987.
84. **Christadoss, P. and Dauphinee, M.J.,** Immunotherapy for myasthenia gravis: a murine model, *J. Immunol.*, 136, 2437, 1986.
85. **Waldor, M.K., Sriram, S., Hardy, R. et al.,** Reversal of experimental allergic encephalomyelitis with monoclonal antibody to a T-cell subset marker, *Science*, 227, 415, 1985.
86. **Koike, T., Itoh, Y. et al.,** Preventive effect of monoclonal anti-L3T4 antibody on development of diabetes in NOD mice, *Diabetes*, 36, 359, 1987.
87. **Nabozny, G.H., Cobbold, S.P., Waldmann, H. et al.,** Suppression in murine experimental autoimmune thyroiditis: in vivo inhibition of CD4+ T-cell mediated resistance by a non-depleting rat CD4 monoclonal antibody, *Cell. Immunol.*, 138, 185, 1991.
88. **Atalla, L., Linker-Israeli, M., Steinman, L., and Rao, N.A.,** Inhibition of autoimmune uveitis by anti-CD4 antibody, *Invest. Ophthalmol. Visual Sci.*, 31, 1264, 1990.
89. **Dalesandro, M.R., Pak, K.-Y., Tam, S. et al.,** In vitro efficacy of a mouse/human chimeric CD4 antibody: functional contributions of isotype and Fc, *J. Cell Biochem.*, (Abstr.) 15E, 179, 1991.
90. **Buchan, G., Barret, K., Turner, M. et al.,** Interleukin-1 and tumor necrosis factor mRNA expression in rheumatoid arthritis prolonged production of IL-1α, *Clin. Exp. Immunol.*, 73, 449, 1988.
91. **Sullivan, G.W., Carper, H.T., Novick, W.J. et al.,** Inhibition of the inflammatory action of interleukin 1 and tumor necrosis factor (alpha) on neutrophil function by pentoxifylline, *Infect. Immun.*, 56, 1722, 1988.
92. **Iigo, Y., Takashi, T., Tamatani, T., Miyasaka, M., Higashida, T., Yagita, H., Okumura, K., and Tsukada, W.,** ICAM-1-dependent pathway is critically involved in the pathogenesis of adjuvant arthritis in rats, *J. Immunol.*, 146, 4167, 1991.

93. **Gundel, R.H., Wegner, C.D., Torcellini, C.A., Clarke, C.C., Haynes, N., Rothlein, R., Smith, C.W., and Letts, L.G.**, Endothelial leukocyte adhesion molecule-1 mediates antigen-induced acute airway inflammation and late-phase airway obstruction in monkeys, *J. Clin. Invest.*, 88, 1407, 1991.
94. **Ma, X., Tsao, P.S., and Lefer, A.M.**, Antibody to CD18 exerts endothelial and cardiac protective effects in myocardial ischemia and reperfusion, *J. Clin. Invest.*, 88, 1237, 1991.
95. **Clark, W.M., Madden, K.P., Rothlein, R., and Zivin, J.A.**, Reduction of central nervous system ischemic injury by monoclonal antibody to intercellular adhesion molecule, *J. Neurosurg.*, 75, 623, 1991.
96. **Cosimi, A.B., Conti, D., Delmonico, F.L., Preffer, F.I., Wee, S., Rothlein, R., Faanes, R., and Colvin, R.B.**, In vivo effects of monoclonal antidy to ICAM-1 (CD54) in nonhuman primates with renal allografts, *J. Immunol.*, 144, 4604, 1990.
97. **Ziegler, E., McCutchan, A., Fierer, J., Glauser, M., Sadoff, J., Douglas, H., and Braude, A.**, Treatment of Gram negative bacteremia and shock with human antiserum to a mutant *Escherichia coli*, *N. Engl. J. Med.*, 307, 1225, 1982.
98. **Teng, N., Kaplan, H., Hebert, J.M. et al.**, Protection against Gram negative bacteria and endotoxin with human monoclonal IgM antibodies, *Proc. Natl. Acad. Sci. USA*, 82, 1790, 1985.
99. **Posner, M.R., Hideshuna, T., Cannon, T. et al.**, An IgG human monoclonal antibody that reacts with HIV-1/GP120, inhibits virus binding to cells, and neutralizes infection, *J. Immunol.*, 146, 4325, 1991.
100. **Aulitzky, W.E., Schulz, T.F., Tilg, H. et al.**, Human monoclonal antibodies neutralizing cytomegalovirus (CMV) for prophylaxis of CMV disease: report of a phase I trial in bone marrow transplant recipients, *J. Infect. Dis.*, 163, 1344, 1991.
101. **Ehrlich, P.**, *Collected Studies on Immunity*, John Wiley & Sons, New York, 1906, 441.
102. **Chaudhary, V.K., Queen, C., Junghans, R.P., Waldmann, T.A., Fitzgerald, D.J., and Pastan, I.**, Recombinant immunotoxin consisting of two antibody variable domains fused to Pseudomonas exotoxin, *Nature*, 339, 394, 1989.
103. **Chaudhary, V.K., Batra, J.K., Gallo, M.G. et al.**, A rapid method of cloning functional variable-region antigen genes in E. coli as a single chain immunotoxin, *Proc. Natl. Acad. Sci. U.S.A.*, 87, 1066, 1990.
104. **Schnee, J.M., Runge, M.S., Matsueda, G.R. et al.**, Construction and expression of a recombinant antibody-targeted plasminogen activator, *Proc. Natl. Acad. Sci. U.S.A.*, 84, 6904, 1987.
105. **LeMaistre, C.F., Meneghetti, C., Rosenblum, M. et al.**, Phase I trial of an interleukin-2 CIL-2 fusion toxin (DAB_{486} IL-2) in hematologic malignancies expressing the IL-2 receptor, *Blood*, 79, 2547, 1992.
106. **Strom, T.B., Anderson, P.L., Rubin-Kelley, V.E. et al.**, Immunotoxins and cytokine toxin fusion proteins, *Ann. N.Y. Acad. Sci.*, 636, 331, 1991.
107. **Sewell, K.L. and Trentham, D.E.**, Improvement in refractory rheumatoid arthritis by interleukin-2 receptor targeted therapy, *Arthritis Rheum.*, 34 (Suppl. 9), 589, 1991.
108. **Strand, V., Lipsky, P.E., Cannon, G. et al.**, Treatment of rheumatoid arthritis with an anti-CD5 immunoconjugate: final results of phase II studies, *Arthritis Rheum.*, 34 (Suppl. 9), A155, 1991.
109. **Wacholtz, M.C., Strand, V., and Lipsky, P.E.**, Treatment of lupus nephritis with CD5 PLUS, an immunoconjugate of anti-CD5 monoclonal antibody and ricin A chain, *Arthritis Rheum.*, 34 (Suppl. 9), 154, 1991.
110. **Larson, S.M., Brown, J.P., Wright, P.W. et al.**, Imaging of melanoma with I-131 labeled monoclonal antibodies, *J. Nucl. Med.*, 24, 123, 1983.
111. **Mach, J.P., Carrel, S., Forni, M. et al.**, Tumor localization of radiolabeled antibodies against carcinoembryonic antigen in patients with carcinoma, *N. Engl. J. Med.*, 303, 5, 1980.
112. **Mach, J.P., Chatal, J.F., Lumbroso, J.D. et al.**, Tumor localization in patients by radiolabeled monoclonal antibodies against colon carcinoma, *Cancer Res.*, 43, 5593, 1983.
113. **Winter G. and Harris, W.J.**, Humanized antibodies, *Trends Pharmacol. Sci.*, 14, 139, 1993.
114. **Waldmann, T.A.**, Genetically engineered monoclonal antibodies armed with radionuclides, *Year Immunol.*, 7, 205, 1993.
115. **Dalesandro, M.R., Pak, K-Y., Tam, S. et al.**, Effects of isotype and Fe region on in vivo function of a mouse/human chimeric CD4 antibody, *Int. Immunol.*, 5, 283, 1993.

Chapter 5

T CELL RECEPTOR-BASED THERAPY IN AUTOIMMUNE DISEASES

Thaila Ramanujam and William V. Williams

CONTENTS

I. INTRODUCTION

T lymphocytes are widely accepted as playing a major role in the pathogenesis of autoimmune diseases. T cells are activated via specific receptors, termed T cell antigen receptors or TCRs, which turn on a cascade of intracellular events culminating in cell activation and

0-8493-9422-8/94/$0.00+$.50

cytokine release that drives the inflammatory response. The antigens (Ag) that trigger the activation of these T cells for many diseases still remain at large. It becomes pertinent that in order to find the criminal we first go to the scene of crime. It is presumed that the unknown antigen is presented to the T cells in conjunction with a major histocompatibility complex (MHC) molecule. Understanding the structure of the T cell receptor and that of the Ag-MHC complex at a molecular level paves the way to developing novel treatment options. Targeting treatment strategies based on interaction of these critical molecules is an area of intense interest and ongoing research. This chapter discusses the molecular structure of T cell receptors, their interaction with major histocompatibility antigens, and the focus of this complex as a target to developing new treatment modalities.

II. THE MOLECULAR BASIS OF T CELL RECOGNITION

Edward Jenner, in his famous experiments demonstrating immunity to cow pox, described the term cell-mediated immunity. The immunity was transferred by a subset of lymphocytes felt to have been processed by the thymus and hence was named T lymphocytes. However, what conferred on these cells their antigen specificity remained a mystery for decades. It became apparent that antibodies and T cells differed in their antigen-binding capacity. Whereas the antibodies could bind an antigen in solution, T cells required that the antigen not only be bound but also be presented in association with a MHC molecule. Monoclonal antibodies have been powerful tools that have aided the definition of T cells into specialized subsets. In humans the antigens CD2 and CD3 are pan T cell markers that are seen in virtually all T cells. CD4 and CD5 are proteins that define helper cells, which are probably responsible for the activation and maturation of B cells and for induction of delayed-type hypersensitivity responses. The CD8 molecule is expressed on cells with the cytotoxic/suppressor phenotype which lyse target cells and controls antigen-specific chronic inflammatory reactions. The CD4 and CD8 molecules form subsidiary links with class II and class I MHC, respectively.[1] While these accessory molecules play a role in T cell activation, specific recognition and triggering is mediated by the T cell receptor (TCR)-CD3 complex. Monoclonal antibodies have greatly contributed to our understanding of the structure of TCR, which is a heterodimer consisting of 42,000 to 45,000 mol wt subunits. The basic structure of the TCR is the same regardless of whether they are expressed in CD4+, CD8+, or CD4-CD8- T cells. There are two chains which form a covalently associated heterodimer and which recognize the Ag-MHC complex. These two chains are noncovalently associated with several smaller proteins that comprise the CD3 complex. The entire TCR-CD3 complex typically consists of seven polypeptide chains. The TCR heterodimer is responsible for Ag-MHC recognition, while the CD3 complex transduces signals into the T cell following specific recognition.

It is now known that there exist two separate types of TCR that are derived from two separate T cell lineages. TCR1 is comprised of a $\gamma + \delta$ heterodimer, and is the first to appear in ontogeny. TCR2 with its α and β chains are found in the cells that generally predominate in adult life.[1] Antigen-MHC recognition by the variable regions of the α and β chains is the best characterized. Experiments done where the TCR genes were transfected from a cytolytic T cell clone to another clone of different specificity demonstrated that the transfected clones were able to lyse the target cells only when both α and β genes were expressed. This confirms Ag-MHC recognition by the TCR, demonstrating also that the signal transduction mediated by the TCR-CD3 complex is sufficient for full expression of functional activity.

TCR proteins were first characterized in 1983 and TCR genes were first cloned in 1984.[2-6] Original studies utilized cDNA clones expressed in T cells and identified rearrangements in various T cell DNAs by screening these clones. The complete primary sequence of these polypeptides was thus obtained. Shortly afterwards, discovery was made of γ and δ TCR which is similarly associated with CD3 as is α and β TCR. One to ten percent of peripheral cells and a vast majority of dendritic T cells in the skin are γ and δ T cells. While the overall structure of the α and β TCR is similar to the γ and δ TCR, they are encoded on genetically distinct loci.

TCR α and β chains are assembled similarly to antibodies. The genes encoding α and β/γ and δ polypeptides are comprised of V (variable), J (joining), and C (constant) regions on their loci, while the β and δ chains also have a D (diversity) region between the V and J regions in addition. These elements are homologous to those found on immunoglobulins. During T cell development, a V region is rearranged adjacent to (D)J region(s) (Figure 1). The V(D)J region is transcribed separated from the C region by an intron, which is spliced out during RNA processing. The fully rearranged/spliced V(D)JC transcript is translated in the endoplasmic reticulum, where assembly of the heterodimer and association with the CD3 complex takes place. The TCR-CD3 complex is transported to the surface where it interacts with Ag-MHC complexes leading to triggering of the T cell.

Mature T cells that bear α and β TCRs generally fall into two categories: CD4+ and CD8+. These accessory molecules impart "restriction" of the T cell either to class II or class I MHC molecules. Interestingly, the antigens presented via class I vs. class II MHC molecules differ. Class II MHC molecules present antigens that have been endocytosed from the outside of the antigen-presenting cell (APC). These endocytosed antigens are subsequently "processed" (broken down into short peptides) in endosomal compartments where they associate with class II MHC molecules, and are expressed on the surface of the APC. In contrast, class I MHC molecules present antigens that are synthesized by the host cell. These antigens (for example, viral proteins produced during infection of the cell) are synthesized on ribosomes either in the cytoplasm or on the rough endoplasmic reticulum. Those in the endoplasmic reticulum are carried into the Golgi apparatus, while those in the cytoplasm are felt to be transported into the Golgi by specific transporter molecules. Once in the Golgi, the antigens are processed and associate with class I MHC molecules. Subsequently, the Ag-MHC complex is transported to the cell surface of the APC. All cells of the body express class I MHC molecules (with the exception of the placenta and certain tumor cells). They serve as the surveillance system for infection or transformation of cells, leading to activation of CD8+ cytotoxic cells. In contrast, only "professional" APC (B cells, monocytes, macrophages, and dendritic cells) and a subset of T cells express class II MHC molecules. These professional APCs stimulate a CD4+ helper T cell response, with subsequent antibody and delayed-type hypersensitivity reactions. The different antigen-processing pathways are shown in Figure 2.

While antigen processing and presentation to class I MHC vs. class II MHC restricted antigens differs, the overall structure of the class I and class II MHC molecules are felt to be similar. Molecules within the MHC complex were initially recognized during the search for factors that caused allogenic graft rejection. While the structure of TCRs remains to be determined, the structure of several class I MHC molecules has been elucidated.[7-12] MHC class I molecules consist of a heavy peptide chain of 43 kDa noncovalently linked to a peptide called β2-microglobulin. MHC class I molecules are comprised of three external domains, the α1, α2, and α3 domains. β2-microglobulin noncovalently associates with the membrane proximal (α3) domain. Both β2-microglobulin and the α3 domain share the overall structure known as the "immunoglobulin fold", which is a beta-barrel structure formed by antiparallel β strands connected by reverse turns. In contrast, the α1 and α2 domains combine to form a pair of α-helices which are positioned on a β-pleated sheet floor. Each domain contributes one helix and half of the β sheet. Between the helices is a "groove" which is the antigen-binding site. Studies of co-crystal structures indicate that the antigens typically assume an extended conformation within the antigen-binding groove, with specific amino acid side chains occupying "pockets" within the groove.[9,10,12,13] These specificity pockets are important in selecting the antigenic peptides presented by the MHC molecule.

The structure of the class II molecule is similar to the crystal structure of a class I molecule.[14] Class II MHC molecules appear to have overall similar structures and peptide selectivity compared with class I MHC molecules.[14-16] For class II MHC molecules, there are

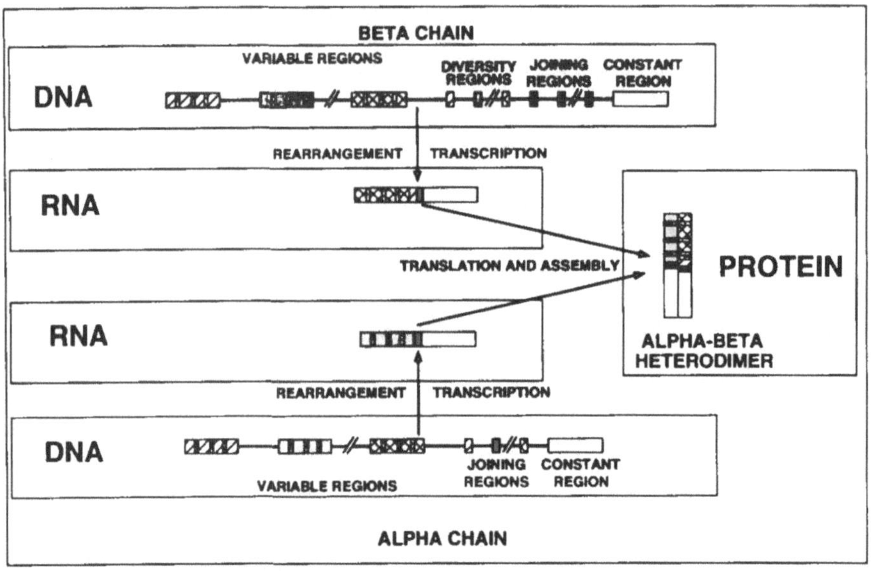

FIGURE 1. Genetic assembly of T cell receptors. The genes for the variable (V), diversity (D), and joining (J) regions are spliced together as DNA in the genome of the immature T cell. RNA processing splices the V(D)J region to the constant (C) region, with the mature V(D)JC transcript translated into protein, which assembles into a functional αβ heterodimer in the endoplasmic reticulum.

two chains, α and β, which each consist of two domains α1/α2 and β1/β2. The α1 and β1 domains combine to form the antigen-binding site, corresponding to the α1 and α2 domains of class I MHC molecules. This is a highly polymorphic system in that marked variability exists between individuals based on multiple allelic forms that are generated by point mutations, recombination, gene conversion, and homologous but unequal crossing over. In the human HLA-DR locus the variability resides in the β chain, while the α chain is invariant. The third hypervariable region of the first domain of the DRβ1 gene is polymorphic as evidenced by DNA sequence analysis. The positions of these polymorphisms are felt to be in the region proposed as the peptide binding groove. Small changes in these regions can greatly influence the involvement of the TCR in any given response. Thus, the structures seen by CD4+ and CD8+ T cells have overall similarities, but differ in the fine structural and chemical aspects of recognition both between these two cell subsets and among different individuals.

TCRs have not been well characterized in terms of their tertiary structures. Sequence homology to immunoglobulin molecules suggests that they have similar structures comprised on immunoglobulin-like domains as noted above. Several hypothetical models have been developed of TCRs based on homology to immunoglobulins.[17,18] These suggest a similar organization of the variable and constant regions as distinct domains, with the variable regions further subdivided into framework and hypervariable regions. The hypervariable regions on immunoglobulins that contact the antigen are called complementarity-determining regions (CDRs). In T cells the regions equivalent to CDR1 and CDR2 are encoded by the V gene and CDR3 equivalent region is formed by the combined efforts of V-(D)-J segments. The dissimilarity between the β chain V region as compared to the V region of immunoglobulin stems from the fact that the Vβ of T cells possess an additional region of amino acid variation. The Wu-Kabat variability coefficient, which is used to describe the susceptibility of an amino acid position to evolutionary replacements, highlights four hypervariable regions which are positioned similar to immunoglobulin CDRs along the chain.[19] The fourth CDR lies in a surface loop which corresponds to the framework 3 region of immunoglobulin V regions. A similar CDR4 may also exist for the α chain of the TCR. A hypothetical model of a TCR Vβ domain is shown in Figure 3.

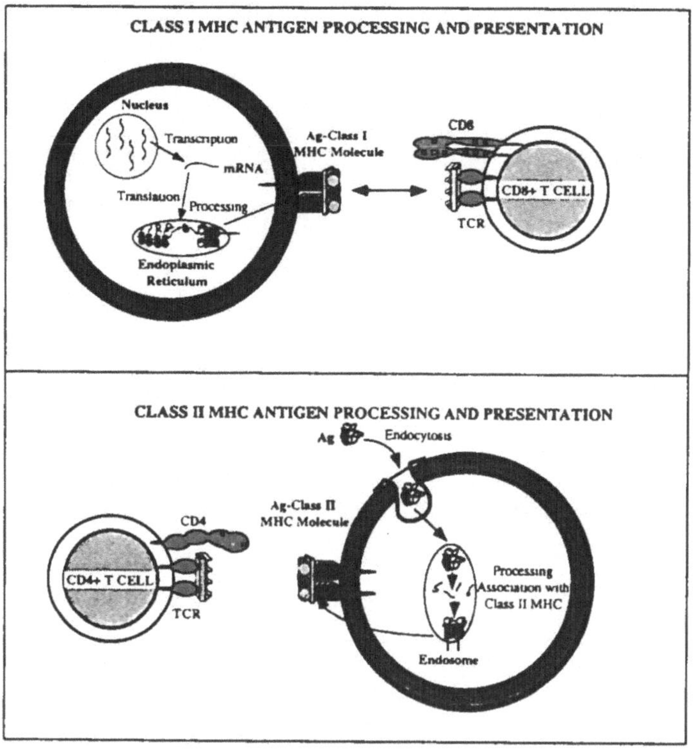

FIGURE 2. Antigen processing and presentation. In the MHC class I-dependent pathway (top), antigens (Ag) are endogenously synthesized in the endoplasmic reticulum. Once synthesized, they are processed into peptide fragments which associate with class I MHC molecules and are transported to the cell surface. This complex of Ag-class I MHC is recognized by CD8+ T cells via their T cell receptors (TCR) in conjunction with the CD8 molecule. In the MHC class II-dependent pathway (bottom), antigens are endocytosed from outside the cell into endosomal vesicles where they are processed into peptides and associate with class II MHC molecules. This Ag-class II MHC complex is transported to the cell surface where it is recognized by the TCRs on CD4+ T cells in conjunction with the CD4 molecule.

The fine specificity of T cells is attributed to the variable region that is found in the amino portions of the TCR polypeptide chains. The diversity of the TCRs is due to both the rearrangement and assembly of germline-encoded somatic elements (Figure 1), as well as the junctional variability between the V and (D)J regions (N region). This N region diversity is felt to be due to the addition of nucleotides prior to rearrangement by terminal deoxynucleotidyl transferase. Functionally, this results in greater diversity for the CDR3 regions compared with the CDR1,2, and 4 regions (Figure 3). Studies of TCR transgenic mice immunized with variant peptides have led to the hypothesis that the CDR3 regions directly contact antigen within the peptide-binding groove of MHC.[20] This would account for the greater diversity of TCR CDR3 regions compared with CDR1, 2, and 4, as the antigen is the most variable component of the Ag-MHC complex.

The human β chain complex is felt to have at least 57 variable gene segments that can be grouped into specific families.[2,21,22] The number of human TCR α chain families now is estimated at >28.[2,22-24] In contrast, the γ and δ TCR chains have a limited number of germline V regions available. 11 human Vγ and 5 Vδ genes have been well characterized thus far.[25-27] These differ from α and β TCRs in that they typically respond to nonpolymorphic antigens such as heat shock proteins. γ/δ-positive T cells tend to be located in the skin (including dendritic epidermal cells) and other epithelial surfaces, and display cytolytic activity when tested against specific targets. Their full role in the immune system has not been fully elucidated.

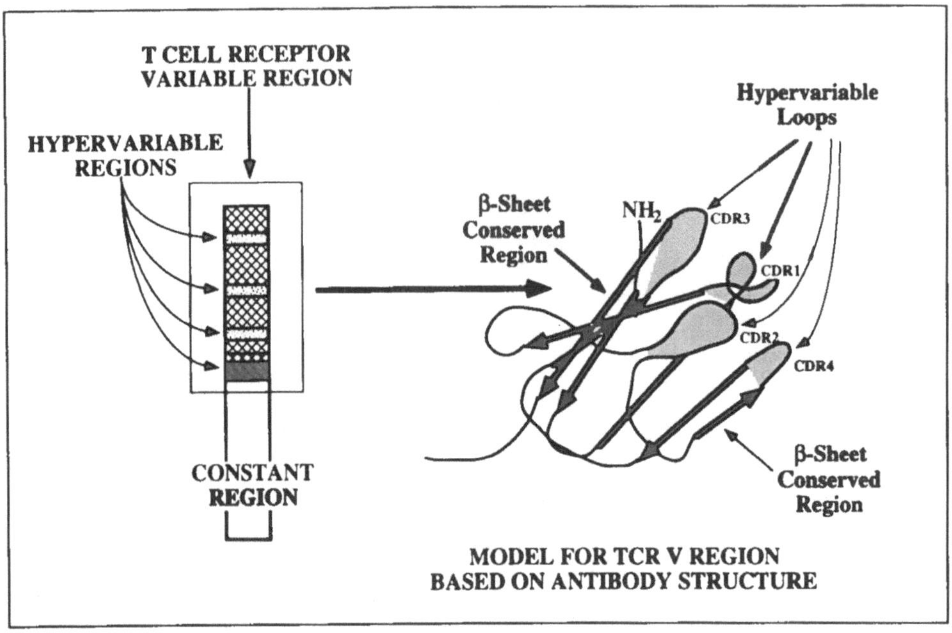

FIGURE 3. Structural model of a TCR variable region. The TCR V region sequence contains regions of hypervariability, also referred to as complementarity-determining regions (CDR1 to 4). These are believed to fold into an immunoglobulin fold analogous to immunoglobulin molecules with a β barrel structure positioning the CDRs on the same face of the molecule where they form reverse turn structures.

Resting lymphocytes undergo little transcription and lay silent until they are activated. The activation of these cells take place when a clonally restricted T cell antigen receptor is signaled through its effective binding to a peptide-MHC molecule on the surface of an APC.[1] TCR chains are thus rendered specific for a particular antigen in association with an MHC. A model of the receptor-ligand interaction that occurs between the TCR and MHC-bound antigen has been proposed. In this the configuration of the TCR is such that the third CDRs are very versatile and are assigned the role of recognizing the peptide that lies sandwiched within the clefts of the MHC molecule. Recent studies with transgenic mice that overexpress specific TCR V regions support recognition of antigen by CDR3 regions.[20,28] A schematic of the TCR → Ag-MHC trimolecular complex is shown in Figure 4.

Recent studies of intermolecular interactions between TCR and Ag-MHC suggest that the α chain of the TCR is primarily involved in MHC recognition.[29] Specific residues were identified that appear to interact with the β chain of class II MHC. This would orient the TCR α chain over the MHC class II β1 domain or the MHC class I α1 domain. While these studies have not yet been generalized to other systems, the overall picture emerging is of CDR3 interaction with Ag and CDR 1 and 2 interaction with MHC.[20]

An additional role has been suggested for the CDR4 region of TCR β chains; that of superantigen recognition. Superantigens are immunostimulatory molecules that activate a wide range of T cells bearing subsets of TCRs.[21,30-32] These include several bacterial toxins such as toxic shock syndrome toxin, staphylococcal enterotoxins, and *Mycoplasma arthritides* superantigen. Superantigens differ from conventional T cell antigens in several respects: they do not require processing by conventional antigen-processing pathways for their effects, they act on a wider range of T cells than conventional antigens, and they are not MHC restricted. Mutagenesis studies suggest that superantigens do not bind to MHC in the same orientation as conventional antigens. Instead, they bind to the "side" of the TCR and MHC molecules[33] (Figure 4). Thus, while superantigens require MHC molecules to stimulate T cells, they bind to nonpolymorphic regions of MHC, thereby bypassing MHC restriction in the classic sense.

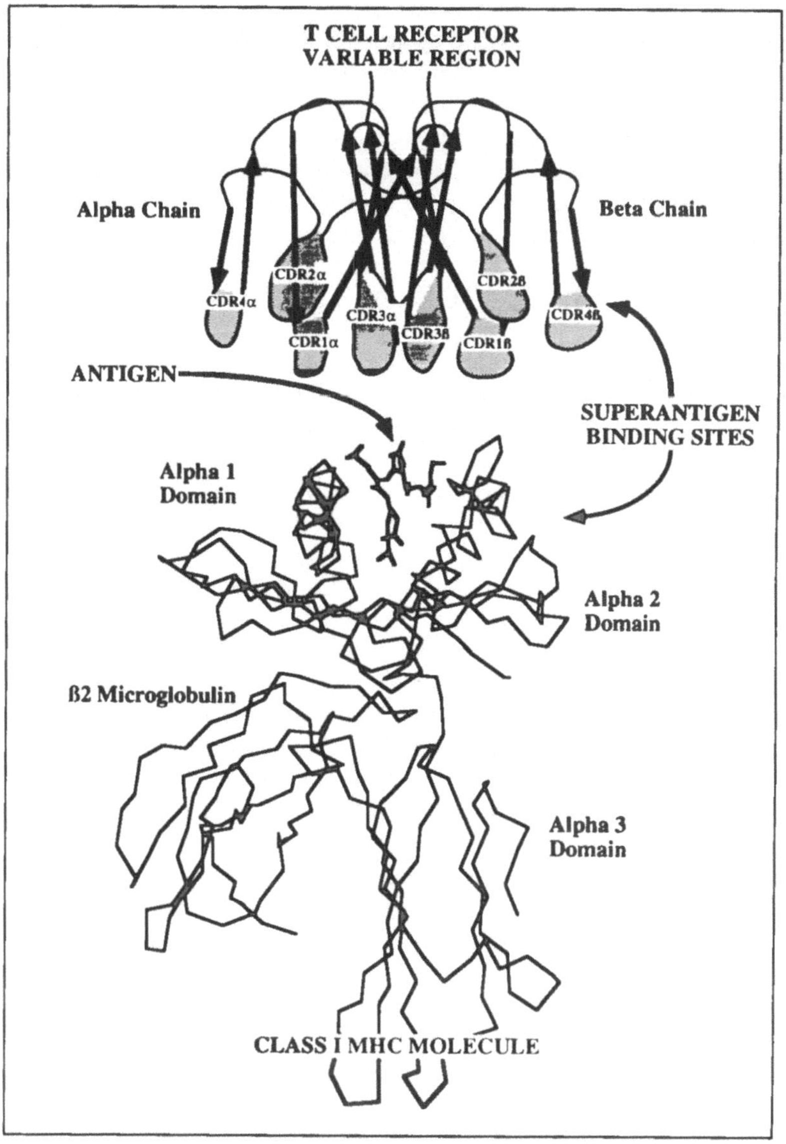

FIGURE 4. Artist's interpretation of TCR interaction with Ag-MHC. This structure of the Ag-MHC complex was derived by superimposing a random short peptide sequence on the antigen-binding groove of the MHC class I molecule HLA-A2[8], which was derived from the Brookhaven Protein Data Base on a Macintosh Quadra 950 computer using the MacImdad program (Molecular Applications Group, Stanford University, Palo Alto, CA). The TCR (artist's representation) is drawn based on immunoglobulin structure, but with the addition of a CDR4 region. There is evidence for this in the β chain,[19,204] whereas for the α chain this remains speculative. The orientation of the CDR3 regions over the antigen is according to Davis and colleagues.[17,20]

The CDR4 region is suggested to contact superantigens in this location. As several different TCRs from related families can share sequence motifs in their CDR4s, all the members of these families may be stimulated by a single superantigen. For example, *Mycoplasma arthritides* superantigen stimulates human T cells bearing Vβ17 and Vβ3 TCRs, which share a common motif in the CDR4 region. Superantigens, by their broad immunostimulatory capacity, have been postulated to play a role in autoimmune disease pathogenesis.

Thus, the interaction between TCR, Ag, and MHC is multifaceted and quite versatile. The regulation of immune responsiveness has evolved to eliminate autoreactive TCRs and to build effective responses against foreign pathogens. It is pertinent to note that studies of transgenic mice that overexpress autoreactive TCRs suggest that most autoreactive T cells are eliminated in the thymus.[34] Those autoreactive cells escaping to the periphery are inactivated and unable to respond (anergic). While several mechanisms exist for breaking tolerance, those active in humans with autoimmunity have not been fully clarified. This will only occur when pathogenic autoreactive cells are studied intensively for cross-reactivity, activation state, and susceptibility to regulation. However, some mechanisms of breaking tolerance have been elucidated in experimental models, and will be discussed below.

III. EXPERIMENTAL MODELS OF AUTOIMMUNE DISEASE

Experimental autoimmunity has been described in a large number of systems. These include organ-specific autoimmune models, such as thyroiditis and arthritis, systemic autoimmune diseases, such as systemic lupus erythematosus (SLE), and transgenic mouse models. The most germane of these with regard to TCR-based therapeutic approaches are the organ-specific autoimmune models. Several of these are reviewed briefly here, focusing on effective therapeutic approaches.

A. EXPERIMENTAL ALLERGIC ENCEPHALOMYELITIS (EAE)

EAE is a T cell-mediated, paralytic, autoimmune demyelinating disease that affects the central nervous system (CNS) of susceptible strains of mice or rats in response to antigens comprising the nerve sheath, such as myelin basic protein (MBP). In mice, the SJL and PL/J strains are susceptible to disease development following immunization with MBP or one of its peptides. The MHC type of the strains determine which determinant of MBP is encephalitogenic. In SJL ($H\text{-}2^s$) mice, the major determinant of disease is contained in amino acids 89-169 of MBP (specifically three peptides 89-100, 92-101, and 96-109 are implicated), while in PL/J mice ($H\text{-}2^u$), amino acids 1-9 are the major determinant.[35] In Lewis rats, the major encephalitogenic determinant is contained in amino acids 68-88 of MBP.[35-37] In all cases, Ia (MHC class II) molecules present the relevant peptides to CD4+ T cells. Thus, peptide selection by MHC molecules appears to play a role in the fine specificity of the autoimmune reaction.

Clones of T cells reactive to MBP are themselves capable of inducing EAE in healthy animals. When these clones were analyzed and their TCRs sequenced it became apparent that these cells utilized two Vβ and two Vα segments along with a limited set of J segments. The rat and mouse TCRs were quite closely related in sequence, comprising Vα2 or Vα4 paired with Vβ8 or Vβ13.[35-37] This finding has been followed by great enthusiasm in developing treatment strategies by using appropriate anti-Vβ monoclonal antibody or immunization with peptides derived from the specific V or J regions to immunize against the disease. Once the T cells are activated a variety of things happen. Critical to its activation is the interaction between class II antigen and the antigenic peptide. In addition, however, there appears to be a need for a simultaneous costimulatory signal from the APC. There are studies that have shown that in the absence of this costimulatory response T cells go into a state of inactivation and antigen-specific tolerance, a phenomenon referred to as clonal anergy.[38-40] Recent studies implicate interactions with the T cell surface antigen CD28 in preventing the anergic state.[41] This property can be utilized to treat autoimmune disease provided the susceptible MHC and the inciting antigen are known.

Recent studies of transgenic mice indicate the critical role of the TCR in EAE pathogenesis. Transgenic mice were developed with a rearranged TCR derived from a myelin basic protein-reactive T cell.[42] These mice expressed autoreactive T cells in the periphery. Activation of these autoreactive T cells by immunization with myelin basic protein and adjuvant plus pertussis toxin resulted in development of EAE. In addition, administration of pertussis toxin alone activated the T cells nonspecifically, with resultant EAE. While transgenic mice housed in sterile facilities were relatively normal, mice housed in nonsterile conditions developed spontaneous EAE, probably as a result of T cell activation in response to external stimuli.[42] This study strengthens the association between specific TCR expression and EAE development.

Various immunotherapies can be developed targeting the interaction of peptide, MHC, and TCR provided that the immune response to MBP was homogeneous in terms of epitope specificity and TCR usage. For example, tolerance can be induced to the major encephalitogenic determinant by neonatal administration of the corresponding peptide.[43] In adult animals, it is possible to treat the disease with antibodies against the implicated TCR V regions.[35,44] Experiments done in animal models used synthetic peptide representing a hypervariable region of the TCR Vβ molecule to immunize these animals. When Vβ8 cells specific to MBP were subsequently introduced, these animals were protected from developing EAE.[45] The TCR Vβ8 region contains a 21-amino acid sequence that includes the second complementarity-determining region (CDR2). This is presumably the region that made these cells immunogenic. The mechanism by which this process offers protection against the disease is by shifting the predominant T cell response away from the encephalitogenic epitope of this antigenic protein.[45] Although this study showed protection against the disease by downregulating the T cell response, other studies have shown upregulation and an enhancement in the disease expression.[46] The EAE model is a prototypic animal model for the human disease multiple sclerosis (MS), which is an inflammatory disease of the CNS characterized by myelin destruction. It has been shown that TCR Vα expression in MS brain lesions is restricted, suggesting that these specific chains might be responding to the epitope of an antigen that is involved in the disease pathogenesis (see below). Thus, these studies open the possibility of peptide immunization or monoclonal antibody treatment to modulate human disease.

B. EXPERIMENTAL AUTOIMMUNE THYROIDITIS (EAT)

In experimental autoimmune thyroiditis CD4+ T cells reactive against specific thyroidal protein (thyroglobulin) are able to transfer disease to naive recipients in experimental models.[47-49] These T cells are restricted by the IA^k determinant and can be blocked specifically by antibodies to IA^k.[49,50] Conversely, these animals can be protected against subsequent development of the disease and disease reversed by treatment with antibodies to the murine CD4 (L3T4) molecule.[51] These observations highlight the importance of interactions between CD4+ T cells and IA+ APCs in disease pathogenesis.

Recent studies point out the importance of T cell-derived cytokines in disease pathogenesis. Murine helper T cells are often subdivided based on the cytokines they produce following activation. TH1 cells produce cytokines including interleukin-2 and γ-interferon in response to stimulation, while TH2 cells do not produce interleukin-2 or γ-interferon, instead producing interleukin-4 and interleukin-5.[1] Interestingly, treatment of thyroglobulin-specific T cells *in vitro* with antibodies to the interleukin-2 receptor or γ-interferon alters the phenotype of the lesion transferred, with greater severity of the thyroiditis and granulomatous inflammation compared with predominately lymphocytic inflammation seen without such treatment.[52,53] These observations are relevant to human autoimmune diseases where granulomas are seen.

C. EXPERIMENTAL AUTOIMMUNE MYASTHENIA GRAVIS (EAMG)

The thymus is an important site of sensitization of autoreactive B and T cells in myasthenia gravis (MG). The acetylcholine receptor (AchR) is the target of antibodies that block acetylcholine binding at the neuromuscular junction, disrupting synaptic transmission and producing muscle weakness. Thus, MG represents a prototypic antibody-mediated autoimmune disease, with EAMG its experimental counterpart. However, T cells are necessary to induce production of the autoantibodies resulting in disease development. This is due to classic T cell-B cell collaboration with CD4+ T cells inducing antigen-specific antibody production. Interestingly, expression of the nicotinic AchR in thymic stromal cells was recently described.[54] As this protein is the product of multiple exons, and alternative splicing of mRNA has been described, exon usage was examined. While the dominant T and B cell epitopes were described in thymic AchR, exon 3A, which is expressed in peripheral muscle, was not detected in thymic stromal AchR. This suggests a role for thymic autoantigen expression in the pathogenesis of MG and EAMG.

In EAMG the autoantigen is structurally and immunologically complex. In spite of this, the TCR repertoire of AchR-specific T cells is dominated by Vβ6, which accounts for up to 75% of AchR-specific TCR Vβ regions in some studies.[55,56] This suggests that TCR-based approaches may also be applicable to this antibody-mediated autoimmune disease.[57]

D. COLLAGEN-INDUCED ARTHRITIS

This is a tissue-specific autoimmune disease that develops following immunization of susceptible strains of mice with type II collagen (which is expressed predominately in cartilage). A destructive arthritis results which mimics human rheumatoid arthritis in many of its aspects. Both antibodies to type II collagen and T cells are involved in disease pathogenesis, although T cells appear to play the predominant role in establishing chronic disease.[58,59] I-A-restricted T cell clones specific for type II collagen are capable of transferring disease.[60,61] Involvement of specific TCR V regions is implicated both by their presence at lesional sites and in draining lymph nodes,[62] and studies of transgenic mice that overexpress TCR V regions from arthritogenic T cell clones.[63] This experimental model, along with adjuvant arthritis, was the first in which T cell-specific disease suppression was demonstrated.[59,64] These studies used vaccination with antigen-specific T cell lines or antiserum to T cells to suppress disease. More specific therapies developed from these early observations. Disease suppression with TCR V region-specific antibodies has been demonstrated, although due to the involvement of multiple TCRs combinations of anti-TCR reagents may be more effective.[61,65,66] This points out the potential utility of this approach even in immunologically complex autoimmune diseases.

IV. PRINCIPLES OF TCR-BASED THERAPY

The lessons learned from the experimental models of autoimmunity suggest several approaches to TCR-based therapy. The general principle is to use our understanding of the TCR gene expression, the structure of the α and β chains and its recognition of a particular Ag-MHC complex to design novel therapies by targeting these structures. The potential targets in this trimolecular interaction are the TCR, the MHC molecule, and the Ag. Each of these targets has been successfully exploited in experimental systems. Recent advances have lead to the characterization of T cell epitopes of antigens that associate with either class I or class II MHC molecules, allowing blocking of the Ag-MHC interaction. Isolation of autoimmune disease-specific T cell clones and TCRs has also progressed recently. This critical understanding of the involvement of the TCR-MHC structure coupled with the results obtained from the prototypic animal studies set the stage for these novel therapies to be translated into the human system. This will lead us to the opportunity to manipulate these immune responses and aid us in developing novel immunotherapies to treat these diseases that have otherwise dismal chances of being cured. Some of the principles behind a few such modalities are listed below.

A. INHIBITORS OF ANTIGEN-MHC INTERACTION

Peptides with high affinity for MHC binding can be designed which have the potential to block MHC presentation of antigens by competitively binding to the antigen-binding cleft of the MHC susceptibility allele. This has recently been the subject of an excellent review.[67] These are, therefore, called MHC antagonists. The core regions of these peptides are typically six to eight amino acids. The relative role of these amino acids are analyzed using single amino acid substitutions. The resulting analogs have been tested for their ability to bind MHC, activate T cells, or induce an immune response. The interaction of class II and these peptides were very permissive and only about three of the amino acids were felt to be crucial for this interaction. As opposed to this, T cells that are very sensitive to amino acid substitutions accept only 10 to 20% of single amino acid substitutions. Therefore, it is relatively straightforward to develop specific MHC-binding peptides that inhibit activation of Ag-MHC-restricted T cells by developing analogs of the Ag that bind the specific MHC but fail to activate the T cell. Such analogs bind to the MHC molecule blocking binding of the antigenic peptide, thereby preventing T cell activation.

Recently, new technologies have been employed to identify peptide sequence motifs for specific MHC molecules. There are three predominant methodologies used to define MHC-binding motifs. The first developed relied on the ability of specific MHC-bearing APCs to present series of peptides to T cells and block presentation of antigenic peptides by competition.[68-70] Next, solid-phase assays were developed using purified MHC molecules and evaluating the ability of specific peptides to bind to them.[71-75] Most recently it has become possible to purify MHC molecules, eluting peptides from them, and subject them to a combination of automated Edman degradation and tandem mass spectrometry to identify shared amino acids at specific positions.[76-82] In addition, advances in X-ray crystallography have allowed elucidation of the structures of MHC molecules co-crystallized with specific antigens.[83-85] These have confirmed prior studies of MHC structures indicating the presence of specific peptide side chain binding "pockets" within the peptide-binding cleft of MHC.[10,86] These pockets are occupied by the side chains of the dominant "motif" amino acids that are selected by the MHC molecule.

This level of understanding of peptide-MHC interactions has allowed the development of specific antagonists of antigenic peptide binding.[87-91] The general scheme is shown in Figure 5. For this scheme to be effective, the disease-associated MHC molecule must be known. Specific peptides that bind to this MHC molecule are developed that inhibit binding of the pathogenic peptide Ag. This blocks binding and prevents activation of the pathogenic T cells. The major advantage of this strategy is that it is relatively specific in that only one MHC allele is inhibited, resulting in minor immunosuppression. The major disadvantage is that it requires repeated dosing with the immunosuppressive peptide. As most peptides are subject to degradation by proteases and peptidases, oral administration is unlikely to be useful. However, peptidomimetics could be developed for this application. It will be interesting to follow additional developments using this technology in the coming years.

B. ANTIBODIES TO SPECIFIC MHC MOLECULES

It has been known for many years that antibodies specific for one MHC molecule will specifically inhibit activation of T cells restricted by that MHC molecule.[1] This is felt to be due to blocking the ability of the TCR to bind to the Ag-MHC complex in the presence of the specific MHC molecule (see Figure 6). This phenomenon is strikingly specific as even closely related MHC-restricted responses are not inhibited by such reagents. However, they are also broad-based as all T cell responses restricted by that MHC molecule are inhibited. Thus, this is an immunosuppressive technique which is relatively specific.[92-94]

Anti-MHC antibodies have been utilized in a number of experimental models of autoimmunity to inhibit activation of pathogenic clones *in vitro* and *in vivo*. This includes several experimental models of diabetes[95-97] where antibodies to class II MHC molecules diminish the incidence of disease in treated animals. This has been demonstrated in the case of the spontaneously diabetic BB rat to require an intact immune system, and in fact to be transferable to naive BB rats by CD4+ T cells, suggesting that complex immunoregulatory systems may be involved in the response. In a related diabetes system, cyclophosphamide-induced and spontaneous diabetes in NOD/Shi/Kbe mice, anti-MHC class I Kd monoclonal antibody also decreases severity of disease.[98] Thus, both class I and class II restricted pathways are likely operative in diabetes development in this system.

In experimental autoimmune thyroiditis, antibodies to class II MHC molecules prevent induction of disease.[50,99] Interestingly, at the induction stage this appears to be due to elimination of I-A-positive cells, as antibodies to related class II MHC molecules expressed on the

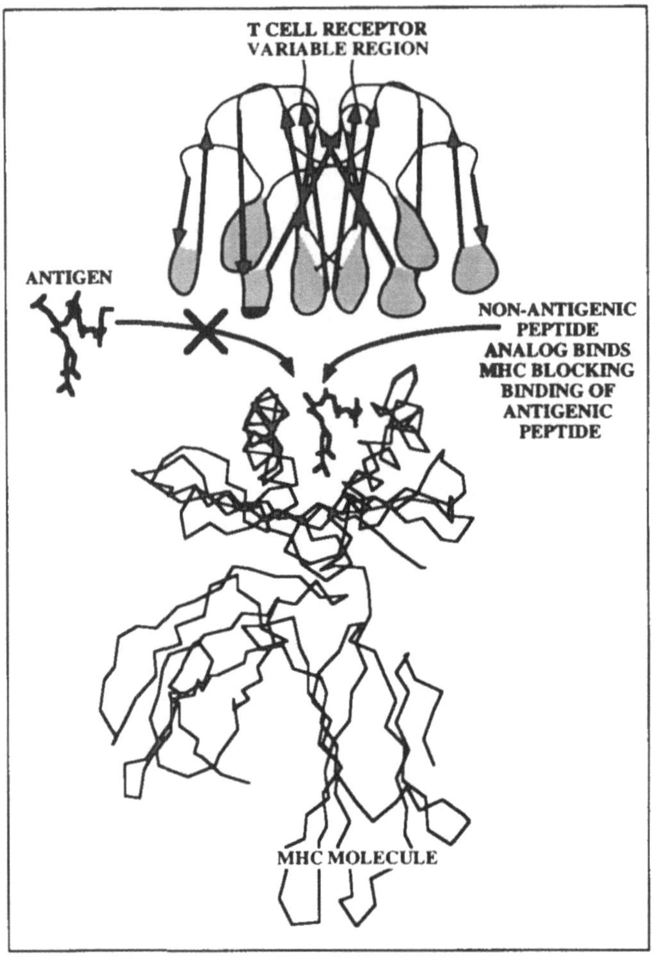

FIGURE 5. Blocking TCR interaction with Ag-MHC by antigen analogs. Labeling is as for Figure 4. In this schematic, an antigen analog binds the MHC molecule with high affinity, blocking binding of the antigen to MHC. This inhibits binding of the Ag-MHC-specific TCR, preventing T cell activation.

same cells in the mice but not genetically linked to disease induction are also effective. At later stages of pathogenesis only antibodies to the class II MHC susceptibility molecule prevent disease induction, and can be effective even if administered following sensitization of the T cells responsible for disease induction.[50] Similar observations have been made in experimental autoimmune uveitis, which is induced by immunization of susceptible rats with S-antigen,[100,101] and collagen-induced arthritis.[102,103] In collagen-induced arthritis, disease susceptibility has been finely mapped to specific residues on the antigen-binding portion of the MHC class II I-A molecule.[60,104] In this disease, treatment with anti-I-A antibodies is effective only if administered during the induction phase of the disease, but ineffective at later stages of disease pathogenesis.[102,103]

The most intensively studied experimental system in evaluating anti-MHC antibody therapy is EAE. In EAE, anti-MHC class II antibodies block *in vitro* activation of MBP-specific T cells and block their ability to transfer disease.[105] *In vivo* administration reverses acute disease and lessens the frequency of relapses in relapsing disease.[106] Suppression of disease was achieved even at late stages of pathogenesis.[107] These observations have been extended to systems employing rhesus monkeys, which develop EAE following subcutaneous immunization with calf brain homogenate in complete Freunds adjuvant.[108] Untreated, these animals invariably

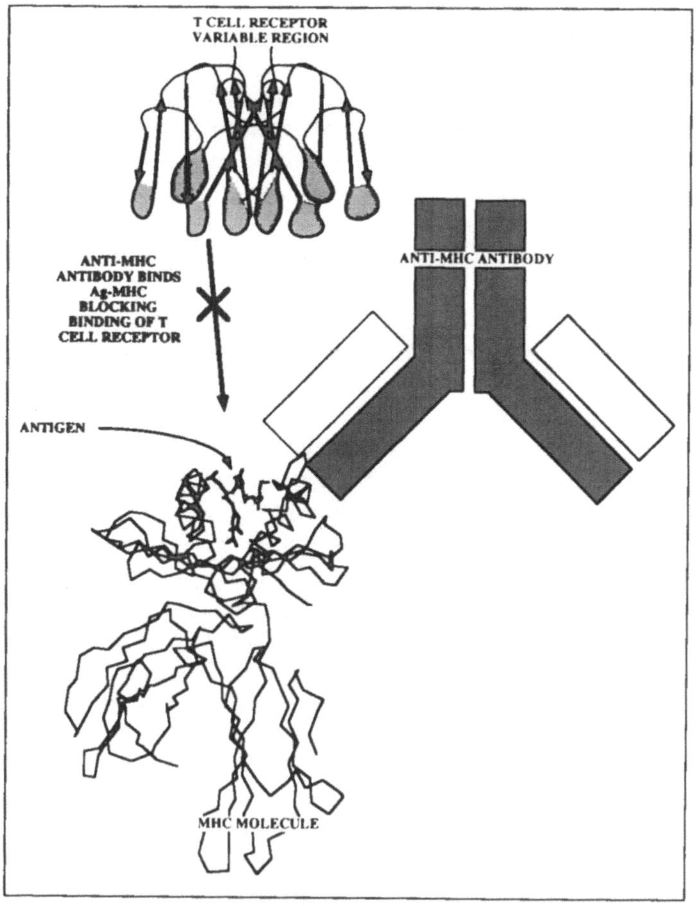

FIGURE 6. Blocking TCR interaction with Ag-MHC by anti-MHC antibodies. Labeling is as for Figure 4. In this schematic, an anti-MHC antibody binds the Ag-MHC complex, blocking binding of the TCR to the Ag-MHC.

die within a few days of disease onset. When treated at the first sign of disease with antibodies to a species cross-reactive antibody to HLA-DQW1 antigen, the treated animals survived significantly longer than untreated control animals. This suggests potential efficacy of this approach in primates.

While this approach is attractive, it does hold the potential for being generally immunosuppressive. Therefore, experiments have been carried out to determine the feasibility of developing monoclonal antibodies specific for Ag-MHC complexes. This has been achieved in the case of EAE where antibodies have been developed specific for the complex of myelin basic protein with the IA^s class II MHC molecule.[109] These antibodies were specific in their inhibition of T cell activation, as only MBP-specific T cell proliferation was blocked, implying specific immunosuppression. These antibodies also inhibited experimental allergic encephalomyelitis in $H\text{-}2^s$ mice. Thus, when the autoantigen and MHC restriction element are known, this technique holds promise for the development of extremely specific immunosuppressive therapy.

C. ANTIBODIES TO SPECIFIC TCR CHAINS

Monoclonal antibodies against particular subsets of lymphocytes that are critical to the disease development can be used to modulate the immune system. Experimental models indicate that antigen-driven autoimmune responses typically involve an oligoclonal expansion of T cells with restricted T cell receptor (TCR) V region usage.[37,44,45,110,111] This has been well documented in several animal models, including collagen-induced arthritis, where I-A-restricted T cell clones specific for type II collagen are capable of transferring disease,[60,61] and experimental autoimmune encephalomyelitis (EAE), where myelin basic protein-specific T cells restricted to specific MHC class II alleles are capable of causing disease on transfer to naive mice.[37] These oligoclonal populations are specific targets for immunotherapy of these autoimmune conditions, and can be targeted in a number of ways. Antibodies to specific TCR chains is one method which has been explored in a number of experimental systems. The interaction of an antibody with a specific TCR chain blocking recognition of Ag-MHC is shown in Figure 7.

In experimental autoimmune thyroiditis, there is evidence that antibodies to T cell subsets are capable of ameliorating disease.[51] Thus, depletion of broad T cell subsets are capable of preventing disease induction and of reversing disease following induction. More specific immunotherapy was evaluated by testing anti-clonotypic antibodies against a thyroglobulin-specific cytolytic T cell clone.[112] An anti-clonotype monoclonal antibody, presumably directed against the TCR of the cytotoxic T cell, was developed. Administration of this antibody 1 d prior to sensitization of susceptible mice prevented induction of disease.

The collagen-induced arthritis system is characterized by oligoclonal expansion of type II collagen-specific T cells.[62,113,114] The restriction in TCR expression is also evident *in vivo* in the joint and draining lymph nodes.[62] Interestingly, strains of mice that bear the susceptible MHC haplotype for collagen arthritis, but lack the capability of producing T cells with specific T cell receptors are resistant to disease induction.[113,115-118] Transgenic mice overexpressing a TCR from an arthritogenic T cell clone show increased susceptibility to disease.[63] In addition, antibodies to T cell surface markers are also capable of ameliorating disease.[119,120] These observations led to the use of antibodies to specific TCR V regions in treating and preventing collagen-induced arthritis. Antibodies to an arthritogenic T cell clone administered to rats just prior to and during induction of collagen-induced arthritis in rats suppressed disease.[61] In a mouse model system, treatment with monoclonal antibodies anti-Vβ8.1,2 or anti-Vβ5.1,2 decreased the incidence of disease, while antibodies to Vβ11 or Vβ6 had no effect and anti-CD4 antibodies completely ameliorated disease.[65] Interestingly, combined treatment with anti-Vβ2 and anti-Vβ5 monoclonal antibody efficiently reduced the development of disease, suggesting that combinations of TCR-specific antibodies can be more effective than monospecific therapy.

The disease-transferring T cells in EAE are oligoclonal, predominantly expressing members of the TCR Vβ8 gene family or Vβ13.[110,111,121-123] Antibodies to Vβ8 are capable of reducing the incidence and severity of disease.[44,45,121,122] Similar to the situation in collagen-induced arthritis, coadministration of antibodies to Vβ8 and Vβ13 are more effective in both preventing disease induction and in reversing established disease.[124] Thus, in many experimental models of human autoimmune disease antibodies to specific TCR chains are capable of both blocking disease induction and ameliorating established disease. This has led to great interest in defining potential oligoclonal expansions in human autoimmunity.

D. INHIBITION OF T CELL ACTIVATION BY Ag-MHC ANALOGS

A similar approach to the utilization of anti-TCR antibodies is to develop other molecules which can bind to the TCR and inhibit its interaction with Ag-MHC. One approach to this is to develop analogs of the Ag-MHC complex. It has been known for many years that T cells do not recognize free Ag with high affinity unless it is processed and bound to MHC. Therefore, antigen analogs are more effective in blocking binding of Ag to MHC than in binding to the TCR. However, all TCRs should have significant contacts with the MHC. Therefore, several investigators have attempted to use soluble analogs of MHC to inhibit T cell activation. This approach is schematized in Figure 8.

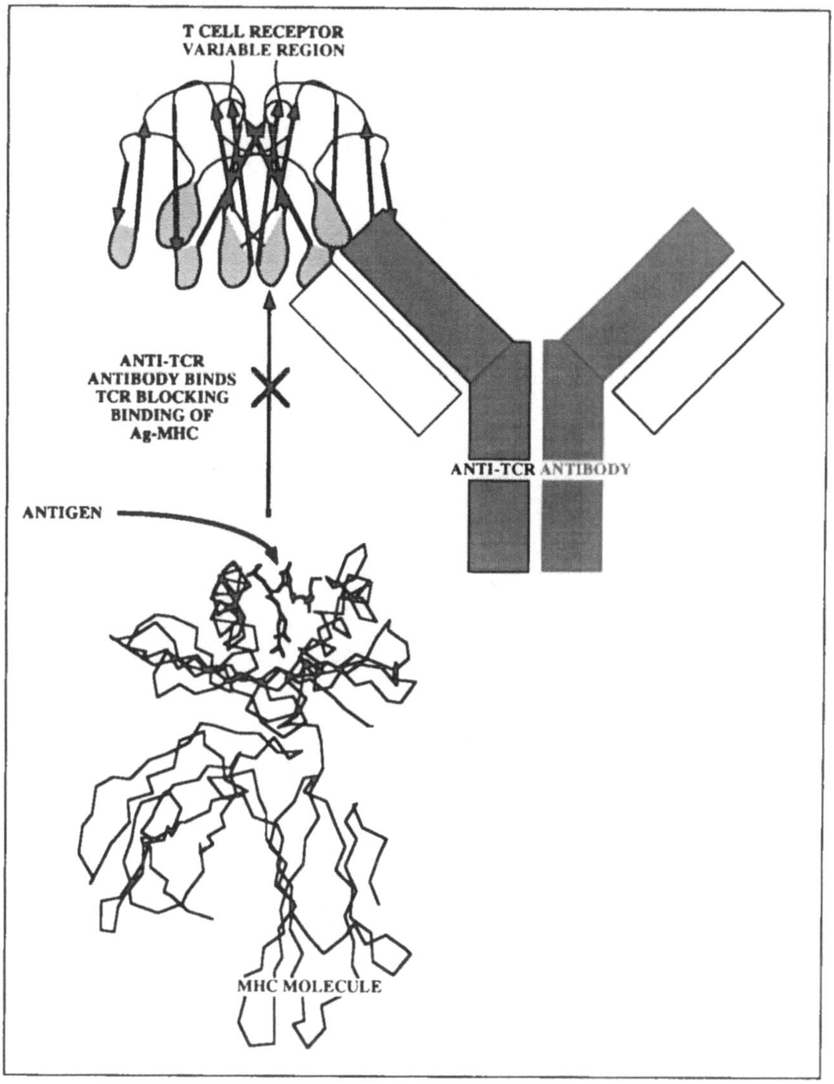

FIGURE 7. Blocking TCR interaction with Ag-MHC by anti-TCR antibodies. Labeling is as for Figure 4. In this schematic, an anti-TCR antibody binds the TCR, blocking binding of the TCR to the Ag-MHC complex.

The first systems used to evaluate the potential of this approach used recognition by T cells of allogenic MHC molecules. Such alloreactive T cells are the major triggers of graft and transplant rejection across MHC types. It was demonstrated in a murine system that an alloreactive cytolytic T cell clone directed against the murine MHC class I molecule H-2K^b was inhibited by a peptide corresponding to amino acids 163-174 of H-2K^b.[125-127] Preincubation experiments suggested that this might be due to interaction of H-2K^b 163-174 with the TCR. However, in a related series of experiments evaluating a distinct H-2K^b restricted cytolytic T cell, it was demonstrated to be inhibited by a peptide from amino acids 111-122.[128] However, it was also demonstrated that the alloreactive T cell also recognized the H-2K^b 111-122 peptide when presented by syngeneic H-2K^d molecules. It was further demonstrated that this resulted in autolysis of the T cells, due to self-presentation of the peptide. Thus, caution in interpreting the mechanism of action induced by these peptides was urged. In fact, several MHC-derived peptides have subsequently been described which bind to self MHC molecules and block antigen presentation by blocking Ag binding to MHC.[69,129]

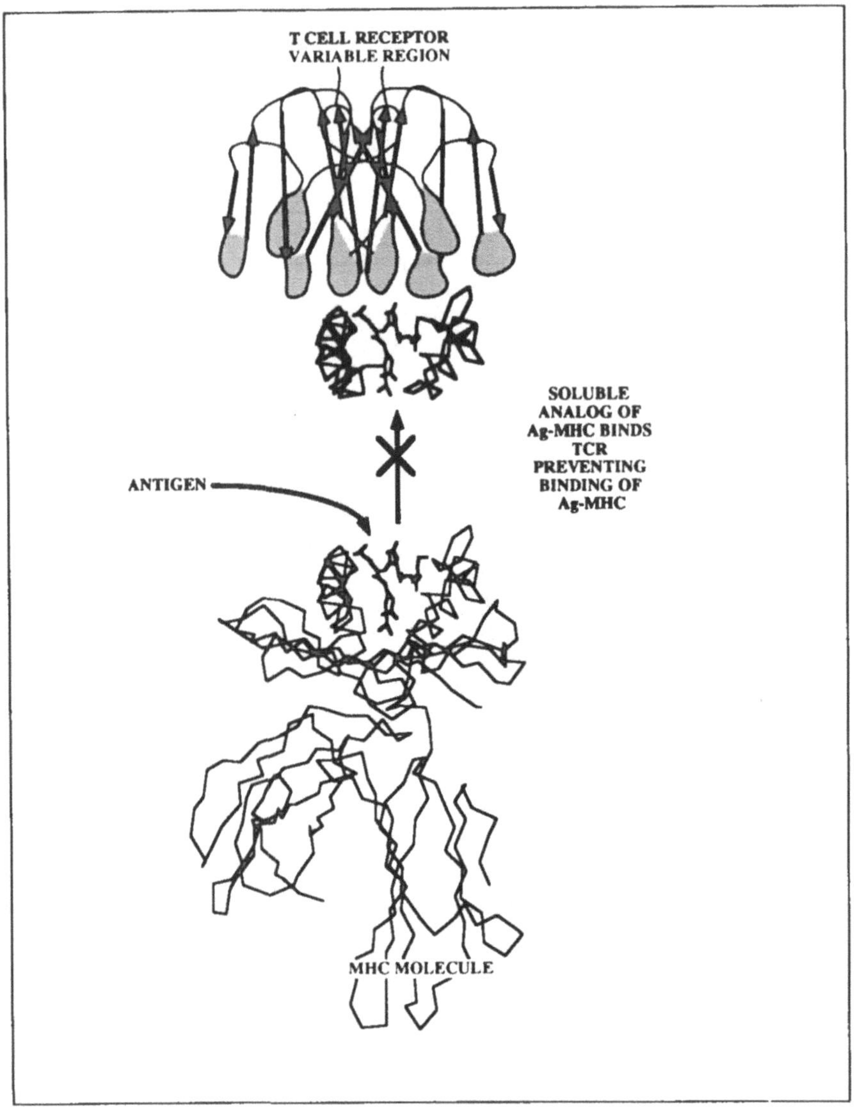

FIGURE 8. Blocking TCR interaction with Ag-MHC by Ag-MHC analogs. Labeling is as for Figure 4. In this schematic, an Ag-MHC analog binds the TCR, blocking binding to the Ag-MHC complex. The Ag-MHC analog could represent an intact MHC molecule, a portion of the MHC molecule, an intact Ag-MHC molecule, or an analog of the Ag-MHC complex.

More recently, this group studied the interaction of a murine helper T cell clone with syngeneic Ag-MHC using a self MHC-derived peptide.[130] These studies addressed the effects of a peptide derived from amino acids 68-83 of the MHC class II IA^k molecule (IA^k 68-83) predicted to represent a portion of an antigen/TCR-binding helix on the $IA^k\beta1$ domain. The IA^k 68-83 peptide was bound by a monoclonal anti-IA^k antibody and inhibited its binding to IA^k-bearing cells. The IA^k 68-83 peptide inhibited the antigen-dependent activation of an IA^k+con-albumin restricted T cell clone. The free peptide had a small effect in limiting binding of anti-clonotypic antibodies to the T cell clone, and a multivalent form bound to bovine serum albumin (BSA) had a more pronounced effect. The BSA-peptide conjugate, when fluoresceinated, specifically stained the T cell clone, and this was specifically competed by unfluoresceinated IA^k 68-83 peptide-BSA conjugate, as well as by anticlonotype. These results suggested that peptides derived from the predicted helical region of MHC class II molecules may have a direct interaction with T cell receptors. Thus, although it cannot be assumed that MHC-derived peptides function solely in binding the TCR and blocking interaction with Ag-MHC, they may also block association of Ag with MHC. Both mechanisms, however, may lead to immune suppression which may be of utility in treating autoimmune diseases.

Larger complexes of Ag-MHC also have been evaluated.[131] A peptide derived from myelin basic protein (MBP 91-103) was complexed to the IA^s molecule. Intravenous injections of 300 μg of MBP 91-103-IA^s complexes were effective in preventing experimental allergic encephalomyelitis. Similarly, administration of 45 μg of I-A^s protein complexed to peptide 139-151 from proteolipoprotein prevented mortality and significantly reduced paralysis induced by immunization with the proteolipoprotein peptide. These studies indicate that treatment with MHC-self-peptide complexes may be of therapeutic efficacy in treating autoimmune diseases when the putative autoantigen and the MHC-restricting elements are known.

E. T CELL VACCINATION

Vaccination against experimental autoimmune diseases using T cells was described in 1983 by Cohen's group.[64,132,133] It was demonstrated that T cell lines derived from rats immunized with Freund's complete adjuvant could be activated *in vitro* with *Mycobacterium tuberculosis* and would transfer arthritis to irradiated recipients.[64] However, nonirradiated recipients failed to develop arthritis, and in fact developed resistance to the subsequent induction of adjuvant arthritis by active immunization to *Mycobacteria*. Further studies indicated that thymus cells obtained from the vaccinated rats could transfer resistance to adjuvant arthritis to naive rats,[134] suggesting that complex immunoregulatory mechanisms are responsible for resistance. Other studies indicated that some arthritogenic T cell lines were ineffective immunogens unless treated with increased hydrostatic pressure, which presumably altered the physical nature of T cell surface proteins, rendering them more effective immunogens.[135]

Similar studies were carried out in the EAE system. Inoculation of rats with attenuated T cell lines specific for myelin basic protein vaccinated them against subsequent attempts to induce active EAE by injection of myelin basic protein in adjuvant.[133] This was demonstrated to be dependent upon the specific T cell epitope on myelin basic protein that the T cell lines were specific for, and suggested that acquired resistance to EAE was directed by the receptor specificity of the autoimmune T cells. When the draining lymph node cells of T cell vaccinated rats were evaluated, two subpopulations were identified. A CD4+ subpopulation, like myelin basic protein itself, stimulated the myelin basic protein-specific vaccinating clone, while the CD8+ subpopulation suppressed the response of the myelin basic protein-specific clone to myelin basic protein.[136,137] Similar observations were made by another group, in both the EAE system and in experimental autoimmune uveitis.[138,139] This indicates complex immunoregulatory events mediating the vaccination process. The means of attenuation are important in these studies, as treatment with increased hydrostatic pressure alone was ineffective as a means of attenuation, and vaccination with pressure-treated T cells actually induced mild signs of EAE.[140] However, a combination of increased hydrostatic pressure with irradiation was effective in attenuating the T cell lines, and such lines were effective vaccines. Interestingly, another model of EAE is also susceptible to modulation by T cell vaccination. In this rat model, hyperacute disease progression and severe demyelination is induced in animals with EAE by injection of a monoclonal antibody specific for a cell surface glycoprotein present on oligodendrocytes.[141] This antibody-hyperacute EAE is also preventable by T cell vaccination with MBP-specific T cell lines. Thus, T cell participation is implicated in this antibody-exacerbated model.

Similar studies were also carried out in experimental autoimmune thyroiditis (EAT). In EAT, thyroglobulin-specific T cell lines transfer disease to naive recipients.[47-49,142] Vaccination of susceptible mice with irradiated thyroglobulin-specific T cell lines prevented disease either by active immunization or passive transfer of the thyroiditogenic T cell lines.[142] In EAT, T cell vaccination induced inhibition of the afferent phase of the response as mediated by both CD4+ and CD8+ T cells, which appeared to function in a cooperative manner.[143] There was also a demonstrated synergism between administration of a low toleragenic dose of thyroglobulin prior to T cell vaccination.[144] Both of these observations suggest complex immunoregulatory phenomena requiring participation of several T cell subpopulations. The molecular basis for such immunoregulatory pathways in experimental autoimmunity remains to be established.

In spite of the successes of T cell vaccination in EAE, EAT, experimental arthritis, and experimental autoimmune uveitis, not all experimental models of autoimmunity have been amenable to this approach. T cell vaccination in experimental autoimmune neuritis did not induce resistance in Lewis rats immunized with P2 protein in complete Freund's adjuvant.[145] Similarly, in the experimental autoimmune myasthenia gravis model, vaccination with acetylcholine receptor-specific T cell lines did not manifest decreased antibody titers to acetylcholine receptor when rats were challenged with acetylcholine receptor. In fact, the antibody response to acetylcholine receptor was potentiated by the vaccine treatment.[146] Thus, protection is not invariably induced by these vaccination protocols. This indicates the need for additional methods of vaccination which may be more effective. One recent approach has been vaccination with T cell receptor-derived peptides.

Peptides made with the sequence of cloned T cells that are capable of transferring disease have been used to immunize against the development of the disease. The short peptides, although unlikely to stimulate B cell responses, should prime antigen-specific T cells as T cell recognition is conformation independent. Subsequent response to the same antigen enables the host to mount an exaggerated response by activating the B cells to turn on their antibody production. This form of prophylactic therapy has found its application in the EAE model.[45,147-149] It had previously been demonstrated that in a rat model of EAE, myelin basic protein-specific T cell clones used common Vβ-Dβ-Jβ and Jα regions (see above). Synthetic peptides were developed based on these shared sequences, and employed to vaccinate rats prior to induction of EAE. As for vaccination with whole T cell lines, vaccinated rats were resistant to induction of EAE.[45,147-149] A reduction in the myelin basic protein-reactive T cells in the CNS and periphery was documented in vaccinated rats.[150] It has been postulated that the mechanism of immunoregulation produced resulted from stimulation of anticlonotypic responses directed at endogenously synthesized TCR peptides presented by class I MHC on the surface of the autoreactive T cells, and further suggested that this mechanism may be part of the natural immunoregulation of T cell responses.[148] However, the results obtained by this group have not been uniformly replicated by others.[46,151] In fact, one study of TCR peptide vaccination in Lewis rats prior to induction of EAE resulted in prevention of disease in some animals, but enhanced disease followed by a prolonged neurologic deficit in others.[46] Such studies point out that when complex immunoregulatory circuits are involved in disease pathogenesis, the outcome of disease modification by immunomodulatory strategies can be difficult to predict.

In spite of these potential problems, vaccination against autoreactive T cell receptors or intact T cells does display the potential to specifically intervene in autoimmune disease pathogenesis. While the best strategy for such vaccination may not yet be established, the approach offers hope of long-lasting disease suppression with relative specificity. The key factor in implementing such a strategy is to understand the autoreactive T cell receptors involved in disease pathogenesis. In recent years, a great deal of progress has been made in characterizing potentially autoreactive T cell receptors in human diseases. These studies should allow implementation of T cell receptor-specific therapy.

V. T CELL RECEPTORS IN HUMAN AUTOIMMUNE DISEASES

Human autoimmune diseases include a spectrum of diseases ranging from organ-specific diseases such as Hashimoto's thyroiditis to the non-organ-specific diseases such as SLE. Many human autoimmune diseases have been linked genetically to specific MHC alleles, suggesting involvement of the TCR-Ag-MHC trimolecular complex in pathogenesis. These diseases appear to represent promising future clinical applications of immunotherapy as described above. The evidence for specific TCR involvement in several human autoimmune diseases is described here, as well as many initial clinical studies of specific immunotherapy. This is not intended as an exhaustive compilation of human autoimmunity, but rather intended to highlight insights from diseases where significant progress has been made.

A. RHEUMATOID ARTHRITIS

Rheumatoid arthritis (RA) is a prototypic autoimmune disorder that has increasing prevalence with advancing age up to the seventh decade of life.[152] The prevalence of "definite" RA increases with increasing age, approaching 2% of all males and 5% of all females over age 55.[153] RA is a major cause of disability in affected individuals, frequently crippling its victims and resulting in impaired function. The etiology of RA is unknown, although many studies have established a genetic predisposition. The variable age of onset of RA implies complex pathogenesis, with genetic and environmental features playing a role.

1. Genetic Predisposition for RA

Immunogenetic analysis reveals that RA is associated with HLA-DR4, and more specifically with glutamine/lysine residues at amino acids 70/71 of the HLA-DRβ chain.[154-159] Of the subtypes of DR-4, Dw4 and Dw14 are linked closely with RA. Seventy percent of all Caucasians with RA are DR4 positive, while the corresponding markers are DR1 for Israeli Jews and DR4 Dw15 for Japanese RA patients. Using alloreactive clones it is possible to identify common determinants in all patients with RA regardless of if they were DR4 positive or not. This implies that the disease susceptibility marker, such as the shared sequence around amino acid 71, may be a common epitope that some of these DR molecules share. Among the HLA haplotypes associated with RA, the DR4+ haplotype Dw10 gene differs from Dw4 and Dw14 by four amino acids clustered on the DRβ1 molecule. The DR4 Dw10 haplotype is not associated with RA, thereby implying that the DRβ1 gene product itself might account for the association with disease on susceptible haplotypes.[156]

Thus, the genetic susceptibility to RA can be mapped to a very well defined region on the polymorphic HLA-DRβ1 domain. This association is reminiscent of similar associations seen in experimental models of autoimmunity, such as those discussed above. Linkage to MHC in these models is due to the function of MHC molecules. These serve as molecular "templates" to which antigenic fragments stick. This antigen (Ag)-MHC complex is recognized by specific receptors on T lymphocytes (T cell receptors or TCRs). Recognition of Ag-MHC by specific TCRs leads to T cell triggering and initiation of an immune response. This is typified in experimental systems by the ability of autoantigen + MHC-specific T cell lines and clones to transfer disease to naive animals.[49,64,160,161] Thus, the immunopathogenic role of MHC in experimental systems of autoimmunity is well characterized. A similar role for HLA-DR4 and related haplotypes is postulated for RA. However, other possibilities exist. For example, it has been demonstrated that the DR4-associated sequence on the DRβ1 domain shares sequence homology with the Epstein-Barr virus gp110 sequence.[159] This raises the possibility that loss of tolerance to this epitope, as might occur following Epstein-Barr virus infection, could induce T cells that react to this HLA-DR epitope acting as the antigen (an MHC antigenic peptide presented by a self MHC molecule). Evidence for this hypothesis or the more standard autoimmune pathogenic schemes should be examined in light of pathologic and immunologic studies of RA.

2. Pathogenesis of RA

Rheumatoid arthritis is characterized pathologically by proliferation of synovial fibroblast-like and macrophage-like cells and infiltration of the synovium with lymphocytes.[162] The steps central to RA pathogenesis have been debated for many years. Early theories were influenced by the characteristic presence of rheumatoid factor in the peripheral blood of RA patients.[162,163] It was postulated that rheumatoid factor production (perhaps locally in the synovium) triggered an immune complex-mediated inflammatory cascade with resultant synovitis. When the HLA-DR associations of RA became clearer, as well as the functions of HLA molecules, these theories were called into question as it was difficult to reconcile an immune complex-mediated disease with an HLA linkage. Also, seronegative rheumatoid arthritis became a better recognized entity, and these patients lack significant quantities of rheumatoid factor. Conversely, many normal individuals express high levels of rheumatoid factor without the development of rheumatoid arthritis.[164] Thus, a role for rheumatoid factor as the sole etiologic agent in RA was called into question.

As the role of MHC antigens in T cell activation became clarified, and the genetic linkage of RA to HLA-DR4 was established, additional theories of pathogenesis arose. These were centered around recognition of Ag-MHC by specific synovial T cells. It was felt that persistent antigenic stimulation might account for both the pathologic and immunogenetic characteristics of RA. As cytokines and lymphokines became better defined, additional studies characterizing their expression in rheumatoid synovial fluid and tissue were performed. In general, these documented high levels of monokines (interleukin-1β, interleukin 6, tumor necrosis factor-α, and granulocyte-macrophage colony stimulating factor), but low levels of lymphokines such as interleukin-2 and γ-interferon.[165-173] Fibroblast-derived cytokines and growth factors also appear to be present.[174-179] These findings have led some to postulate that the T cell response and T cell infiltration may not be central in the perpetuation of synovitis.[165] The suggestion was made that an ongoing interaction between type I macrophage-like synoviocytes and monokines produced by them stimulate type II fibroblast-like synoviocytes to produce cytokines and growth factors which then stimulate the type I synoviocytes in a vicious cycle. These factors would in turn stimulate endothelial expression of cell adhesion molecules, which would selectively result in T cell accumulation in the synovium.[165] While this hypothesis may account for the ongoing synovial proliferation and destructive aspects of rheumatoid arthritis, it does not address either the role of HLA-DR antigens or the inciting factors that initiate disease. In addition, synovial T cells do express message for a number of cytokines,[180] indicating that they are activated *in vivo*.

Rheumatoid synovial T cells are predominantly of the helper (CD4+) phenotype, more specifically the CD4+CDw29+ subset.[181-185] Such CD4+ T cells are typically activated by an antigenic peptide complexed with class II MHC molecules (HLA-DR/DP/DQ). Many studies indicate high levels of HLA-DR expression in rheumatoid synovium.[162,185] The high DR expression suggests persistent antigen presentation and stimulation of the T cell infiltrates. An autoimmune cycle of persistent antigen presentation, T cell stimulation, cytokine secretion, synovial cell activation, and tissue destruction may result. T cell activation is probably an early event in this cycle.

3. T Cell Receptors in RA

Several studies have attempted to address the potential antigen specificity of rheumatoid synovial T cells by seeking evidence of a restricted TCR repertoire. Early studies of RA synovial T cell populations provided evidence both for and against the presence of oligoclonality.[154,186-195] These studies generally employed Southern analysis searching for restriction fragment length polymorphisms (RFLPs) to determine the oligoclonality of the populations analyzed. More recent studies have utilized DNA amplification via the polymerase chain reaction (PCR) in conjunction with family-specific oligonucleotide primers to assess the T cell populations present in RA synovial fluid[190,196-199] and tissue.[200-203] In this technique, synovial RNA is extracted and complementary DNA (cDNA) synthesized by reverse transcription (RT). The cDNA serves as a template for DNA amplification with oligonucleotide primers specific for the different TCR families. This "RT-PCR" technique allows evaluation of the TCR families present, as well as providing a source of TCR fragments for cloning and evaluation of the heterogeneity of the T cell response. This is important as T cell responses that are antigen-driven tend to also exhibit oligoclonality. An example of the family-specific amplification of TCRs from rheumatoid synovial tissue is shown in Figure 9. In this figure, the family specific oligonucleotides were used to direct amplification of synovial tissue cDNA with detection utilizing a radiolabeled internal constant region probe. As can be seen, the heterogeneity varies widely from patient to patient, with some quite diverse and some quite restricted. It is noteworthy that these studies utilized synovial tissue obtained at the time of joint surgery, indicating chronic disease. Thus, the finding of limited heterogeneity in any of these cases strongly implies an antigen-driven process.

Several studies have found some evidence of oligoclonality in rheumatoid synovial T cells, with the most extensive analysis having been performed on TCR Vβ genes. Paliard et al. compared the frequency of TCR Vβ transcripts present in RA synovial fluid and blood of the same individuals.[196] Their studies focused attention on the Vβ14 family, as Vβ14 expression was demonstrated to be higher in synovial fluid from these individuals. Sequence analysis of the TCR Vβ14 PCR products after cloning revealed oligoclonality.[196] Sioud et al. found similar results with elevated synovial:peripheral Vβ14 in rheumatoid arthritis patients.[199] Howell et al. studied TCR Vβ regions in rheumatoid synovial tissue T cells, specifically those T cells which expressed interleukin-2 receptor and therefore represented *in vivo* activated cells.[200] They found frequent expression of Vβ17, and the Vβ17 PCR products also showed evidence of oligoclonality. Studies from our group demonstrated a higher prevalence of Vβ12, Vβ14, and Vβ17 in rheumatoid synovium compared with the other TCR families.[201] More recently, these have been demonstrated to be oligoclonal on sequence analysis.[204] While other studies, most of which examined material from relatively few patients, have not confirmed the potential involvement of these specific TCRs,[190,198,202,203] four studies implicate members of the Vβ3-Vβ14-Vβ17 "extended family" of TCRs.[196,199-201] These TCRs are interesting as they have related sequences, and have been characterized as responsive to specific "superantigens".[30,205] Thus, the most recent evidence indicates an oligoclonal response in RA, linked to TCRs characterized by common superantigen reactivity.

When the sequences of the rheumatoid synovial TCRs are examined, several additional insights are obtained. The previously published sequences of several Vβ3, Vβ14, and Vβ17 TCRs[196,200,201] have been listed with the V-D-J sequences in Table 1. It is apparent that only a few J regions (Jβ1.1, 1.2, 2.1, 2.3, and 2.7) account for the vast majority of J sequences. When the NDβN regions of these receptors are analyzed within each of these Jβ families, some recurrent motifs are seen. For the Jβ1.1 TCRs, the NDβN region has at least one positive charge in 5/9 clones, and this always includes the last or second to last position in the NDβN region. For the Jβ1.2 TCRs, the NDβN region has at least one positive charge in 4/4 sequences, and this occurs at the last NDβN residue in 3/4 sequences including the sequences of 2/2 "dominant" clones. Similarly, for Jβ2.1 the NDβN sequences display a positive charge in 7/12, including 3/4 dominant clones. The Jβ2.3 related NDβN sequences have a positive charge in 6/9 including all three dominant clones, with 5/9 having an arginine residue at the second to last position including 3/3 dominant clones. The frequent finding of positive charges at fixed positions in relation to the J region usage in the dominant clones is reminiscent of the T cell receptor contacts with antigen recently described by Jorgensen et al.[20] They studied TCR transgenic mice in which the T cells all expressed a common transgenic α chain and these mice were immunized with variants of a peptide that the transgenic TCR was specific for. It was

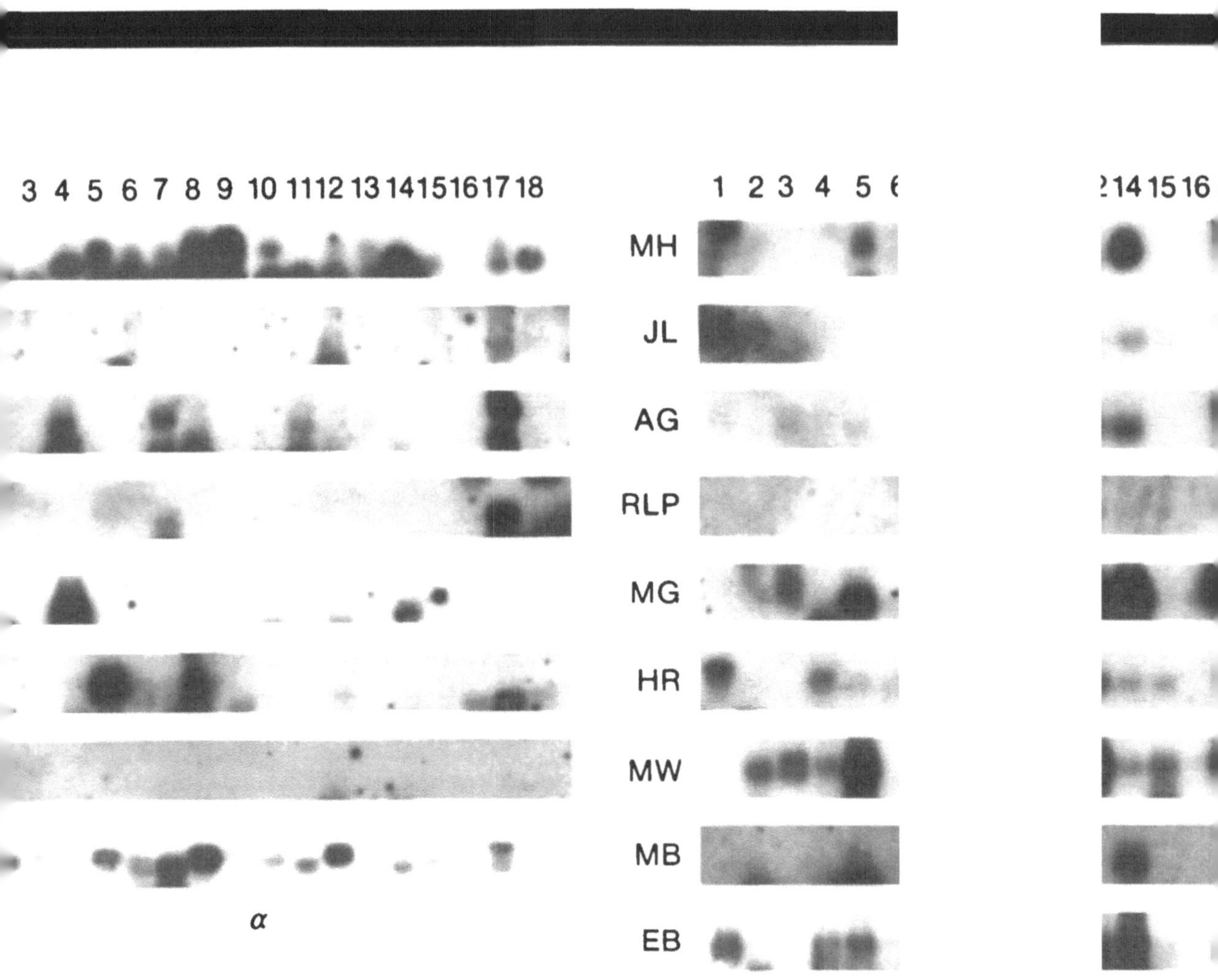

:R expression in rheumatoid synovium. Reverse transcription-polymerase chain reaction (RT-PCR) of TCR V
d detection by Southern blotting is as previously described.[201] The TCR Vα and Vβ families are shown along the
erage expression of TCR Vα regions was approximately half that of Vβ regions per synovium in this study, w
d.

eotides for spe
for the individ
l Vα1 and 17

TABLE 1
V-D-J Sequences of Rheumatoid Synovial T Cell Receptor β Chains

	% of Clones	V seq	$ND_{\beta}N$	J Sequence	J Region
Paliard[196]					
RA-2 Vβ14:	61%	YFCASSL	SRP	DTQYFGPGTRLTVL	Jβ2.3
	11%	YFCASSL	YGTRN	TQYFGPGTRLTVL	Jβ2.3
RA-1 Vβ14:	62%	YFCASS	TG	NTEAFFGQGTRLVV	Jβ1.1
	10%	YFCAS	RLAS	NEQFFGPGTRLTVL	Jβ2.1
RA-5 Vβ14:	32%	YFCAS	NPGGV	NTEAFFGQGTRLVV	Jβ1.1
	14%	YFCASS	PRGAY	TQYFGPGTRLTVL	Jβ2.3
Howell[200]					
1012 Vβ17	5/11	YLCASS	ISSG	SYNEQFFGPGTRLTVL	Jβ2.1
	5/11	YLCASS	PIGTGIH	GYTFGSGTRLTVV	Jβ1.2
	1/11	YLCASS	IIEDSAG	EKLFFGSGTQLSVL	Jβ1.4
1012 Vβ3	2/6	YLCASS	RM	NTEAFFGQGTRLVV	Jβ1.1
	2/6	YLCASS	HLGHP	NTEAFFGQGTRLVV	Jβ1.1
	1/6	YLCASS	FRTTI	GYTFGSGTRLTVV	Jβ1.2
	1/6	YLCASS	QDRTTL	TGELFFGEGSRLTVL	Jβ2.2
1012 Vβ14	2/7	YFCASS	LGGAV	SYNEQFFGPGTRLTVL	Jβ2.1
	2/7	YFCASS	LASGGAV	SYNEQFFGPGTRLTVL	Jβ2.1
	1/7	YFCASS	RFGGDG	SYEQYFGPGTRLTVT	Jβ2.7
	1/7	YFCASS	PLAGV	NTGELFFGEGSRLTVL	Jβ2.2
	1/7	YFCASS	LSQATPLR		
1013 Vβ17	13/13	YLCAS	KGRDEPFF	YNEQFFGPGTRLTVL	Jβ2.1
1013 Vβ3	5/5	YLCASS	LGGE	ETQYFGPGTRLLVL	Jβ2.5
1014 Vβ17	Direct	YLCAS	VRDRR	NYGYTFGSGTRLTVV	Jβ1.2
1014 Vβ3	3/3	YLCASS	NRLR	QFFGPGTRLTVL	Jβ2.1
1015 Vβ17	Direct	YLCASS	SIDS	SYEQYFGPGTRLTVT	Jβ2.7
1015 Vβ3A	1/3	YLCASS	FSRGGTRI	TQYFGPGTRLTVL	Jβ2.3
1015 Vβ3B	1/3	YLCAS	TDS	STDTQYFGPGTRLTVL	Jβ2.3
	1/3	YLCAS	VVGIPPRTSD	NEQFFGPGTRLTVL	Jβ2.1
1015 Vβ14	6/6	YFCASS	LSFGGRMA	NEQFFGPGTRLTVL	Jβ2.1
1020 Vβ17	2/3	YLCASS	IVTGTT	YNEQFFGPGTRLTVL	Jβ2.1
	1/3	YLCAS	TAAGGA	DTQYFGPGTRLTVL	Jβ2.3
1020 Vβ3	5/7	YLCASS	LGLAGRP	DTQYFGPGTRLTVL	Jβ2.3
	1/7	YLCASS	LSGQGR	YNEQFFGPGTRLTVL	Jβ2.1
	1/7	YL	SSGSFG	SPLHFGNGTRLTVT	Jβ1.6
1020 Vβ14	1/3	YFCAS	RDFKGGR	NTEAFFGQGTRLVV	Jβ1.1
	1/3	YFCASS	FGEV	TEAFFGQGTRLVV	Jβ1.1
	1/3	YFCA	THPRDRH	TEAFFGQGTRLVV	Jβ1.1
Williams[204]					
Pt2 β14a	1/2	YFCASS	RQS	SGNTIYFGEGSWLTVV	Jβ1.3
Pt2 β14b	1/2	YFCASS	SVGSR	FGPGTRLTVT	Jβ2.7
Pt3 β3.1a	1/2	YLCASS	PTRQGAK	YFGPGTRLTVT	Jβ2.7
Pt3 β3.1b	1/2	YLCA	AEGNRRHKR	SYEQYFGPGTRLTVT	Jβ2.7
Pt3 β14a	1/2	YFCA	AALRHRARGGSTFRTS	AGTRLSVL	Jβ2.4
Pt3 β14b	1/2	YFCASS	LLGTGDLWPA	QHFGDGTRLSIL	Jβ1.5
Pt5 β3.1a	1/6	YLCASS	LTSV	TDTQYFGPGTRLTVL	Jβ2.3
Pt5 β3.1b	4/6	YLCASS	LLQRT	TTDTQYFGPGTRLTVL	Jβ2.3
Pt5 β3.1f	1/6	YLCASS	LDRG	EQYFGPGTRLTVT	Jβ2.7
Pt6 β3.1a	1/4	YLCASS	WG	TEAFFGQGTRLTVV	Jβ1.1
Pt6 β3.1b	1/4	YLCASS	PGRY	TEAFFGQGTRLTVV	Jβ1.1
Pt6 β3.1c	1/4	YLCASS	SQKPNSK	TFGSGTRFSVV	Jβ1.2
Pt6 β3.1d	1/4	YLCAS	RLGQGD	QPQHFGDGTRLSIL	Jβ1.5
Pt6 β14a	4/7	YFCASS	FEQG	YEQYFGPGTRLTVT	Jβ2.7
Pt6 β14e	1/7	YFCAS	TLGGGN	EQYFGPGTRLTVR	Jβ2.7
Pt6 β14f	1/7	YFCASS	LGGT	YNEQFFGPGTRLTVL	Jβ2.1

TABLE 1 (Continued)
V-D-J Sequences of Rheumatoid Synovial T Cell Receptor β Chains

	% of Clones	V seq	$ND_{\beta}N$	J Sequence	J Region
Pt6 β14g	1/7	YFCASS	PFSRAS	YGYTFGSGTRLTVV	Jβ1.2
Pt6 β17a	1/3	YLCASS	IGGQGLTG	AKNIQYFGAGTRPSVL	Jβ2.4
Pt6 β17b	1/3	YLCAS	RALLG	SYNEQFFGPGTRLTVL	Jβ2.1
Pt6 β17c	1/3	YLCASS	RLGA	SPSILVMGLDSPIL	Jβ1.5

noted that charge substitutions in the TCR contacting regions of the antigen often elicited reciprocal changes in the CDR3 regions of the TCR β chain. The charged residues which were presumably contacting antigen were typically seen in the NDβN region. Thus, the finding of recurrent positively charged residues in RA TCR NDβN regions suggests a negatively charged antigen.

It is also notable that the diversity of RA TCR α chains in general appears to be more limited than the β chains expressed,[201,202,206] although again there is not universal agreement on this point.[190,203] This is of particular interest, as recent studies map the MHC interaction site of TCRs to the α chain in some systems.[29] The genetic linkage of RA to sequence motifs in the HLA-DRβ1 domain could be "mirrored" by this restriction in α chain usage. Sequence analysis of α chains in RA has not progressed as rapidly as β chain sequence information,[206] and therefore the insights are more limited.

In spite of these advances, several features of RA pathogenesis remain unclear. If there is an antigen- or superantigen-driven response, what is the antigen responsible? Interestingly, both Vβ17 and Vβ3 have been reported as expressed on T cells activated by *Mycoplasma arthritides* superantigen.[200,205] Whether this superantigen plays a role in RA remains to be seen, although several clinical studies over the years have suggested a potential role for mycoplasma in RA pathogenesis.[207,208] The staphylococcal enterotoxin superantigens SEB and SEC2 also stimulate human Vβ12-, 14-, and 17-bearing T cells.[30] It is noteworthy that rheumatoid factors (IgM anti-IgG) bind the identical site on IgG molecules that interact with staphylococcal protein A.[209] A variety of other potential infectious agents have been associated with RA over the years.[163] Clear-cut evidence of intra-articular chronic infection, however, has not been established. This suggests other possibilities. For example, an acute or subacute infection could activate T cell clones that are cross-reactive with self proteins present in the synovium when presented by the appropriate MHC. In this instance, there may be an evolution of the immune response, from antigen-specific to autoreactive. The antigen-specific T cells should be present early in disease pathogenesis, with autoreactive T cells dominating later stages. Understanding the T cell receptors present on synovial T cells early during the pathogenesis of synovitis should allow analysis of the interaction of these TCRs with the inciting antigen-MHC complex.

A. TCR-BASED THERAPY IN RA

While the potential for TCR-based therapeutic approaches in RA is obvious, relatively few studies have been performed to date. Monoclonal antibodies to broad T cell subsets (CD4+ cells) have been attempted in RA with some efficacy,[210,211] indicating that therapy aimed at broad T cell subsets can be of some utility. Early attempts at T cell vaccination in RA[212] have not been fully reported in the literature, although the results will be of great interest.

Future investigations into TCR-based therapy of RA are likely to proceed in multiple directions. The well-defined HLA-DR linkage of disease makes RA an excellent target for MHC-blocking peptide therapy.[67] Recent studies have begun to dissect the MHC-interaction sites of HLA-DR binding peptides.[72,74,78,213] These studies have not yet exhaustively examined binding motifs to the RA-associated HLA-DR molecules, but this data should soon be available and allow development of specific antagonists based on competition for binding to

HLA-DR. T cell receptor vaccination studies using peptides derived from the CDR regions of the Vβ3/14/17 "superfamily" are a logical extension of the work to date. Additional vaccination approaches may also be contemplated, as well as development of monoclonal antibody-based therapeutic approaches. As of yet, monoclonals to Vβ17 have been developed,[205] but Vβ3 and Vβ14 are not recognized by these reagents, and they are murine monoclonals. They need to be humanized prior to their therapeutic application.

B. MULTIPLE SCLEROSIS

Multiple sclerosis (MS) is an autoimmune demyelinating disease of the central nervous system. Clinically, MS is characterized by progressive motor dysfunction, which evolves in a patchy distribution, and typically has a waxing and waning course. Pathologically, MS is characterized by inflammatory demyelinating lesions in the central nervous system. These MS lesions are called plaques and consist of large numbers of T cells. In addition to the brain, T cell infiltration is also seen in the cerebrospinal fluid (CSF). These T cells are felt to represent a very important aspect of MS pathogenesis in a fashion similar to the synovial-infiltrating T cells of rheumatoid synovitis. Activation of these T cells is central to development of the MS lesion.

1. Immunogenetics in Multiple Sclerosis

The Ag-MHC specificity of the MS plaque-infiltrating T cells has been the subject of intensive investigation. Genetically, MS has been linked to the MHC class II alleles HLA-DR2 and HLA-DQw1.[214,215] The DQ susceptibility has also been suggested to be linked to a glutamine residue in the DQα chain, although this may be due to linkage dysequilibrium.[215] Additional genetic susceptibility has been mapped to TCR loci, including the TCR α chain locus in,[216,217] a Cβ[218] and a Vβ8-Vβ11 related RFLP haplotype.[219,220] An interaction between HLA-DR2 and TCR α chain appears to confer additional susceptibility.[214] However, TCR α and β locus-linked susceptibility has been disputed in some studies.[221-224] Genetic linkage to both MHC class II and TCR loci has obvious implications for MS pathogenesis.

2. Antigen Specificity of T Cells in Multiple Sclerosis

In addition to these features, MS is also characterized by T cell reactivity to myelin basic protein and perhaps an additional protein expressed in nerve sheaths, proteolipid protein.[225-230] Epitope mapping of T cells responsive to myelin basic protein has implicated two regions with immunodominant epitopes including amino acids 84-102/89-106,[226,230] and 139-153/143-168/149-170.[228-230] These include both cytotoxic and helper T cell epitopes, and the HLA-DR restriction elements of myelin basic protein antigen presentation are over-represented in MS populations.[226] Thus, it has been postulated that the pathogenesis of MS closely parallels that of the mouse model EAE with myelin basic protein-reactive T cells infiltrating brain tissue, triggering inflammatory episodes with consequent demyelination. This has raised the potential of applying TCR-based therapeutic modalities that have been effective in EAE to therapy of MS. For this to be successful, the TCRs involved in development of MS should be characterized.

3. T Cell Receptors in Multiple Sclerosis

Studies of TCRs in MS were among the first to apply PCR technology to human autoimmune disease. In 1990, Oksenberg et al. reported a restricted heterogeneity of TCR α chains present in MS plaques.[231] They demonstrated a narrow restriction of only two to four rearranged TCR Vα transcripts in three MS brains. Vα12.1 transcripts were expressed with a limited number of Jα segments. Similar studies reveal that TCR expression in active lesions appears broader than in inactive, chronic lesions.[232]

Myelin basic protein-specific T cell clones from MS patients express a restricted usage of TCR Vβ genes, with some clones predominating in individuals (e.g., 75% of clones from one

MS patient expressed Vβ15).[225] Similarly, T cell clones derived from cerebrospinal fluid of MS patients are often oligoclonal without antigen stimulation.[233] RT-PCR analysis of 83 myelin basic protein-reactive T cell lines from MS patients and normal subjects revealed common usage of Vβ17 and Vβ12.[230] Vβ17-positive clones typically reacted with peptides corresponding to amino acids 84-102 of myelin basic protein, but Vβ17 expression was infrequent in T cell lines responding to a distinct epitope corresponding to amino acids 143-168.[230] However, other studies of myelin basic protein-reactive T cell clones, even those restricted by the same epitope, expressed multiple TCRs.[228]

Quantitative PCR analysis has indicated a skewing of the peripheral blood TCR β chain repertoire in peripheral blood of MS patients.[234] In some patients, brain tissue also revealed a preponderance of Vβ12 expression. Skewing has also been observed in myelin basic protein-reactive T cells from peripheral blood of MS patients,[227] but in this case the skewing was toward Vβ5.2 and, to a lesser extent, Vβ6.1. Vβ5.2 was also prominent in myelin basic protein-reactive T cell clones from MS patients restricted by HLA-DR2.[229] Recently, Vβ5.2 expression was detected in MS brain plaques from all patients with the HLA haplotype DRB1*1501, DQA1*0102, DQB1*0602, DPB1*0401.[235] Vβ5.2-Dβ-Jβ sequences described from the MS brain plaques encoded identical CDR3 regions as a Vβ5.2 T cell clone specific for myelin basic protein amino acids 89-106 derived from an individual with the HLA-DRB*1501, DQB*0602, DPB*0401 phenotype.[235] The same CDR3 sequence motif had been reported in myelin basic protein-reactive T cells from animals with EAE. This strongly supports the contention that such Vβ5.2-expressing T cells present in the MS brain plaques are specifically responding to myelin basic protein in the context of the specific MHC class II antigens, and are etiologic for the disease. Thus, molecular understanding of the TCR expression in human autoimmune disease can elucidate aspects of antigen specificity involved in autoimmune pathogenesis.

4. TCR-Based Approaches to Therapy of Multiple Sclerosis

The above observations have led to several potential approaches to immunotherapy of multiple sclerosis which exploit a molecular understanding of immunopathogenesis. Vaccination with attenuated T cell clones derived from cerebrospinal fluid of MS patients is being attempted.[236] Preliminary results suggest safety in this approach, but it remains too early to evaluate efficacy.

A related strategy is to develop suppressor T cells that will regulate autoreactive T cells. This has been performed *in vitro* with myelin basic protein-specific T cells.[237] Such suppressor T cells inhibit the activation of myelin basic protein-specific T cells. While such *in vitro* generated suppressor cells have not been administered to MS patients, an alternative strategy of developing T cell suppression has been evaluated. In this approach, oral administration of the antigen (myelin antigens) generates tolerance to that antigen. This has been evaluated recently as a potential therapy in MS.[238] In this preliminary trial, 6/15 individuals treated for 1 year with oral capsules of bovine myelin had at least one major exacerbation, compared with 12/15 individuals in the control group. This therapy reduced myelin basic protein-reactive T cells. This supports the role of myelin-reactive T cells in MS pathogenesis, and suggests one method for antigen-specific effective immunotherapy.

Perhaps the most theoretically ambitious TCR-based therapy of MS being attempted at present is vaccination against peptides derived from the TCR.[239] While these trials are still in progress, preliminary results indicate that anti-TCR immunity can be boosted efficiently and safely, with concomitant loss of myelin basic protein reactivity. The outcome of these limited trials will be important predominately for establishing the safety of these potentially specific approaches to therapy. Efficacy will not be readily evaluable until many trials targeting appropriate TCRs have been conducted, probably with several vaccination protocols.

C. DIABETES

Type I or insulin-dependent diabetes mellitus (IDDM) develops due to destruction of the insulin-secreting β cells of the pancreas. The islets of Langerhans are the portions of the pancreas that contain the β cells, and these are infiltrated with lymphocytes during the development of IDDM. The infiltration and subsequent destruction is extremely specific, as the exocrine portion of the pancreas is unaffected in IDDM, with only the islets suffering from damage.

A number of studies indicate a genetic linkage of IDDM with specific MHC haplotypes.[240-251] Prominent among the associations described is the finding of absence of aspartic acid at position 57 on the DQβ chain (DQβ 57 Asp-) and/or the presence of arginine at position 52 on the DQα chain (DQα 52 Arg+) in Caucasians with IDDM.[243,244,250,252] The combination of DQβ57 Asp-/DQα52 Arg+ may account for the greater prevalence of IDDM in heterozygotes due to transcomplementation.[244] While the HLA-IDDM associations in the Japanese are not explained by this model, these observations point out the central role of HLA in IDDM pathogenesis.

There have also been many studies searching for associations of IDDM with T cell haplotypes.[253-264] There has been evidence presented both for and against such an association. However, direct examination of islet-infiltrating lymphocytes in human IDDM is less well investigated. Activated T cells are present in the peripheral blood of newly diagnosed IDDM patients.[265] These are often oligoclonal in their TCR cell surface phenotype, although different Vβ families appeared augmented in individual patients. Examination of pancreatic tissue from IDDM patients reveals elevated Vβ8 expression, as well as increased expression of intercellular adhesion molecule-1 on vascular endothelium, which typically increases endothelial adhesion of mononuclear cells, increasing their accumulation in tissues.[257] Islet-reactive T cells are also obtained from the peripheral blood of newly diagnosed IDDM patients, probably representing autoreactive cells.[265] Thus, involvement of TCR-Ag-MHC is strongly implicated in the development of IDDM. While the HLA susceptibility appears relatively well defined, many studies remain to define the relevant TCRs and antigen(s).

D. OTHER AUTOIMMUNE DISEASES

Autoimmune destruction of the thyroid gland with resultant hypothyroidism occurs in autoimmune thyroiditis, a category which includes both Graves' disease and Hashimoto's disease. T cell receptor expression of thyroid-infiltrating lymphocytes has been analyzed in these diseases by RT-PCR with V region-specific oligonucleotides.[266-268] While the TCRs examined predominately represented polyclonal populations, there was evidence for restricted α-chain expression. Five of the 18 Vα genes were expressed by intrathyroidal T cells, compared with 17 Vα genes expressed in peripheral blood T cells from the same patients.[266] While the predominantly expressed Vα genes differed from patient to patient, the restricted number of α chains seen raises the potential for TCR-based therapeutic approaches.

Myasthenia gravis is a neuromuscular disease caused by autoimmune destruction of acetylcholine receptors at the neuromuscular junction. While autoantibodies play a major role in pathogenesis of this disease, their production is likely dependent on acetylcholine receptor-specific T cells which provide T cell help for autoantibody production. Thus, identification of autoreactive TCRs to the acetylcholine receptor offers a potential avenue for therapeutic intervention. Acetylcholine receptor-reactive T and B cells are demonstrable in the peripheral blood of myasthenia gravis patients at an elevated frequency.[269] T cell epitopes on the acetylcholine receptor have been identified on both the α and δ subunits.[270,271] Abnormal TCR V region usage in the peripheral blood of myasthenia gravis patients has also been observed.[272] Additional studies are needed to further clarify the TCRs used in recognition of acetylcholine receptor in this disease.

Many other autoimmune diseases are potential targets for TCR-based therapeutic approaches. These include diseases such as psoriasis, scleroderma, polymyositis, dermatomyositis, ankylosing spondylitis, Crohn's disease, ulcerative colitis, sarcoidosis, pulmonary fibrosis, temporal arteritis, and primary biliary cirrhosis to name only a few. The involvement of lymphocytic infiltrates including T cells in these and other diseases indicates the potentially central role specific TCRs play in pathogenesis. As additional tools for examining the T cell repertoire in these diseases become available, this potential will be further clarified.

VI. SUMMARY

The engagement of a specific TCR by a specific Ag-MHC complex remains one of the most highly specific interactions in immunology. The recent strides made in understanding this trimolecular complex has allowed a number of strategies for inhibiting this interaction to be developed. Deleting the autoreactive T cells by either vaccination or anti-TCR reagents is perhaps the most actively pursued at this time. Blocking antigen binding to MHC or inhibiting the interaction between TCR and Ag-MHC with reagents directed at the MHC also show considerable promise. It remains unclear at this time which one or which combination of these strategies will be most beneficial in the treatment of human autoimmune diseases. However, it is clear that these strategies offer the potential for effective, specific therapy with few side effects. These should be welcomed by sufferers of these chronic conditions as well as their physicians. More importantly, by attempting these therapies we will all learn a great deal about the etiology and pathogenesis of these diseases, and about the normal and abnormal functioning of the immune system. With greater understanding, improved therapeutic approaches will become feasible.

REFERENCES

1. **Paul, W.,** *Fundamental Immunology,* Raven Press, New York, 1989.
2. **Toyonaga, B. and Mak, T.W.,** Genes of the T-cell antigen receptor in normal and malignant cells, *Annu. Rev. Immunol.,* 5, 585, 1987.
3. **Davis, M.M. and Bjorkman, P.J.,** T-cell antigen receptor genes and T-cell recognition, *Nature,* 334, 395, 1988.
4. **Haskins, K., Kubo, R., White, J., Pigeon, M., Kappler, J., and Marrack, P.,** The major histocompatibility complex-restricted antigen receptor on T cells. I. Isolation with a monoclonal antibody, *J. Exp. Med.,* 157, 1149, 1983.
5. **Meuer, S.C., Fitzgerald, K.A., Hussey, R.E., Hodgdon, J.C., Schlossman, S.F., and Reinherz, E.L.,** Clonotypic structures involved in antigen-specific human T-cell function. Relationship to the T3 molecular complex, *J. Exp. Med.,* 157, 705, 1983.
6. **Hedrick, S.M., Cohen, D.I., Nielsen, D.A., and Davis, M.M.,** Isolation of cDNA clones encoding T cell-specific membrane-associated proteins, *Nature,* 308, 149, 1984.
7. **Bjorkman, P.J., Saper, M.A., Samraoui, B., Bennett, W.S., Strominger, J.L., and Wiley, D.C.,** The foreign antigen binding site and T cell recognition regions of class I histocompatibility antigens, *Nature,* 329, 512, 1987.
8. **Bjorkman, P.J., Saper, M.A., Samraoui, B., Bennett, W.S., Strominger, J.L., and Wiley, D.C.,** Structure of the human class I histocompatibility antigen, HLA-A2, *Nature,* 329, 506, 1987.
9. **Garrett, T.P., Saper, M.A., Bjorkman, P.J., Strominger, J.L., and Wiley, D.C.,** Specificity pockets for the side chains of peptide antigens in HLA-Aw68 [see comments], *Nature,* 342, 692, 1989.
10. **Madden, D.R., Gorga, J.C., Strominger, J.L., and Wiley, D.C.,** The structure of HLA-B27 reveals nonamer self-peptides bound in an extended conformation, *Nature,* 353, 321, 1991.
11. **Madden, D.R., Gorga, J.C., Strominger, J.L., and Wiley, D.C.,** The three-dimensional structure of HLA-B27 at 2.1 Å resolution suggests a general mechanism for tight peptide binding to MHC, *Cell,* 70, 1035, 1992.
12. **Garboczi, D.N., Hung, D.T., and Wiley, D.C.,** HLA-A2-peptide complexes: refolding and crystallization of molecules expressed in Escherichia coli and complexed with single antigenic peptides, *Proc. Natl. Acad. Sci. U.S.A.,* 89, 3429, 1992.

13. **Parker, K.C., Silver, M.L., and Wiley, D.C.**, An HLA-A2/beta 2-microglobulin/peptide complex assembled from subunits expressed separately in Escherichia coli, *Mol. Immunol.*, 29, 371, 1992.
14. **Brown, J.H., Jardetzky, T.S., Gerga, J.C., Stern, L.J., Urban, R.G., Strominger, J.L., and Wiley, D.C.**, Three-dimensional structure of the human class II antigen HLA-DR1, *Nature*, 364, 33, 1993.
15. **Gorga, J.C., Brown, J.H., Jardetzky, T., Wiley, D.C., and Strominger, J.L.**, Crystallization of HLA-DR antigens, *Res. Immunol.*, 142, 401, 1991.
16. **Jardetzky, T.S., Gorga, J.C., Busch, R., Rothbard, J., Strominger, J.L., and Wiley, D.C.**, Peptide binding to HLA-DR1: a peptide with most residues substituted to alanine retains MHC binding, *EMBO J.*, 1797, 1990.
17. **Davis, M.M. and Bjorkman, P.J.**, A model for T cell receptor and MHC/peptide interaction, *Adv. Exp. Med. Biol.*, 254, 13, 1989.
18. **Bjorkman, P.J. and Davis, M.M.**, Model for the interaction of T-cell receptors with peptide/MHC complexes, *Cold Spring Harbor Symp. Quant. Biol.*, 1, 365, 1989.
19. **Jores, R., Alzari, P.M., and Meo, T.**, Resolution of hypervariable regions of T-cell receptor β chains by a modified Wu-Kabat index of amino acid diversity, *Proc. Natl. Acad. Sci. U.S.A.*, 87, 9138, 1990.
20. **Jorgensen, J.L., Esser, U., de St Groth, B.F., Reay, P.A., and Davis, M.M.**, Mapping T-cell receptor-peptide contacts by variant peptide immunization of single-chain transgenics, *Nature*, 355, 224, 1992.
21. **Choi, Y., Kotzin, B., Herron, L., Callahan, J., Marrack, P., and Kappler, J.**, Interaction of Staphylococcus aureus toxin "superantigens" with human T cells, *Proc. Natl. Acad. Sci. U.S.A.*, 86, 8941, 1989.
22. **Kabat, E.A., Wu, T.T., Perry, H.M., Gottesman, K.S., and Foeller, C.**, *Sequences of Proteins of Immunological Interest*, U.S. Department of Health and Human Services, Bethesda, MD, 1991, 2597.
23. **Uematsu, Y., Wege, H., Straus, A., Ott, M., Bannwarth, W., Lanchbury, J., Panayi, G., and Steinmetz, M.**, The T-cell-receptor repertoire in the synovial fluid of a patient with rheumatoid arthritis is polyclonal, *Proc. Natl. Acad. Sci. U.S.A.*, 88, 8534, 1991.
24. **Yoshikai, Y., Kimura, N., Toyonaga, B., and Mak, T.W.**, Sequences and repertoire of human T cell receptor α chain variable regions in mature T lymphocytes, *J. Exp. Med.*, 164, 90, 1986.
25. **Loh, E.Y., Elliott, J.F., Cwirla, S., Lanier, L.L., and Davis, M.M.**, Polymerase chain reaction with single-sided specificity: analysis of T cell receptor lambda chain, *Science*, 243, 217, 1989.
26. **Kabelitz, D.**, Function and specificity of human gamma/delta-positive T cells, *Crit. Rev. Immunol.*, 11, 281, 1992.
27. **Allison, J.P. and Havran, W.L.**, The immunobiology of T cells with invariant gamma delta antigen receptors, *Annu. Rev. Immunol.*, 9, 679, 1991.
28. **Jorgensen, J.L., Reay, P.A., Ehrich, E.W., and Davis, M.M.**, Molecular components of T-cell recognition, *Annu. Rev. Immunol.*, 10, 835, 1992.
29. **Hong, S.-C., Chelouche, A., Lin, R., Shaywitz, D., Braunstein, N.S., Glimcher, L., and Janeway, C.A.**, An MHC interaction site maps to the amino-terminal half of the T cell receptor α chain variable domain, *Cell*, 69, 999, 1992.
30. **Marrack, P. and Kappler, J.**, The staphylococcal enterotoxins and their relatives, *Science*, 248, 705, 1990.
31. **DerSimonian, H., Sugita, M., Glass, D.N., Maier, A.L., Weinblatt, M.E., Reme, T., and Brenner, M.B.**, Clonal V alpha 12.1+ T cell expansions in the peripheral blood of rheumatoid arthritis patients, *J. Exp. Med.*, 177, 1623, 1993.
32. **Kappler, J., Kotzin, B., Herron, L., Gelfand, E.W., Bigler, R.D., Boylston, A., Carrel, S., Posnett, D.N., Choi, Y., and Marrack, P.**, V beta-specific stimulation of human T cells by staphylococcal toxins, *Science*, 244, 811, 1989.
33. **Pullen, A.M., Wade, T., Marrack, P., and Kappler, J.W.**, Identification of the region of T cell receptor β chain that interacts with the self-superantigen MLS-1^a, *Cell*, 61, 1365, 1990.
34. **von Boehmer, H.**, Positive and negative selection of the alpha beta T-cell repertoire in vivo, *Curr. Opin. Immunol.*, 3, 210, 1991.
35. **Heber-Katz, E. and Acha-Orbea, H.**, The V-region disease hypothesis: evidence from autoimmune encephalomyelitis, *Immunol. Today*, 10, 164, 1989.
36. **Heber-Katz, E.**, The autoimmune T cell receptor: epitopes, idiotopes, and malatopes, *Clin. Immunol. Immunopathol.*, 55, 1, 1990.
37. **Beraud, E., Resshef, T., Vandenbark, A.A., Offner, H., Friz, R., Chou, C.-H. J., Bernard, D., and Cohen, I.R.**, Experimental autoimmune encephalomyelitis mediated by T lymphocyte lines: genotype of antigen-presenting cells influences immunodominant epitope of basic protein, *J. Immunol.*, 136, 511, 1986.
38. **Jenkins, M.K., Pardoll, D.M., Mizuguchi, J., Quill, H., and Schwartz, R.H.**, T-cell unresponsiveness in vivo and in vitro: fine specificity of induction and molecular characterization of the unresponsive state, *Immunol. Rev.*, 95, 113, 1987.
39. **Schwartz, R.H., Mueller, D.L., Jenkins, M.K., and Quill, H.**, T-cell clonal anergy, *Cold Spring Harbor Symp. Quant. Biol.*, 2, 605, 1989.
40. **Quill, H., Riley, M.P., Cho, E.A., Casnellie, J.E., Reed, J.C., and Torigoe, T.**, Anergic Th1 cells express altered levels of the protein tyrosine kinases p56lck and p59fyn, *J. Immunol.*, 149, 2887, 1992.
41. **Harding, F.A., McArthur, J.G., Gross, J.A., Raulet, D.H., and Allison, J.P.**, CD28-mediated signalling co-stimulates murine T cells and prevents induction of anergy in T-cell clones, *Nature*, 356, 607, 1992.

42. **Goverman, J., Woods, A., Larson, L., Weiner, L.P., Hood, L., and Zaller, D.M.**, Transgenic mice that express a myelin basic protein-specific T cell receptor develop spontaneous autoimmunity, *Cell*, 72, 551, 1993.
43. **Clayton, J.P., Gammon, G.M., Ando, D.G., Kono, D.H., Hood, L., and Sercarz, E.E.**, Peptide-specific prevention of experimental allergic encephalomyelitis. Neonatal tolerance induced to the dominant T cell determinant of myelin basic protein, *J. Exp. Med.*, 169, 1681, 1989.
44. **Hashim, G., Vandenbark, A., Galang, A., Diamanduros, T., Carvalho, E., Srinivasan, J., Jones, R., Vainiene, M., Morrison, W., and Offner, H.**, Antibodies specific for Vβ8 receptor peptide suppress experimental autoimmune encephalomyelitis, *J. Immunol.*, 144, 4621, 1990.
45. **Vandenbark, A., Hashim, G., and Offner, H.**, Immunization with a synthetic T-cell receptor V-region peptide protects against experimental autoimmune encephalomyelitis, *Nature*, 341, 541, 1989.
46. **Desquenne-Clark, L., Esch, T.R., Otvos, L.J., and Heber-Katz, E.**, T-cell receptor peptide immunization leads to enhanced and chronic experimental allergic encephalomyelitis, *Proc. Natl. Acad. Sci. U.S.A.*, 88, 7219, 1991.
47. **Braley, M.H., Johnson, M., Sharp, G.C., and Kyriakos, M.**, Induction of experimental autoimmune thyroiditis in mice with in vitro activated splenic T cells, *Cell. Immunol.*, 93, 132, 1985.
48. **Williams, W.V., Kyriakos, M., Sharp, G.C., and Braley-Mullen, H.**, The role of cellular proliferation in the induction of experimental autoimmune thyroiditis in mice, *Cell. Immunol.*, 103, 96, 1986.
49. **Williams, W.V., Kyriakos, M., Sharp, G.C., and Braley-Mullen, H.**, The cellular basis for the Ia restriction in murine experimental autoimmune thyroiditis, *Cell. Immunol.*, 110, 35, 1987.
50. **Stull, S.J., Kyriakos, M., Sharp, G.C., Bickel, J.T., and Braley, M.H.**, Effects of anti-I-A and anti-I-E monoclonal antibodies on the induction and expression of experimental autoimmune thyroiditis in mice, *Autoimmunity*, 6, 23, 1990.
51. **Stull, S.J., Kyriakos, M., Sharp, G.C., and Braley, M.H.**, Prevention and reversal of experimental autoimmune thyroiditis (EAT) in mice by administration of anti-L3T4 monoclonal antibody at different stages of disease development, *Cell. Immunol.*, 117, 188, 1988.
52. **Braley, M.H., Sharp, G.C., Bickel, J.T., and Kyriakos, M.**, Induction of severe granulomatous experimental autoimmune thyroiditis in mice by effector cells activated in the presence of anti- interleukin 2 receptor antibody, *J. Exp. Med.*, 173, 899, 1991.
53. **Stull, S.J., Sharp, G.C., Kyriakos, M., Bickel, J.T., and Braley, M.H.**, Induction of granulomatous experimental autoimmune thyroiditis in mice with in vitro activated effector T cells and anti-IFN-gamma antibody, *J. Immunol.*, 149, 2219, 1992.
54. **Wheatley, L.M., Urso, D., Tumas, K., Maltzman, J., Loh, E., and Levinson, A.I.**, Molecular evidence for the expression of nicotinic acetylcholine receptor alpha-chain in mouse thymus, *J. Immunol.*, 148, 3105, 1992.
55. **Krco, C.J., David, C.S., and Lennon, V.A.**, Mouse T lymphocyte response to acetylcholine receptor determined by T cell receptor for antigen V beta gene products recognizing Mls-1a, *J. Immunol.*, 147, 3303, 1991.
56. **Infante, A.J., Levcovitz, H., Gordon, V., Wall, K.A., Thompson, P.A., and Krolick, K.A.**, Preferential use of a T cell receptor V beta gene by acetylcholine receptor reactive T cells from myasthenia gravis-susceptible mice, *J. Immunol.*, 148, 3385, 1992.
57. **Steinman, L. and Mantegazza, R.**, Prospects for specific immunotherapy in myasthenia gravis, *FASEB J.*, 4, 2726, 1990.
58. **Holmdahl, R., Klareskog, L., Rubin, K., Larsson, E., and Wigzell, H.**, T lymphocytes in collagen II-induced arthritis in mice. Characterization of arthritogenic collagen II-specific T-cell lines and clones, *Scand. J. Immunol.*, 22, 295, 1985.
59. **Brahn, E. and Trentham, D.E.**, Effect of antithymocyte serum on collagen arthritis in rats: evidence that T cells are involved in its pathogenesis, *Cell. Immunol.*, 86, 421, 1984.
60. **Holmdahl, R., Karlsson, M., Andersson, M.E., Rask, L., and Andersson, L.**, Localization of a critical restriction site on the I-A beta chain that determines susceptibility to collagen-induced arthritis in mice, *Proc. Natl. Acad. Sci. U.S.A.*, 86, 9475, 1989.
61. **Peacock, D.J., Ku, G., Banquerigo, M.L., and Brahn, E.**, Suppression of collagen arthritis with antibodies to an arthritogenic, oligoclonal T cell line, *Cell. Immunol.*, 140, 444, 1992.
62. **Haqqi, T.M., Anderson, G.D., Banerjee, S., and David, C.S.**, Restricted heterogeneity in T-cell antigen receptor V beta gene usage in the lymph nodes and arthritic joints of mice, *Proc. Natl. Acad. Sci. U.S.A.*, 89, 1253, 1992.
63. **Mori, L., Loetscher, H., Kakimoto, K., Bluethmann, H., and Steinmetz, M.**, Expression of a transgenic T cell receptor beta chain enhances collagen-induced arthritis, *J. Exp. Med.*, 176, 381, 1992.
64. **Holoshitz, J., Naparstek, Y., Ben-Nun, A., and Cohen, I.R.**, Lines of T lymphocytes induce or vaccinate against autoimmune arthritis, *Science*, 219, 56, 1983.
65. **Chiocchia, G., Boissier, M.C., and Fournier, C.**, Therapy against murine collagen-induced arthritis with T cell receptor V beta-specific antibodies, *Eur. J. Immunol.*, 21, 2899, 1991.

66. **Goldschmidt, T.J., Jansson, L., and Holmdahl, R.**, In vivo elimination of T cells expressing specific T-cell receptor V beta chains in mice susceptible to collagen-induced arthritis, *Immunology*, 69, 508, 1990.
67. **Sette, A., Lamont, A.G., and Grey, H.M.**, The design of MHC binding peptides, in *Biologically Active Peptides: Design, Synthesis and Utilization*, Williams, W.V. and Weiner, D.B., Eds., Technomic, Lancaster, PA, 1992, 289.
68. **Townsend, A.R., Rothbard, J., Gotch, F.M., Bahadur, G., Wraith, D., and McMichael, A.J.**, The epitopes of influenza nucleoprotein recognized by cytotoxic T lymphocytes can be defined with short synthetic peptides, *Cell*, 44, 959, 1986.
69. **Rosloniec, E.F., Vitez, L.J., Buus, S., and Freed, J.H.**, MHC class II-derived peptides can bind to class II molecules, including self molecules, and prevent antigen presentation, *J. Exp. Med.*, 171, 1419, 1990.
70. **Natarajan, K., Burstyn, D., and Zauderer, M.**, Major histocompatibility complex determinants select T-cell receptor alpha chain variable region dominance in a peptide-specific response, *Proc. Natl. Acad. Sci. U.S.A.*, 89, 8874, 1992.
71. **Parker, K.C., Bednarek, M.A., Hull, L.K., Utz, U., Cunningham, B., Zweerink, H.J., Biddison, W.E., and Coligan, J.E.**, Sequence motifs important for peptide binding to the human MHC class I molecule, HLA-A2, *J. Immunol.*, 149, 3580, 1992.
72. **O'Sullivan, D., Sidney, J., Appella, E., Walker, L., Phillips, L., Colon, S.M., Miles, C., Chesnut, R.W., and Sette, A.**, Characterization of the specificity of peptide binding to four DR haplotypes, *J. Immunol.*, 145, 1799, 1990.
73. **Bouillot, M., Choppin, J., Cornille, F., Martinon, F., Papo, T., Gomard, E., Fournie, Z.M., and Levy, J.P.**, Physical association between MHC class I molecules and immunogenic peptides, *Nature*, 339, 473, 1989.
74. **Sidney, J., Oseroff, C., Southwood, S., Wall, M., Ishioka, G., Koning, F., and Sette, A.**, DRB1*0301 molecules recognize a structural motif distinct from the one recognized by most DBβ_1 alleles, *J. Immunol.*, 149, 2634, 1992.
75. **Schumacher, T.N., Heemels, M.T., Neefjes, J.J., Kast, W.M., Melief, C.J., and Ploegh, H.L.**, Direct binding of peptide to empty MHC class I molecules on intact cells and in vitro, *Cell*, 62, 563, 1990.
76. **Rudensky, A.Y.U., Preston, H.P., al Ramadi, B.K., Rothbard, J., and Janeway, C.A.J.**, Truncation variants of peptides isolated from MHC class II molecules suggest sequence motifs, *Nature*, 359, 429, 1992.
77. **Hunt, D.F., Michel, H., Dickinson, T.A., Shabanowitz, J., Cox, A.L., Sakaguchi, K., Appella, E., Grey, H.M., and Sette, A.**, Peptides presented to the immune system by the murine class II major histocompatibility complex molecule I-Ad, *Science*, 256, 1817, 1992.
78. **Chicz, R.M., Urban, R.G., Lane, W.S., Gorga, J.C., Stern, L.J., Vignali, D.A., and Strominger, J.L.**, Predominant naturally processed peptides bound to HLA-DR1 are derived from MHC-related molecules and are heterogeneous in size, *Nature*, 358, 764, 1992.
79. **Corr, M., Boyd, L.F., Frankel, S.R., Kozlowski, S., Padlan, E.A., and Margulies, D.H.**, Endogenous peptides of a soluble major histocompatibility complex class I molecule, H-2Lds: sequence motif, quantitative binding, and molecular modeling of the complex, *J. Exp. Med.*, 176, 1681, 1992.
80. **Falk, K., Rotzschke, O., Stevanovic, S., Jung, G., and Rammensee, H.G.**, Allele-specific motifs revealed by sequencing of self-peptides eluted from MHC molecules, *Nature*, 351, 290, 1991.
81. **Wei, M.L. and Cresswell, P.**, HLA-A2 molecules in an antigen-processing mutant cell contain signal sequence-derived peptides, *Nature*, 356, 443, 1992.
82. **van Bleek, G.M. and Nathenson, S.G.**, The structure of the antigen-binding groove of major histocompatibility complex class I molecules determines specific selection of self-peptides, *Proc. Natl. Acad. Sci. U.S.A.*, 88, 11032, 1991.
83. **Fremont, D.H., Matsumura, M., Stura, E.A., Peterson, P.A., and Wilson, I.A.**, Crystal structures of two viral peptides in complex with murine MHC class I H-2Kb, *Science*, 257, 919, 1992.
84. **Stura, E.A., Matsumura, M., Fremont, D.H., Saito, Y., Peterson, P.A., and Wilson, I.A.**, Crystallization of murine major histocompatibility complex class I H- 2Kb with single peptides, *J. Mol. Biol.*, 228, 975, 1992.
85. **Zhang, W., Young, A.C., Imarai, M., Nathenson, S.G., and Sacchettini, J.C.**, Crystal structure of the major histocompatibility complex class I H- 2Kb molecule containing a single viral peptide: implications for peptide binding and T-cell receptor recognition, *Proc. Natl. Acad. Sci. U.S.A.*, 89, 8403, 1992.
86. **Matsui, M., Hioe, C.E., and Frelinger, J.A.**, Roles of the six peptide-binding pockets of the HLA-A2 molecule in allorecognition by human cytotoxic T-cell clones, *Proc. Natl. Acad. Sci. U.S.A.*, 90, 674, 1993.
87. **Guery, J.C., Sette, A., Leighton, J., Dragomir, A., and Adorini, L.**, Selective immunosuppression by administration of major histocompatibility complex (MHC) class II-binding peptides. I. Evidence for in vivo MHC blockade preventing T cell activation, *J. Exp. Med.*, 175, 1345, 1992.
88. **Lamont, A.G., Powell, M.F., Colon, S.M., Miles, C., Grey, H.M., and Sette, A.**, The use of peptide analogs with improved stability and MHC binding capacity to inhibit antigen presentation in vitro and in vivo, *J. Immunol.*, 144, 2493, 1990.
89. **Muller, S., Adorini, L., Juretic, A., and Nagy, Z.A.**, Selective in vivo inhibition of T cell activation by class II MHC-binding peptides administered in soluble form, *J. Immunol.*, 145, 4006, 1990.

90. **Adorini, L., Appella, E., Doria, G., Cardinaux, F., and Nagy, Z.A.**, Competition for antigen presentation in living cells involves exchange of peptides bound by class II MHC molecules, *Nature*, 342, 800, 1989.
91. **Sakai, K., Zamvil, S.S., Mitchell, D.J., Hodgkinson, S., Rothbard, J.B., and Steinman, L.**, Prevention of experimental encephalomyelitis with peptides that block interaction of T cells with major histocompatibility complex proteins, *Proc. Natl. Acad. Sci. U.S.A.*, 86, 9470, 1989.
92. **McDevitt, H.O., Perry, R., and Steinman, L.A.**, Monoclonal anti-Ia antibody therapy in animal models of autoimmune disease, *Ciba Found. Symp.*, 129, 184, 1987.
93. **Steinman, L., Waldor, M.K., Zamvil, S.S., Lim, M., Herzenberg, L., Herzenberg, L., McDevitt, H.O., Mitchell, D., and Sriram, S.**, Therapy of autoimmune diseases with antibody to immune response gene products or to T-cell surface markers, *Ann. N.Y. Acad. Sci.*, 475, 274, 1986.
94. **Steinman, L.**, Therapy of autoimmune disease with monoclonal antibodies to class II gene products of the major histocompatibility complex, *Prog. Allergy*, 45, 161, 1988.
95. **Boitard, C., Michie, S., Serrurier, P., Butcher, G.W., Larkins, A.P., and McDevitt, H.O.**, In vivo prevention of thyroid and pancreatic autoimmunity in the BB rat by antibody to class II major histocompatibility complex gene products, *Proc. Natl. Acad. Sci. U.S.A.*, 82, 6627, 1985.
96. **Boitard, C., Bendelac, A., Richard, M.F., Carnaud, C., and Bach, J.F.**, Prevention of diabetes in nonobese diabetic mice by anti-I-A monoclonal antibodies: transfer of protection by splenic T cells, *Proc. Natl. Acad. Sci. U.S.A.*, 85, 9719, 1988.
97. **Kiesel, U., Oschilewski, M., Taniguchi, M., and Kolb, H.**, Modulation of low-dose streptozotocin-induced diabetes in mice by administration of antibodies to I-A, I-E and I-J determinants, *Diabetologia*, 32, 173, 1989.
98. **Taki, T., Nagata, M., Ogawa, W., Hatamori, N., Hayakawa, M., Hari, J., Shii, K., Baba, S., and Yokono, K.**, Prevention of cyclophosphamide-induced and spontaneous diabetes in NOD/Shi/Kbe mice by anti-MHC class I Kd monoclonal antibody, *Diabetes*, 40, 1203, 1991.
99. **Vladutiu, A.O. and Steinman, L.**, Inhibition of experimental autoimmune thyroiditis in mice by anti-I-A antibodies, *Cell. Immunol.*, 109, 169, 1987.
100. **Wetzig, R., Hooks, J.J., Percopo, C.M., Nussenblatt, R., Chan, C.C., and Detrick, B.**, Anti-Ia antibody diminishes ocular inflammation in experimental autoimmune uveitis, *Curr. Eye Res.*, 7, 809, 1988.
101. **Rao, N.A., Atalla, L., Linker, I.M., Chen, F.Y., George, F. 4th, Martin, W.J., and Steinman, L.**, Suppression of experimental uveitis in rats by anti-I-A antibodies, *Invest. Ophthalmol. Vis. Sci.*, 30, 2348, 1989.
102. **Cooper, S.M., Sriram, S., and Ranges, G.E.**, Suppression of murine collagen-induced arthritis with monoclonal anti- Ia antibodies and augmentation with IFN-gamma, *J. Immunol.*, 141, 1958, 1988.
103. **Wooley, P.H., Luthra, H.S., Lafuse, W.P., Huse, A., Stuart, J.M., and David, C.S.**, Type II collagen-induced arthritis in mice. III. Suppression of arthritis by using monoclonal and polyclonal anti-Ia antisera, *J. Immunol.*, 134, 2366, 1985.
104. **Gustafsson, K., Karlsson, M., Andersson, L., and Holmdahl, R.**, Structures on the I-A molecule predisposing for susceptibility to type II collagen-induced autoimmune arthritis, *Eur. J. Immunol.*, 20, 2127, 1990.
105. **Offner, H., Brostoff, S.W., and Vandenbark, A.A.**, Antibodies against I-A and I-E determinants inhibit the activation and function of encephalitogenic T-lymphocyte lines, *Cell. Immunol.*, 100, 364, 1986.
106. **Sriram, S., Topham, D.J., and Carroll, L.**, Haplotype-specific suppression of experimental allergic encephalomyelitis with anti-IA antibodies, *J. Immunol.*, 139, 1485, 1987.
107. **Sriram, S., Topham, D.J., and Carroll, L.**, Haplotype-specific suppression of experimental allergic encephalomyelitis with anti-IA antibodies, *J. Immunol.*, 139, 1485, 1987.
108. **Jonker, M., van, L.R., Mitchell, D.J., Durham, S.K., and Steinman, L.**, Successful treatment of EAE in rhesus monkeys with MHC class II specific monoclonal antibodies, *J. Autoimmun.*, 1, 399, 1988.
109. **Aharoni, R., Teitelbaum, D., Arnon, R., and Puri, J.**, Immunomodulation of experimental allergic encephalomyelitis by antibodies to the antigen-Ia complex, *Nature*, 351, 147, 1991.
110. **Burns, F.R., Li, X., Shen, N., Offner, H., Chou, Y.K., Vandenbark, A.A., and Heber-Katz, E.**, Both rat and mouse T cell receptors specific for the encephalitogenic determinant of myelin basic protein use similar Vα and Vβ chain genes even though the major histocompatibility complex and encephalitogenic determinants being recognized are different, *J. Exp. Med.*, 169, 27, 1989.
111. **Saki, K., Sinha, A.A., Mitchell, D.J., Zamvil, S.S., Rothbard, J.B., McDevitt, H.O., and Steinman, L.**, Involvement of distinct murine T-cell receptors in the autoimmune encephalitogenic response to nested epitopes of myelin basic protein, *Proc. Natl. Acad. Sci. U.S.A.*, 85, 8608, 1988.
112. **Texier, B., Bedin, C., Roubaty, C., Brezin, C., and Charreire, J.**, Protection from experimental autoimmune thyroiditis conferred by a monoclonal antibody to T cell receptor from a cytotoxic hybridoma specific for thyroglobulin, *J. Immunol.*, 148, 439, 1992.
113. **Haqqi, T.M. and David, C.S.**, T-cell receptor V beta genes repertoire in mice. Possible role in resistance and susceptibility to type II collagen-induced arthritis, *J. Autoimmun.*, 3, 113, 1990.
114. **Andersson, M., Jansson, L., and Holmdahl, R.**, Role for T-cell receptor Vb genes in collagen induced arthritis [letter], *Immunogenetics*, 35, 71, 1992.

115. **Anderson, G.D., Banerjee, S., Luthra, H.S., and David, C.S.,** Role of Mls-1 locus and clonal deletion of T cells in susceptibility to collagen-induced arthritis in mice, *J. Immunol.*, 147, 1189, 1991.
116. **Banerjee, S., Haqqi, T.M., Luthra, H.S., Stuart, J.M., and David, C.S.,** Possible role of V beta T cell receptor genes in susceptibility to collagen-induced arthritis in mice, *J. Exp. Med.*, 167, 832, 1988.
117. **David, C.S.,** Genes for MHC, TCR and Mls determine susceptibility to collagen induced arthritis, *Apmis*, 98, 575, 1990.
118. **Haqqi, T.M., Banerjee, S., Jones, W.L., Anderson, G., Behlke, M.A., Loh, D.Y., Luthra, H.S., and David, C.S.,** Identification of T-cell receptor V beta deletion mutant mouse strain AU/ssJ (H-2q) which is resistant to collagen-induced arthritis, *Immunogenetics*, 29, 180, 1989.
119. **Yoshino, S., Cleland, L.G., and Mayrhofer, G.,** Treatment of collagen-induced arthritis in rats with a monoclonal antibody against the alpha/beta T cell antigen receptor, *Arthritis Rheum.*, 34, 1039, 1991.
120. **Yoshino, S., Schlipkoter, E., Kinne, R., Hunig, T., and Emmrich, F.,** Suppression and prevention of adjuvant arthritis in rats by a monoclonal antibody to the alpha/beta T cell receptor, *Eur. J. Immunol.*, 20, 2805, 1990.
121. **Acha-Orbea, H., Mitchell, D.J., Timmermann, L., Wraith, D.C., Tausch, G.S., Waldor, M.K., Zamvil, S.S., McDevitt, H.O., and Steinman, L.,** Limited heterogeneity of T cell receptors from lymphocytes mediating autoimmune encephalomyelitis allows specific immune intervention, *Cell*, 54, 263, 1988.
122. **Zamvil, S.S., Mitchell, D.J., Lee, N.E., Moore, A.C., Waldor, M.K., Sakai, K., Rothbard, J.B., McDevitt, H.O., Steinman, L., and Acha-Orbea, H.,** Predominant expression of a T cell receptor V beta gene subfamily in autoimmune encephalomyelitis, *J. Exp. Med.*, 167, 1586, 1988.
123. **Heber-Katz, E., Owhashi, M., Happ, M.P., Burns, F., Shen, N., and Li, X.,** Clonal modulation of experimental allergic encephalomyelitis by a monoclonal antibody directed to the T-cell receptor, *Ann. N.Y. Acad. Sci.*, 540, 576, 1988.
124. **Zaller, D.M., Osman, G., Kanagawa, O., and Hood, L.,** Prevention and treatment of murine experimental allergic encephalomyelitis with T cell receptor V beta-specific antibodies, *J. Exp. Med.*, 171, 1943, 1990.
125. **Munitz, T.I., Schneck, J., Coligan, J.E., Maloy, W.L., Henrich, J.P., Sharrow, S.O., Margulies, D.H., and Singer, A.,** A peptide derived from the alpha-helical region of class I MHC blocks CTL engagement of the class I MHC molecule, *Cold Spring Harbor Symp. Quant. Biol.*, 1, 557, 1989.
126. **Schneck, J., Maloy, W.L., Coligan, J.E., and Margulies, D.H.,** Inhibition of an allospecific T cell hybridoma by soluble class I proteins and peptides: estimation of the affinity of a T cell receptor for MHC, *Cell*, 56, 47, 1989.
127. **Schneck, J., Munitz, T., Coligan, J.E., Maloy, W.L., Margulies, D.H., and Singer, A.,** Inhibition of allorecognition by an H-2Kb-derived peptide is evidence for a T-cell binding region on a major histocompatibility complex molecule, *Proc. Natl. Acad. Sci. U.S.A.*, 86, 8516, 1989.
128. **Heath, W.R., Vitiello, A., and Sherman, L.A.,** Mapping of epitopes recognized by alloreactive cytotoxic T lymphocytes using inhibition by MHC peptides, *J. Immunol.*, 143, 1441, 1989.
129. **Harris, P.E., Liu, Z., and Suciu-Foca, N.,** MHC class II binding of peptides derived from HLA-DR 1, *J. Immunol.*, 148, 2169, 1992.
130. **Williams, W.V., Weiner, D.B., Borofsky, M.A., Yui, K., Rubin, D., and Greene, M.I.,** Modulation of T cell responses with MHC derived peptides, *Immunol. Res.*, 11, 11, 1992.
131. **Sharma, S.D., Nag, B., Su, X.M., Green, D., Spack, E., Clark, B.R., and Sriram, S.,** Antigen-specific therapy of experimental allergic encephalomyelitis by soluble class II major histocompatibility complex-peptide complexes, *Proc. Natl. Acad. Sci. U.S.A.*, 88, 11465, 1991.
132. **Naparstek, Y., Ben, N.A., Holoshitz, J., Reshef, T., Frenkel, A., Rosenberg, M., and Cohen, I.R.,** T lymphocyte lines producing or vaccinating against autoimmune encephalomyelitis (EAE). Functional activation induces peanut agglutinin receptors and accumulation in the brain and thymus of line cells, *Eur. J. Immunol.*, 13, 418, 1983.
133. **Holoshitz, J., Frenkel, A., Ben, N.A., and Cohen, I.R.,** Autoimmune encephalomyelitis (EAE) mediated or prevented by T lymphocyte lines directed against diverse antigenic determinants of myelin basic protein. Vaccination is determinant specific, *J. Immunol.*, 131, 2810, 1983.
134. **Holoshitz, J., Matitiau, A., and Cohen, I.R.,** Role of the thymus in induction and transfer of vaccination against adjuvant arthritis with a T lymphocyte line in rats, *J. Clin. Invest.*, 75, 472, 1985.
135. **Lider, O., Karin, N., Shinitzky, M., and Cohen, I.R.,** Therapeutic vaccination against adjuvant arthritis using autoimmune T cells treated with hydrostatic pressure, *Proc. Natl., Acad. Sci. U.S.A.*, 84, 4577, 1987.
136. **Lider, O., Reshef, T., Beraud, E., Ben, N.A., and Cohen, I.R.,** Anti-idiotypic network induced by T cell vaccination against experimental autoimmune encephalomyelitis, *Science*, 239, 181, 1988.
137. **Lider, O., Beraud, E., Reshef, T., Friedman, A., and Cohen, I.R.,** Vaccination against experimental autoimmune encephalomyelitis using a subencephalitogenic dose of autoimmune effector T cells. II. Induction of a protective anti-idiotypic response, *J. Autoimmun.*, 2, 87, 1989.
138. **Beraud, E., Kotake, S., Caspi, R.R., Oddo, S.M., Chan, C.C., Gery, I., and Nussenblatt, R.B.,** Control of experimental autoimmune uveoretinitis by low dose T cell vaccination, *Cell. Immunol.*, 140, 112, 1992.
139. **Beraud, E.,** T cell vaccination in autoimmune diseases, *Ann. N.Y. Acad. Sci.*, 636, 124, 1991.

140. **Offner, H., Jones, R., Celnik, B., and Vandenbark, A.A.**, Lymphocyte vaccination against experimental autoimmune encephalomyelitis: evaluation of vaccination protocols, *J. Neuroimmunol.*, 21, 13, 1989.
141. **Schluesener, H.J. and Meyermann, R.**, T cell vaccination in monoclonal antibody-induced hyperacute experimental allergic encephalomyelitis, *J. Neuroimmunol.*, 24, 233, 1989.
142. **Maron, R., Zerubavel, R., Friedman, A., and Cohen, I.R.**, T lymphocyte line specific for thyroglobulin produces or vaccinates against autoimmune thyroiditis in mice, *J. Immunol.*, 131, 2316, 1983.
143. **Flynn, J.C. and Kong, Y.C.**, In vivo evidence for CD4+ and CD8+ suppressor T cells in vaccination-induced suppression of murine experimental autoimmune thyroiditis, *Clin. Immunol. Immunopathol.*, 60, 484, 1991.
144. **Nabozny, G.H., Flynn, J.C., and Kong, Y.C.**, Synergism between mouse thyroglobulin- and vaccination-induced suppressor mechanisms in murine experimental autoimmune thyroiditis, *Cell. Immunol.*, 136, 340, 1991.
145. **Jung, S., Schluesener, H.J., Toyka, K., and Hartung, H.P.**, T cell vaccination does not induce resistance to experimental autoimmune neuritis, *J. Neuroimmunol.*, 35, 1, 1991.
146. **Kahn, C.R., McIntosh, K.R., and Drachman, D.B.**, T-cell vaccination in experimental myasthenia gravis: a double-edged sword, *J. Autoimmun.*, 3, 659, 1990.
147. **Howell, M.D., Winters, S.T., Olee, T., Powell, H.C., Carlo, D.J., and Brostoff, S.W.**, Vaccination against experimental allergic encephalomyelitis with T cell receptor peptides, *Science*, 246, 668, 1989.
148. **Brostoff, S.W. and Howell, M.D.**, Immunoregulation of autoimmune disease by vaccination with T cell receptor peptides, *Ann. N.Y. Acad. Sci.*, 636, 71, 1991.
149. **Stevens, D.B., Karpus, W.J., Gould, K.E., and Swanborg, R.H.**, Studies of V beta 8 T cell receptor peptide treatment in experimental autoimmune encephalomyelitis, *J. Neuroimmunol.*, 37, 123, 1992.
150. **Vandenbark, A.A., Vainiene, M., Celnik, B., Hashim, G., and Offner, H.**, TCR peptide therapy decreases the frequency of encephalitogenic T cells in the periphery and the central nervous system, *J. Neuroimmunol.*, 39, 251, 1992.
151. **Kawano, Y., Sasamoto, Y., Kotake, S., Thurau, S.R., Wiggert, B., and Gery, I.**, Trials of vaccination against experimental autoimmune uveoretinitis with a T-cell receptor peptide, *Curr. Eye Res.*, 10, 789, 1991.
152. **Harris, E.D., Jr.**, Rheumatoid arthritis: the clinical spectrum, in *Textbook of Rheumatology*, 2nd ed., Kelley, W.N., Harris, J. E.D., Ruddy, S., and Sledge, C.B., Eds., W.B. Saunders, Philadelphia, 1985, 915.
153. **Medsger, T.A., Jr., and Masi, A.T.**, Epidemioloy of the rheumatic sideases, in *Arthritis and Allied Conditions*, 10th ed., McCarty, D.J., Ed., Lea & Febiger, Philadelphia, 1985, 9.
154. **Gao, X., Ball, E., Dombrausky, L., Olsen, N., Pincus, T., Kahn, M., and Wolfe, F.**, Class II human leukocyte antigen genes and T cell receptor polymorphisms in patients with rheumatoid arthritis, *Am. J. Med.*, 85, 14, 1988.
155. **Goronzy, J., Weyand, C.M., and Fathman, C.G.**, Shared T cell recognition sites on human histocompatibility antigen class II molecules of patients with seropositive rheumatoid arthritis, *J. Clin. Invest.*, 77, 1042, 1986.
156. **Gregersen, P., Silver, J., and Winchester, R.**, Genetic susceptibility to rheumatoid arthritis and human leukocyte antigen polymorphism. The role of shared conformational determinants, *Am. J. Med.*, 85, 17, 1988.
157. **Merryman, P., Crapper, R., Lee, S., Gregersen, P., and Winchester, R.**, Class II major histocompatibility complex gene sequences in rheumatoid arthritis, *Arthritis Rheum.*, 32, 251, 1989.
158. **Nepom, G., Hansen, J., and Nepom, B.**, The molecular basis for HLA class II association with rheumatoid arthritis, *J. Clin. Immunol.*, 7, 1, 1987.
159. **Roudier, J., Petersen, J., Rhodes, G., Luka, J., and Carson, D.**, Susceptibility to rheumatoid arthritis maps to a T-cell epitope shared by the HLA-Dw4 DR β-1 chain and the Epstein-Barr virus glycoprotein gp110, *Proc. Natl. Acad. Sci. U.S.A.*, 86, 5104, 1989.
160. **Holoshitz, J., Matitiau, A., and Cohen, I.R.**, Arthritis induced in rats by cloned T lymphocytes responsive to mycobacteria but not to collagen type II, *J. Clin. Invest.*, 73, 211, 1984.
161. **van Eden, W., Holoshitz, J., Nevo, Z., Frenkel, A., Klajman, A., and Cohen, I.R.**, Arthritis induced by a T-lymphocyte clone that responds to Mycobacterium tuberculosis and to cartilage proteoglycans, *Proc. Natl. Acad. Sci. U.S.A.*, 82, 5117, 1985.
162. **Harris, E.D., Jr.**, Pathogenesis of rheumatoid arthritis, in *Textbook of Rheumatology*, 2nd ed., Kelley, W.N., Harris, E.D., Jr., Ruddy, S., and Sledge, C.B., Eds., W.B. Saunders, Philadelphia, 1985, 886.
163. **Bennett, J.C.**, The etiology of rheumatoid arthritis, in *Textbook of Rheumatology*, 2nd ed., Kelley, W.N., Harris, E.D., Jr., Ruddy, S., and Sledge, C.B., Eds., W.B. Saunders, Philadelphia, 1985, 879.
164. **Carson, D.A.**, Rheumatoid factor, in *Textbook of Rheumatology*, 2nd ed., Kelley, W.N., Harris, E.D., Jr., Ruddy, S., and Sledge, C.B., W.B. Saunders, Philadelphia, 1985, 664.
165. **Firestein, G.S. and Zvaifler, N.J.**, How important are T cells in chronic rheumatoid synovitis?, *Arthritis Rheum.*, 33, 768, 1990.
166. **Kahle, P., Saal, J.G., Schaudt, K., Zacher, J., Fritz, P., and Pawelec, G.**, Determination of cytokines in synovial fluids: correlation with diagnosis and histomorphological characteristics of synovial tissue, *Ann. Rheum. Dis.*, 51, 731, 1992.

167. **Goddard, D.H.**, Regulation of synovial cell growth by polypeptide growth factors, DNA *Cell Biol.*, 11, 259, 1992.
168. **Westacott, C.I., Whicher, J.T., Barnes, I.C., Thompson, D., Swan, A.J., and Dieppe, P.A.**, Synovial fluid concentration of five different cytokines in rheumatic diseases [see comments], *Ann. Rheum. Dis.*, 49, 676, 1990.
169. **Chu, C.Q., Field, M., Allard, S., Abney, E., Feldmann, M., and Maini, R.N.**, Detection of cytokines at the cartilage/pannus junction in patients with rheumatoid arthritis: implications for the role of cytokines in cartilage destruction and repair, *Br. J. Rheumatol.*, 31, 653, 1992.
170. **Bucala, R., Ritchlin, C., Winchester, R., and Cerami, A.**, Constitutive production of inflammatory and mitogenic cytokines by rheumatoid synovial fibroblasts, *J. Exp. Med.*, 173, 569, 1991.
171. **Alvaro, G.J., Zvaifler, N.J., and Firestein, G.S.**, Cytokines in chronic inflammatory arthritis. V. Mutual antagonism between interferon-gamma and tumor necrosis factor-alpha on HLA-DR expression, proliferation, collagenase production, and granulocyte macrophage colony-stimulating factor production by rheumatoid arthritis synoviocytes, *J. Clin. Invest.*, 86, 1790, 1990.
172. **Alvaro, G.J., Zvaifler, N.J., Brown, C.B., Kaushansky, K., and Firestein, G.S.**, Cytokines in chronic inflammatory arthritis. VI. Analysis of the synovial cells involved in granulocyte-macrophage colony-stimulating factor production and gene expression in rheumatoid arthritis and its regulation by IL-1 and tumor necrosis factor-alpha, *J. Immunol.*, 146, 3365, 1991.
173. **Haworth, C., Brennan, F.M., Chantry, D., Turner, M., Maini, R.N., and Feldmann, M.**, Expression of granulocyte-macrophage colony-stimulating factor in rheumatoid arthritis: regulation by tumor necrosis factor-alpha, *Eur. J. Immunol.*, 21, 2575, 1991.
174. **Baker, D.G., Krakauer, K.A., Tate, G., Laposata, M., and Zurier, R.B.**, Suppression of human synovial cell proliferation by dihomogammalinolenic acid, *Arthritis Rheum.*, 32, 1273, 1989.
175. **Butler, D.M., Leizer, T., and Hamilton, J.A.**, Stimulation of human synovial fibroblast DNA synthesis by platelet-derived growth factor and fibroblast growth factor. Differences to the activation by IL-1, *J. Immunol.*, 142, 3098, 1989.
176. **Lafyatis, R., Thompson, N.L., Remmers, E.F., Flanders, K.C., Roche, N.S., Kim, S.J., Case, J.P., Sporn, M.B., Roberts, A.B., and Wilder, R.L.**, Transforming growth factor-beta production by synovial tissues from rheumatoid patients and streptococcal cell wall arthritic rats. Studies on secretion by synovial fibroblast-like cells and immunohistologic localization, *J. Immunol.*, 143, 1142, 1989.
177. **Melnyk, V.O., Shipley, G.D., Sternfeld, M.D., Sherman, L., and Rosenbaum, J.T.**, Synoviocytes synthesize, bind, and respond to basic fibroblast growth factor, *Arthritis Rheum.*, 33, 493, 1990.
178. **Remmers, E.F., Lafyatis, R., Kumkumian, G.K., Case, J.P., Roberts, A.B., Sporn, M.B., and Wilder, R.L.**, Cytokines and growth regulation of synoviocytes from patients with rheumatoid arthritis and rats with streptococcal cell wall arthritis, *Growth Factors*, 2, 179, 1990.
179. **Shiozawa, S., Shiozawa, K., Tanaka, Y., Morimoto, I., Uchihashi, M., Fujita, T., Hirohata, K., Hirata, Y., and Imura, S.**, Human epidermal growth factor for the stratification of synovial lining layer and neovascularisation in rheumatoid arthritis, *Ann. Rheum. Dis.*, 48, 820, 1989.
180. **Waalen, K., Sioud, M., Natvig, J.B., and Forre, O.**, Spontaneous in vivo gene transcription of interleukin-2, interleukin-3, interleukin-4, interleukin-6, interferon-gamma, interleukin-2 receptor (CD25) and proto-oncogene c-myc by rheumatoid synovial T lymphocytes, *Scand. J. Immunol.*, 36, 865, 1992.
181. **Duke, O., Panayi, G.S., Janossy, G., and Poulter, L.W.**, An immunohistological analysis of lymphocyte subpopulations and their microenvironment in the synovial membranes of patients with rheumatoid arthritis using monoclonal antibodies, *Clin. Exp. Immunol.*, 49, 22, 1982.
182. **Nakao, H., Eguchi, K., Kawakami, A., Migita, K., Otsubo, T., Yueki, Y., Shimomura, C., Tezuka, H., Matsunaga, M., Maeda, K., and Nagataki, S.**, Phenotypic characterization of lymphocytes infiltrating synovial tissue from patients with rheumatoid arthritis: analysis of lymphocytes isolated from minced synovial tissue by dual immunofluorescent staining, *J. Rheumatol.*, 17, 142, 1990.
183. **Ranki, A., Paavonen, T., Tolvanen, E., Kankaanpaa, U., and Hayry, P.**, T lymphocyte subclasses in rheumatoid synovia as analysed with monoclonal antibodies and functional in vitro tests, *Scand. J. Rheumatol.*, 13, 67, 1984.
184. **Lapadula, G., Covelli, M., Numo, R., Tricarico, G., Amendoni, G., and Berlingerio, C.**, Monoclonal antibody investigation in rheumatoid arthritis: presence of a T cell subpopulation bearing a double marker, *Clin. Rheumatol.*, 3, 137, 1984.
185. **Firestein, G. and Zvaifler, N.**, The pathogenesis of rheumatoid arthritis, in *Immunology of Rheumatic Diseases*, Pisetsky, D. and Snyderman, R., Eds., W.B. Saunders, Philadelphia, 1987, 447.
186. **van Laar, J.M., Miltenburg, A., Verdonk, M., Daha, M., Vries, R.D., Elsen, P.V.D., and Breedveld, F.**, Lack of T cell oligoclonality in enzyme-digested synovial tissue and in synovial fluid in most patients with rheumatoid arthritis, *Clin. Exp. Immunol.*, 83, 352, 1991.
187. **Miltenburg, A., Laar, J.V., Daha, M., Vries, R.D., Elsen, P.V.D., and Breedveld, F.**, Dominant T-cell receptor beta-chain gene rearrangements indicate clonal expansion in the rheumatoid joint, *Scand. J. Immunol.*, 31, 121, 1990.

188. **Duby, A., Sinclair, A., Osborne-Lawrence, S., Zeldes, W., Kan, L., and Fox, D.,** Clonal heterogeneity of synovial fluid T lymphocytes from patients with rheumatoid arthritis, *Proc. Natl. Acad. Sci. U.S.A.*, 86, 6206, 1989.
189. **Stamenkovic, I., Stegagno, M., Wright, K.A., Krane, S.M., Amento, E.P., Colvin, R.B., Duquesnoy, R.J., and Kurnick, J.T.,** Clonal dominance among T-lymphocyte infiltrates in arthritis, *Proc. Natl. Acad. Sci. U.S.A.*, 85, 1179, 1988.
190. **Sottini, A., Imberti, L., Gorla, R., Cattaneo, R., and Primi, D.,** Restricted expression of T cell receptor V beta but not V alpha genes in rheumatoid arthritis, *Eur. J. Immunol.*, 21, 461, 1991.
191. **Savill, C.M., Delves, P.J., Kioussis, D., Walker, P., Lydyard, P.M., Colaco, B., Shipley, M., and Roitt, I.M.,** A minority of patients with rheumatoid arthritis show a dominant rearrangement of T-cell receptor beta chain genes in synovial lymphocytes, *Scand. J. Immunol.*, 25, 629, 1987.
192. **Stamenkovic, I., Stegagno, M., Wright, K.A., Krane, S.M., Amento, E.P., Colvin, R.B., Duquesnoy, R.J., and Kurnick, J.T.,** T lymphocyte infiltrates in inflammatory synovia are oligoclonal, *Transplant. Proc.*, 20, 315, 1988.
193. **Malhotra, U. and Concannon, P.,** T cell receptor beta gene polymorphism and rheumatoid arthritis, *Autoimmunity*, 12, 75, 1992.
194. **Lu, Y., Kim, B.S., and Pope, R.M.,** Clonal heterogeneity of synovial fluid T lymphocytes in inflammatory synovitis, *Clin. Immunol. Immunopathol.*, 63, 28, 1992.
195. **van Laar, J.M., Miltenburg, A.M., Verdonk, M.J., Daha, M.R., de Vries, R.R., van den Elsen, P.J., and Breedveld, F.C.,** T-cell receptor beta-chain gene rearrangements of T-cell populations expanded from multiple sites of synovial tissue obtained from a patient with rheumatoid arthritis, *Scand. J. Immunol.*, 35, 187, 1992.
196. **Paliard, X., West, S., Lafferty, J., Clements, J., Kappler, J., Marrack, P., and Kotzin, B.,** Evidence for the effects of a superantigen in rheumatoid arthritis, *Science*, 253, 325, 1991.
197. **Sioud, M., Kjeldsen-Kragh, J., Suleyman, S., Vinje, O., Natvig, J.B., and Forre, O.,** Limited heterogeneity of T cell receptor variable region gene usage in juvenile rheumatoid arthritis synovial T cells, *Eur. J. Immunol.*, 22, 2413, 1992.
198. **Pluschke, G., Ricken, G., Taube, H., Kroninger, S., Melchers, I., Peter, H.H., Eichmann, K., and Krawinkel, U.,** Biased T cell receptor V alpha region repertoire in the synovial fluid of rheumatoid arthritis patients, *Eur. J. Immunol.*, 21, 2749, 1991.
199. **Sioud, M., Kjeldsen-Kragh, J., Quayle, A.J., Wiker, H.G., Sorskaar, D., Natvig, J.B., and Forre, O.,** Immune responses to 18.6 and 30-kDa mycobacterial antigens in rheumatoid patients, and V beta usage by specific synovial T-cell lines and fresh T cells, *Scand. J. Immunol.*, 34, 803, 1991.
200. **Howell, M.D., Diveley, J.P., Lundeen, K.A., Esty, A., Winters, S.T., Carlo, D.J., and Brostoff, S.W.,** Limited T-cell receptor β-chain heterogeneity among interleukin 2 receptor-positive synovial T cells suggests a role for superantigen in rheumatoid arthritis, *Proc. Natl. Acad. Sci. U.S.A.*, 88, 10921, 1991.
201. **Williams, W.V., Fang, Q., Demarco, D., VonFeldt, J., Zurier, R.B., and Weiner, D.B.,** Restricted heterogeneity of T cell receptor transcripts in rheumatoid synovium, *J. Clin. Invest.*, 90, 326, 1992.
202. **Bucht, A., Oksenberg, J.R., Lindblad, S., Grönberg, A., Steinman, L., and Klareskog, L.,** Characterization of T-cell receptor αβ repertoire in synovial tissue from different temporal phases of rheumatoid arthritis, *Scand. J. Immunol.*, 35, 159, 1992.
203. **Olive, C., Gatenby, P.A., and Serjeantson, S.W.,** Analysis of T cell receptor V alpha and V beta gene usage in synovia of patients with rheumatoid arthritis, *Immunol. Cell Biol.*, 69, 349, 1991.
204. **Williams, W.V., Kieber-Emmons, T., Fang, Q., Von Feldt, J., Wang, B., Ramanujam, T., and Weiner, D.B.,** Conserved motifs in rheumatoid arthritis synovial tissue T cell receptor beta chains, *DNA Cell Biol.*, 12, 425, 1993.
205. **Friedman, S.M., Crow, M.K., Tumang, J.R., Tumang, M., Xu, Y., Hodtsev, A.S., Cole, B.C., and Posnett, D.N.,** Characterization of human T cells reactive with the *Mycoplasma arthritidis*-derived superantigen (MAM): generation of a monoclonal antibody against Vβ17, the T cell receptor gene product expressed by a large fraction of MAM-reactive human T cells, *J. Exp. Med.*, 174, 891, 1991.
206. **Pulschke, G., Ricken, G., Taube, H., Kroninger, S., Melchers, I., Peter, H.H., Eichmann, K., and Krawinkel, U.,** Biased T cell receptor Vα region repertoire in the synovial fluid of a rheumatoid arthritis patient, *Eur. J. Immunol.*, 21, 2749, 1991.
207. **Taylor-Robinson, D. and Taylor, G.,** Do mycoplasmas cause rheumatic disease?, in *Infection and Immunology in the Rheumatic Diseases*, Dumonde, D.C., Ed., Blackwell Scientific Publications, Oxford, 1976, 177.
208. **Cassell, G.H. and Cole, B.C.,** Mycoplasmas as agents of human disease, *N. Engl. J. Med.*, 304, 80, 1981.
209. **Nardella, F.A., Teller, D.C., Barber, C.V., and Mannik, M.,** IgG rheumatoid factors and and staphylococcal protein A bind to a common molecular site on IgG, *J. Exp. Med.*, 162, 1811, 1985.
210. **Wendling, D., Wijdenes, J., and Racadot, E.,** Utilisation therapeutique d'un anticorps monoclonal anti-CD4 dans la polyarthrite rhumatoide réfractaire. Résultats preéliminaires, *Rev. Rhum. Mal Osteoartic*, 58, 13, 1991.
211. **Wendling, D., Wijdenes, J., Racadot, E., and Morel-Fourrier, B.,** Therapeutic use of monoclonal anti-CD4 antibody in rheumatoid arthritis, *J. Rheumatol.*, 18, 325, 1991.

212. **van Laar, J.M., Miltenburg, A.M., Verdonk, M.J., Daha, M.R., de Vries, R.R., and Breedveld, F.C.,** T cell vaccination in rheumatoid arthritis, *Br. J. Rheumatol.*, 2, 28, 1991.
213. **Barber, L.D., Bal, V., Lamb, J.R., O'Hehir, R.E., Yendle, J., Hancock, R.J., and Lechler, R.I.,** Contribution of T-cell receptor-contacting and peptide-binding residues of the class II molecule HLA-DR4 Dw10 to serologic and antigen-specific T-cell recognition, *Hum. Immunol.*, 32, 110, 1991.
214. **Sherritt, M.A., Oksenberg, J., de Rosbo N.K., and Bernard, C.C.,** Influence of HLA-DR2, HLA-DPw4, and T cell receptor alpha chain genes on the susceptibility to multiple sclerosis, *Int. Immunol.*, 4, 177, 1992.
215. **Olerup, O. and Hillert, J.,** HLA class II-associated genetic susceptibility in multiple sclerosis: a critical evaluation, *Tissue Antigens*, 38, 1, 1991.
216. **Oksenberg, J.R., Sherritt, M., Begovich, A.B., Erlich, H.A., Bernard, C.C., Cavalli, S.L., and Steinman, L.,** T-cell receptor V alpha and C alpha alleles associated with multiple sclerosis and myasthenia gravis, *Proc. Natl. Acad. Sci. U.S.A.*, 86, 988, 1989.
217. **Ransohoff, R.M.,** T-cell receptor germline genes and multiple sclerosis susceptibility: an unfinished tale [editorial], *Neurology*, 42, 714, 1992.
218. **Seboun, E., Robinson, M.A., Doolittle, T.H., Ciulla, T.A., Kindt, T.J., and Hauser, S.L.,** A susceptibility locus for multiple sclerosis is linked to the T cell receptor beta chain complex, *Cell*, 57, 1095, 1989.
219. **Beall, S.S., Concannon, P., Charmley, P., McFarland, H.F., Gatti, R.A., Hood, L.E., McFarlin, D.E., and Biddison, W.E.,** The germline repertoire of T cell receptor beta-chain genes in patients with chronic progressive multiple sclerosis, *J. Neuroimmunol.*, 21, 59, 1989.
220. **Charmley, P., Beall, S.S., Concannon, P., Hood, L., and Gatti, R.A.,** Further localization of a multiple sclerosis susceptibility gene on chromosome 7q using a new T cell receptor beta-chain DNA polymorphism, *J. Neuroimmunol.*, 32, 231, 1991.
221. **Lynch, S.G., Rose, J.W., Petajan, J.H., Stauffer, D., Kamerath, C., and Leppert, M.,** Discordance of T-cell receptor beta-chain genes in familial multiple sclerosis, *Ann. Neurol.*, 30, 402, 1991.
222. **Lynch, S.G., Rose, J.W., Petajan, J.H., and Leppert, M.,** Discordance of the T-cell receptor alpha-chain gene in familial multiple sclerosis, *Neurology*, 42, 839, 1992.
223. **Hashimoto, L.L., Mak, T.W., and Ebers, G.C.,** T cell receptor alpha chain polymorphisms in multiple sclerosis, *J. Neuroimmunol.*, 40, 41, 1992.
224. **Hillert, J., Leng, C., and Olerup, O.,** T-cell receptor alpha chain germline gene polymorphisms in multiple sclerosis, *Neurology*, 42, 80, 1992.
225. **Ben Nun, A., Liblau, R.S., Cohen, L., Lehmann, D., Tournier, L.E., Rosenzweig, A., Zhang, J.W., Raus, J.C., and Bach, M.A.,** Restricted T-cell receptor V beta gene usage by myelin basic protein-specific T-cell clones in multiple sclerosis: predominant genes vary in individuals, *Proc. Natl. Acad. Sci. U.S.A.*, 88, 2466, 1991.
226. **Martin, R., Howell, M.D., Jaraquemada, D., Flerlage, M., Richert, J., Brostoff, S., Long, E.O., McFarlin, D.E., and McFarland, H.F.,** A myelin basic protein peptide is recognized by cytotoxic T cells in the context of four HLA-DR types associated with multiple sclerosis, *J. Exp. Med.*, 173, 19, 1991.
227. **Kotzin, B.L., Karuturi, S., Chou, Y.K., Lafferty, J., Forrester, J.M., Better, M., Nedwin, G.E., Offner, H., and Vandenbark, A.A.,** Preferential T-cell receptor beta-chain variable gene use in myelin basic protein-reactive T-cell clones from patients with multiple sclerosis, *Proc. Natl. Acad. Sci. U.S.A.*, 88, 9161, 1991.
228. **Giegerich, G., Pette, M., Meinl, E., Epplen, J.T., Wekerle, H., and Hinkkanen, A.,** Diversity of T cell receptor alpha and beta chain genes expressed by human T cells specific for similar myelin basic protein peptide/major histocompatibility complexes, *Eur. J. Immunol.*, 22, 753, 1992.
229. **Chou, Y.K., Henderikx, P., Vainiene, M., Whitham, R., Bourdette, D., Chou, C.H., Hashim, G., Offner, H., and Vandenbark, A.A.,** Specificity of human T cell clones reactive to immunodominant epitopes of myelin basic protein, *J. Neurosci. Res.*, 28, 280, 1991.
230. **Wucherpfennig, K.W., Ota, K., Endo, N., Seidman, J.G., Rosenzweig, A., Weiner, H.L., and Hafler, D.A.,** Shared human T cell receptor Vβ usage to immunodominant regions of myelin basic protein, *Science*, 248, 1016, 1990.
231. **Oksenberg, J.R., Stuart, S., Begovich, A.B., Bell, R.B., Erlich, H.A., Steinman, L., and Bernard, C.C.A.,** Limited heterogeneity of rearranged T-cell receptor Vα transcripts in brains of multiple sclerosis patients, *Nature*, 345, 344, 1990.
232. **Wucherpfennig, K.W., Newcombe, J., Li, H., Keddy, C., Cuzner, M.L., and Hafler, D.A.,** T cell receptor V alpha-V beta repertoire and cytokine gene expression in active multiple sclerosis lesions, *J. Exp. Med.*, 175, 993, 1992.
233. **Hafler, D.A., Duby, A.D., Lee, S.J., Benjamin, D., Seidman, J.G., and Weiner, H.L.,** Oligoclonal T lymphocytes in the cerebrospinal fluid of patients with multiple sclerosis, *J. Exp. Med.*, 167, 1313, 1988.
234. **Birnbaum, G. and van Ness, B.,** Quantitation of T-cell receptor V beta chain expression on lymphocytes from blood, brain, and spinal fluid in patients with multiple sclerosis and other neurological diseases, *Ann. Neurol.*, 32, 24, 1992.

235. **Oksenberg, J.R., Panzara, M.A., Begovich, A.B., Mitchell, D., Ehrlich, H.A., Murray, R.S., Shimonkevitz, R., Sherritt, M., Rothbard, J., Bernard, C.C.A., and Steinman, L.**, Selection of Vβ-Dβ-Jβ gene rearrangements for a myelin basic protein peptide in brain lesions of multiple sclerosis, *Nature*, 362, 68, 1993.
236. **Hafler, D.A., Cohen, I., Benjamin, D.S., and Weiner, H.L.**, T cell vaccination in multiple sclerosis: a preliminary report, *Clin. Immunol. Immunopathol.*, 62, 307, 1992.
237. **Zhang, J.W., Schreurs, M., Medaer, R., and Raus, J.C.**, Regulation of myelin basic protein-specific helper T cells in multiple sclerosis: generation of suppressor T cell lines, *Cell. Immunol.*, 139, 118, 1992.
238. **Weiner, H.L., Mackin, G.A., Matsui, M., Orav, E.J., Khoury, S.J., Dawson, D.M., and Hafler, D.A.**, Double-blind pilot trial of oral tolerization with myelin antigens in multiple sclerosis, *Science*, 259, 1321, 1993.
239. **Vandenbark, A.**, Strategies to treat neurologic disease based on TCR peptides, American College of Rheumatology 56th Annual Meeting, October 12, 1992.
240. **Nepom, G.T.**, Mutagenesis and expression of putative class II susceptibility genes: a "reverse immunogenetics" approach to analysis of HLA and disease, *Autoimmunity*, 7, 189, 1990.
241. **Nepom, G.T. and Erlich, H.**, MHC class-II molecules and autoimmunity, *Annu. Rev. Immunol.*, 9, 493, 1991.
242. **Nerup, J., Christy, M., Kromann, H., Platz, P., Ryder, L.P., Thomsen, M., and Svejgaard, A.**, HLA and insulin-dependent diabetes mellitus, *Postgrad. Med. J.*, 2, 8, 1979.
243. **Aparicio, J.M.**, HLA and non-HLA genetic factors in Japanese IDDM, *Hokkaido Igaku Zasshi*, 66, 780, 1991.
244. **Deschamps, I., Beressi, J.P., Khalil, I., Robert, J.J., and Hors, J.**, The role of genetic predisposition to type I (insulin-dependent) diabetes mellitus, *Ann. Med.*, 23, 427, 1991.
245. **Erlich, H.A.**, HLA class II sequences and genetic susceptibility to insulin dependent diabetes mellitus, *Baillieres Clin. Endocrinol. Metab.*, 5, 395, 1991.
246. **Ito, M., Tanimoto, M., Kamura, H., Yoneda, M., Morishima, Y., Takatsuki, K., Itatsu, T., and Saito, H.**, Association of HLA-DR phenotypes and T-lymphocyte-receptor beta-chain-region RFLP with IDDM in Japanese, *Diabetes*, 37, 1633, 1988.
247. **Rubinstein, P.**, HLA and IDDM: facts and speculations on the disease gene and its mode of inheritance, *Hum. Immunol.*, 30, 270, 1991.
248. **Sheehy, M.J.**, T cell defined HLA epitopes and T cell receptor polymorphism in insulin dependent diabetes mellitus, *Baillieres Clin. Endocrinol. Metab.*, 5, 341, 1991.
249. **Sheehy, M.J.**, HLA and insulin-dependent diabetes. A protective perspective, *Diabetes*, 41, 123, 1992.
250. **Tait, B.D.**, Genetic susceptibility to type I diabetes: a review, *J. Autoimmun.*, 1, 3, 1990.
251. **Tuomilehto, W.E. and Tuomilehto, J.**, HLA antigens in insulin-dependent diabetes mellitus, *Ann. Med.*, 23, 481, 1991.
252. **Thorsby, E., Gjertsen, H.A., Lundin, K.E., and Ronningen, K.S.**, Insulin dependent diabetes mellitus susceptibility or protection may be determined by certain HLA-DQ molecules, *Baillieres Clin. Endocrinol. Metab.*, 5, 361, 1991.
253. **al Sakkaf, L., Pozzilli, P., Bingley, P.J., Lowdell, M.W., Thomas, J.M., Bonifacio, E., Gale, E.A., and Bottazzo, G.F.**, Early T-cell defects in pre-type 1 diabetes, *Acta Diabetol.*, 28, 189, 1992.
254. **Bhatia, E., Buse, J.B., and Jackson, R.A.**, T-cell antigen receptor alpha chain polymorphisms in insulin-dependent diabetes, *J. Autoimmun.*, 1, 389, 1988.
255. **Boehm, B.O., Manfras, B.J., Rosak, C., Kuehnl, P., Schoffling, K., and Trucco, M.**, TcR-alpha and TcR-beta dialellic RFLPs in insulin-dependent (type I) Caucasian diabetic patients, *Diabetes Res.*, 15, 63, 1990.
256. **Concannon, P., Wright, J.A., Wright, L.G., Sylvester, D.R., and Spielman, R.S.**, T-cell receptor genes and insulin-dependent diabetes mellitus (IDDM): no evidence for linkage from affected sib pairs, *Am. J. Hum. Genet.*, 47, 45, 1990.
257. **Hanninen, A., Jalkanen, S., Salmi, M., Toikkanen, S., Nikolakaros, G., and Simell, O.**, Macrophages, T cell receptor usage, and endothelial cell activation in the pancreas at the onset of insulin-dependent diabetes mellitus, *J. Clin. Invest.*, 90, 1901, 1992.
258. **Hibberd, M.L., Millward, B.A., Wong, F.S., and Demaine, A.G.**, T-cell receptor constant beta chain polymorphisms and susceptibility to type 1 diabetes, *Diabetes Med.*, 9, 929, 1992.
259. **Offner, H., Buenafe, A.C., Vainiene, M., Celnik, B., Weinberg, A.D., Gold, D.P., Hashim, G., and Vandebark, A.A.** Where, when, and how to detect biased expression encephalomyelitis, *J. Immunol.*, 151, 506, 1993.
260. **Martinez, N.E., Coto, E., Gutierrez, V., Urra, J.M., Setien, F., Dominguez, O., Hood, L.E., and Lopez, L.C.**, Germline repertoire of T-cell receptor beta-chain genes in patients with insulin-dependent diabetes mellitus, *Hum. Immunol.*, 31, 77, 1991.
261. **Millward, B.A., Welsh, K.I., Leslie, R.D., Pyke, D.A., and Demaine, A.G.**, T cell receptor beta chain polymorphisms are associated with insulin-dependent diabetes, *Clin. Exp. Immunol.*, 70, 152, 1987.
262. **Reijonen, H., Silvennoinen, K.S., Ilonen, J., and Knip, M.**, Lack of association of T cell receptor beta-chain constant region polymorphism with insulin-dependent diabetes mellitus in Finland, *Clin. Exp. Immunol.*, 81, 396, 1990.

263. **Sheehy, M.J., Meske, L.M., Emler, C.A., Rowe, J.R., Neme de Gimenez, M.H., Ingle, C.A., Chan, A., Trucco, M., and Mak, T.W.,** Allelic T-cell receptor alpha complexes have little or no influence on susceptibility to type 1 diabetes, *Hum. Immunol.*, 26, 261, 1989.
264. **Sheehy, M.J.,** T cell defined HLA epitopes and T cell receptor polymorphism in insulin dependent diabetes mellitus, *Baillieres Clin. Endocrinol. Metab.*, 5, 341, 1991.
265. **Kontiainen, S., Toomath, R., Lowder, J., and Feldmann, M.,** Selective activation of T cells in newly diagnosed insulin-dependent diabetic patients: evidence for heterogeneity of T cell receptor usage, *Clin. Exp. Immunol.*, 83, 347, 1991.
266. **Davies, T.F., Martin, A., Concepcion, E.S., Graves, P., Cohen, L., and Ben, N.A.,** Evidence of limited variability of antigen receptors on intrathyroidal T cells in autoimmune thyroid disease, *N. Engl. J. Med.*, 325, 238, 1991.
267. **Davies, T.F., Martin, A., Concepcion, E.S., Graves, P., Lahat, N., Cohen, W.L., and Ben, N.A.,** Evidence for selective accumulation of intrathyroidal T lymphocytes in human autoimmune thyroid disease based on T cell receptor V gene usage, *J. Clin. Invest.*, 89, 157, 1992.
268. **Lipoldova, M., Londei, M., Grubeck, L.B., Feldmann, M., and Owen, M.J.,** Analysis of T-cell receptor usage in activated T-cell clones from Hashimoto's thyroiditis and Graves' disease, *J. Autoimmun.*, 2, 1, 1989.
269. **Link, H., Olsson, O., Sun, J., Wang, W.Z., Andersson, G., Ekre, H.P., Brenner, T., Abramsky, O., and Olsson, T.,** Acetylcholine receptor-reactive T and B cells in myasthenia gravis and controls, *J. Clin. Invest.*, 87, 2191, 1991.
270. **Ahlberg, R., Yi, Q., Eng, H., Pirskanen, R., and Lefvert, A.K.,** T-cell epitopes on the human acetylcholine receptor alpha-subunit residues 10-84 in myasthenia gravis, *Scand. J. Immunol.*, 36, 435, 1992.
271. **Protti, M.P., Manfredi, A.A., Wu, X.D., Moiola, L., Howard, J.J., and Conti, T.B.,** Myasthenia gravis. T epitopes on the delta subunit of human muscle acetylcholine receptor, *J. Immunol.*, 146, 2253, 1991.
272. **Grunewald, J., Ahlberg, R., Lefvert, A.K., DerSimonian, H., Wigzell, H., and Janson, C.H.,** Abnormal T-cell expansion and V-gene usage in myasthenia gravis patients, *Scand. J. Immunol.*, 34, 161, 1991.

Chapter 6

OLIGOSACCHARIDE PHARMACEUTICALS

Stephen Roth and David Zopf

CONTENTS

I. INTRODUCTION

The study of the complex carbohydrates has a long and fascinating history. Although oligosaccharides have been the target of some of the most systematic, meticulous, and elegant structural studies in all of biochemistry, functional analyses still suffer from under-experimentation and over-interpretation. Perhaps the most extreme example of this dichotomy resides with the human blood group antigens, A, B, and H. The structures of these oligosaccharidic antigens have been determined. Even the molecular genetics and population genetics of the enzymes that make them are well understood. Yet we know nothing about the function of the blood group substances. Fortunately, however, the functions of other cell surface oligosaccharides are becoming more and more clear.

In general, complementary molecular interactions between proteins and carbohydrates are mechanisms for effecting specific recognition events at several levels of biological organization. At the molecular level, for example, glycoproteins can be targeted to specific sites according to the nature of their oligosaccharide side chains. For example, serum glycoproteins are cleared from the circulation by liver cell surface receptors that recognize β-linked galactosides;[1] lysosomal enzymes have, as oligosaccharide addresses, terminal mannose-6-PO_4 residues;[2] the circulatory half-life of human gonadotrophins depends on sulfated galactosaminides;[3] and human IgA is marked for secretion into milk, saliva, and other fluids by incomplete galactosylation.[4]

0-8493-9422-8/94/$0.00+$.50

At the cellular level, specific adhesions among cells often occur, at least initially, also as a result of the interactions between particular surface complex carbohydrates and proteins that recognize them on apposing cells. This mechanism is responsible not only for recognition between eukaryotic cells, but also for the specific attachment of bacteria, viruses, and fungi to host mammalian cells. From some of the earliest cell adhesion studies[5] to the most recent,[6] however, the protein portion of the carbohydrate-protein pair has typically received the most attention; the reason for this asymmetry is that our abilities to analyze and synthesize the complex carbohydrates have lagged far behind our similar abilities with the other biological polymers — nucleic acids and proteins. There are two reasons, in turn, for the relative weakness in synthetic carbohydrate biochemistry. One is the absence, until recently, of a clear notion of oligosaccharide function. And the second reason is the very diverse nature of the oligosaccharides themselves.

The inability to manufacture specific, human oligosaccharides in large amounts and at reasonable cost is the sole reason that these compounds have not yet been tested as pharmaceuticals. There is no question that oligosaccharides have potential as anti-infectives, anti-inflammatories, diagnostics, and drug delivery aids, all with a presumed lack of toxicity. Until recently, however, there has been no method for obtaining amounts of human oligosaccharides sufficient even for safety tests in animals, much less efficacy tests in humans. As the synthesis hurdle is overcome, the true worth of these natural antibiotics and recognition molecules will be rigorously tested. Many scientists believe that the result will be an entirely new class of potent, safe, and highly manipulable pharmaceuticals.

II. THE NATURE OF OLIGOSACCHARIDES

Complex carbohydrates are polymers of monosaccharides. The polymers may be unbranched homopolymers, like cellulose, containing thousands of repeats of the same monosaccharide, or branched homopolymers, like glycogen. Others are copolymers that consist largely of thousands of disaccharide repeats, like hyaluronic acid and the chondroitin sulfates.

This chapter will concentrate on the most complex of the complex carbohydrates — the heteropolymers. Compared to homopolymers and repeating copolymers, animal heteropolymers are small, rarely containing more than 30 monosaccharidic units. But, taken together, these chains may contain seven different monosaccharides, six different branch points, and dozens of different glycosidic linkages. Such structures are typically attached to lipids or proteins, and are classified according to the nature of these covalent attachments. Most glycoproteins consist of carbohydrate heteropolymers attached to peptide backbones by any of three linkages: *N*-acetylglucosamine-asparagine ("N" linkages), *N*-acetylgalactosamine-serine or -threonine ("*O*" linkages), and most recently, *N*-acetylglucosamine-serine or -threonine, which is most often found within nuclei. Heteropolymer attachment to lipids occurs either through a glucose-ceramide linkage, or a glycoside-phosphoinositol linkage.

The nature of sugar linkages allows the complex carbohydrates to be the most diverse of all biological polymers. Two different amino acids, or two different nucleic acids, can be attached to one another in only two ways: AB or BA. By contrast, two simple hexoses can form 21 different disaccharides. The reducing, aldehydic carbon (C1) of either monosaccharide can form an ester linkage with any of the five nonreducing carbon atoms of the other monosaccharide. Because each linkage formed can be either α or β, the result is ten possible AB molecules, and ten possible BA molecules. Also, the two sugars can be joined C1 to C1, forming two nonreducing disaccharides. If this progression is expanded to include not two monosaccharides, but the eight most commonly found in animals, and not a polymer that is two sugars long, but, e.g., 30 sugars long, then the number of different polysaccharides possible is essentially infinite.

Interestingly, although the diversity of the complex carbohydrates is theoretically enormous, they tend to fall into a relatively small number of polymer types and patterns. The following figures and tables illustrate some of the oligosaccharide patterns that occur in glycolipids, in two types of glycoproteins, and in some of the glycosaminoglycans. These patterns are those that exist in mammalian systems. In lower vertebrates, the oligosaccharide patterns are similar, although they tend to be truncated at the nonreducing ends. Invertebrates and primitive eukaryotes can have patterns that differ very significantly from one another, and from vertebrates, whereas prokaryotes and plants can contain complex carbohydrate polymers with monosaccharide units that are completely absent in animals.

A. GLYCOLIPIDS

In cells of most vertebrates as well as some invertebrates, the glycolipids that occur most commonly in cell membranes are built up sequentially from a precursor containing the disaccharide lactose (galactose β1-4glucose) linked to a lipid moiety, ceramide. The position and anomeric linkage for each of the simple sugars, or monosaccharide units, is specified by a glycosyltransferase. Several different glycosyltransferases can utilize lactosyl ceramide as an acceptor. Subsequent enzymatic additions of monosaccharides to form four-sugar backbone structures and longer sugar chains of each gycolipid family are carried out by glycosyltransferases highly specific for the terminal, nonreducing structure of the growing sugar chains. Thus, the structural diversity among completed glycolipid chains results from the relative efficiencies and copy numbers of a set of highly specific enzymes that are competing for common acceptor substrates.

Figure 1 illustrates the diversities and similarities that are present simultaneously in the core tetrasaccharide structures of the six glycolipid families commonly found in vertebrate tissues.

B. GLYCOPROTEINS

Glycoproteins, or proteins with oligosaccharide side chains, are split into groups according to the nature of covalent linkage between the oligosaccharide moiety and the peptide moiety. The mucin-type linkages are characterized by an *N*-acetylgalactosamine that is O-linked to a serine or threonine residue of the protein backbone. The N-linked glycoproteins have a core *N*-acetylglucosamine that is linked to asparagine amino groups.

Mucins are highly glycosylated, high-molecular-weight glycoproteins that often contain hundreds of O-linked oligosaccharide chains. Such O-linked oligosaccharides share a few common core structures near the linkage region (Figure 2). Oligosaccharide chains in some mucins are short, containing only two to four simple sugars. Mucins from other tissues may contain elongated and branched oligosaccharides. The disaccharide sequence Galβ1-4GlcNAcβ1-3 ... occurs at or near the termini of many sugar chains found on mucins and can occur as repeating subunits, forming "polylactosamine" chains. Certain "terminating" sugars typically are added at or near the ends of polylactosamine chains. For example, fucosyl, sialyl, galactosyl, and *N*-acetylgalactosaminyl residues are added in various combinations to form the heritable ABO and Lewis blood group antigens (Figure 3).

Soluble and cell membrane-bound glycoproteins often contain N-linked oligosaccharides. These fall into two broad categories, termed "high mannose" and "complex". Both types of chains contain a conserved oligosaccharide core N-glycosidically linked via asparagine to the peptide chain. High mannose chains, as illustrated in Figure 4, contain almost exclusively mannosyl residues linked in a characteristic branching pattern to the N-linked core. Complex chains, an example of which is shown in Figure 5, contain two or more antennary branches linked to the mannosyl residues of the N-linked core. The antennary chains frequently terminate in sialic acid linked to one or several lactosamine units. A variety of other terminating structures are known, however, including those that form the ABO and Lewis antigens

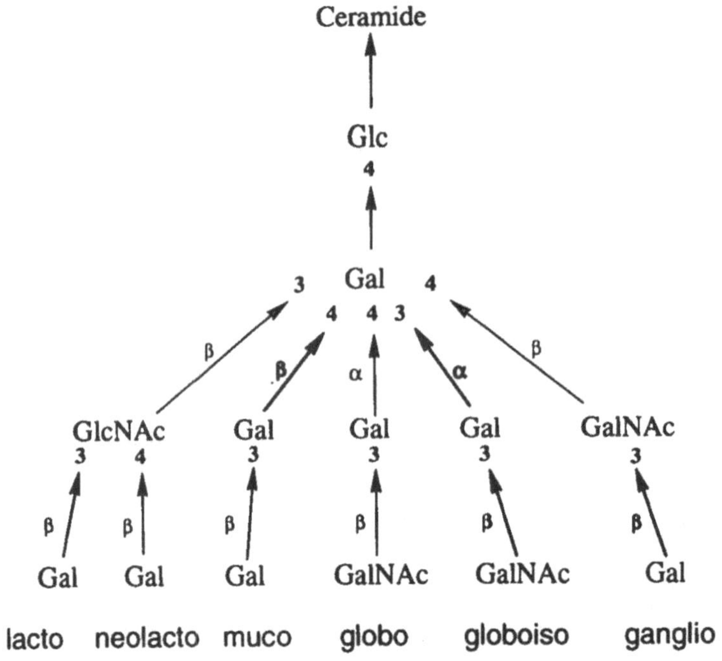

FIGURE 1. The majority of mammalian glycolipids has a core tetrasaccharide structure that falls into one of these six series. Each series is further modified by sugar additions, yielding a very large, but unknown, number of glycolipids. For example, the ganglio series is characterized by the presence of at least one sialic acid residue. The human ABO(O) blood group antigens are built on the lacto- (Type I) or neolacto- (Type II) series, and contain, minimally, a fucose residue on the β-linked, terminal galactoside shown.

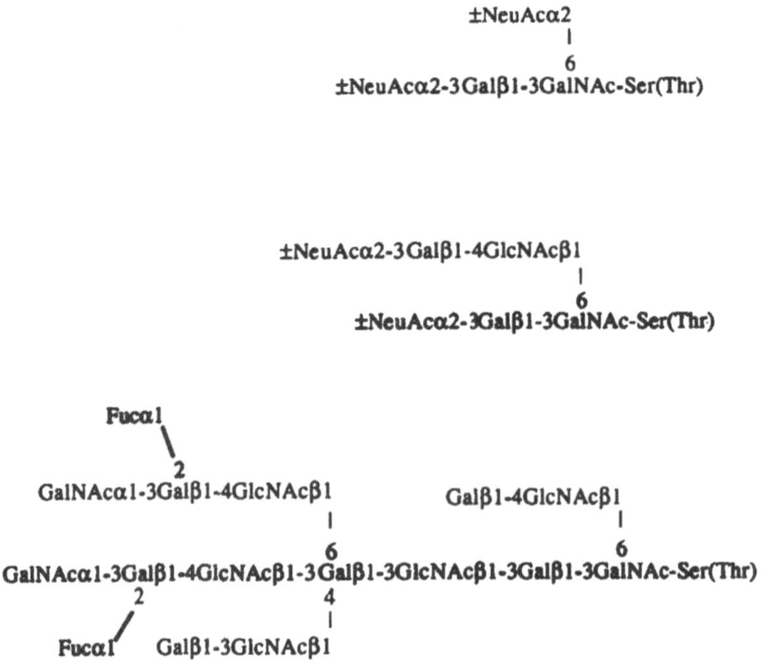

FIGURE 2. Glycoproteins are classified according to nature of the covalent linkage between the oligosaccharide and peptide chains. Typical *O*-linked glycoproteins (referred to in the older literature as mucin-type glycoproteins) have an *N*-acetylgalactosamine linked to the protein backbone through a hydroxyl group on a serine or threonine residue. Three examples of *O*-linked oligosaccharides are illustrated.

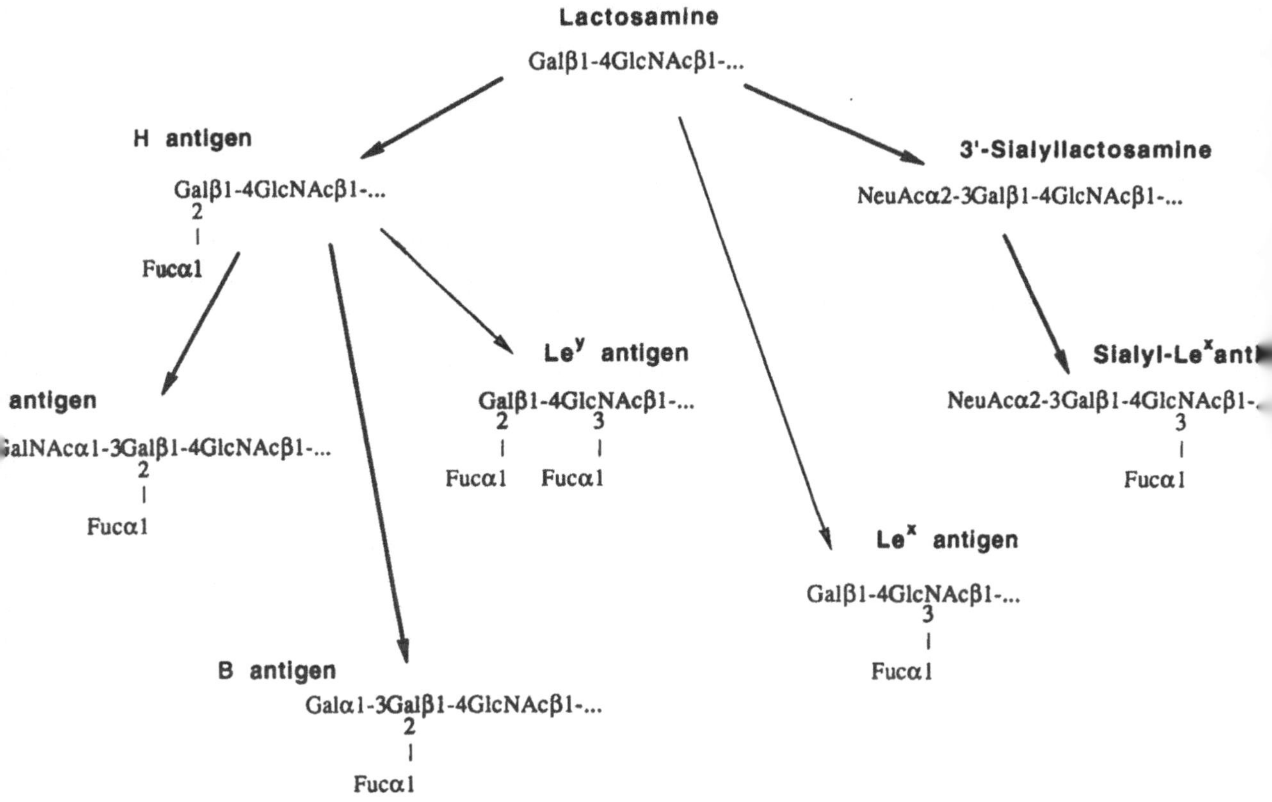

E 3. In humans, the major ABH(O) and Lewis blood group determinants are oligosaccharides, as shown. Inheritance of these determinants occurs onl ce of the glycosyltransferases that catalyze the synthesis of each, specific product. Because the oligosaccharides themselves are not encoded in the humar often termed indirect gene products. For clarity, only Type II structures are illustrated. Most of these structures have been found on glycoproteins and gl

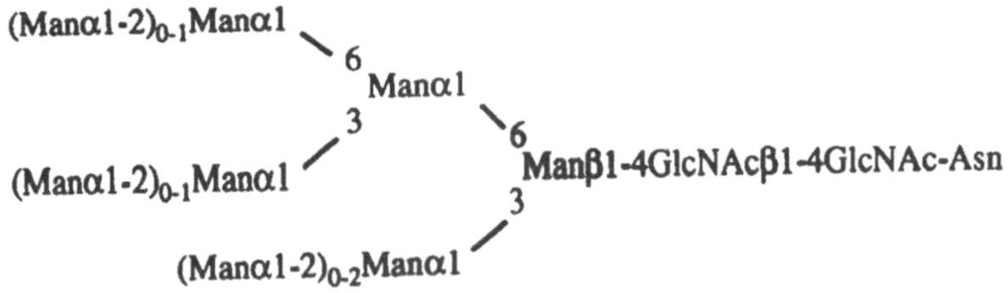

FIGURE 4. *N*-linked glycoproteins are typified by an *N*-acetylglucosamine linked to the amino nitrogen of an asparagine residue in the protein backbone. Such *N*-linked oligosaccharide chains can have branching mannose residues, both of whose nonreducing termini typically end with a sialyllactosamine-type trisaccharide motif. The number of chains, or antennae, found on a single, *N*-linked oligosaccharide is variable. A triantennary compound is illustrated.

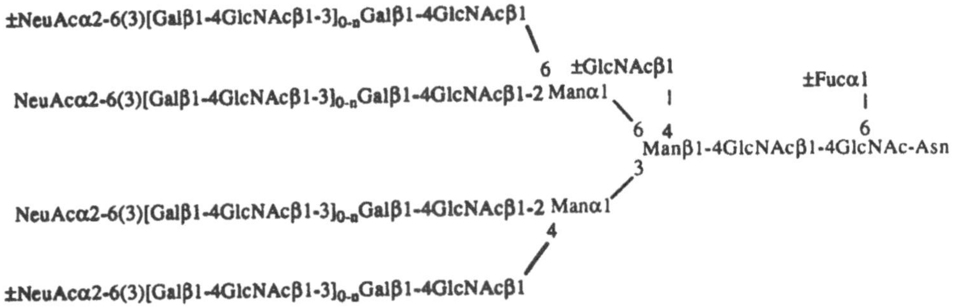

FIGURE 5. A more complex, tetra-antennary, *N*-linked oligosaccharide. The ± indicates that the designated sugar may or may not be found in that position.

(see Figure 3) as well as sulfated, *N*-acetylgalactosaminyl, xylosyl, and α-linked galactosyl residues.

Interestingly, certain carbohydrate epitopes — functionally recognized groups of sugars stereospecifically linked in a specific sequence — can occur at termini of glycolipids and N-linked and O-linked oligosaccharide chains. For example, the sialyl Lewis^x determinant, which is thought to play a key role in the earliest adhesion events involved in leukocyte passage across endothelia, has been found in all three classes of glycoconjugates, as shown in Table 1.

Some proteins may have only mucin-type oligosaccharides, such as ovine submaxillary mucin; some proteins have only N-linked oligosaccharides, such as human α1 acid glycoprotein (often called orosomucoid); and some proteins, like the calf blood protein fetuin, have both kinds of oligosaccharide linkages. Most recently, O-linked *N*-acetylglucosamine residues have been discovered among glycoproteins on the cytoplasmic face of the plasma membrane, and on the nuclear membrane.

Regardless of the diversity of the complex carbohydrates, however, all are assembled by a class of enzymes termed the glycosyltransferases. These enzymes all transfer sugars as monosaccharides, or, as in the case of the core region of the N-linked oligosaccharides, *en bloc*, from high-energy sugar donors to acceptors. The enzymes are typified by very high specificities for both their sugar donors and their sugar acceptors. With only two exceptions, every glycosyltransferase so far described catalyzes the synthesis of only one glycosidic linkage. Although the number of different glycosyltransferases that exist in a single mammalian species is not known, if there are approximately as many different enzymes as different glycosidic linkages, then the number of transferases must be very large.

Table 1

	Reference	Structure
	(7)	**Fucα1** **|** **3** **Neu5Acα2-3Galβ1-4GlcNAcβ1**-3Galβ1-4Glc
ic ma	(8)	**Fucα1** Fucα1 **|** | **3** 3 **Neu5Acα2-3Galβ1-4GlcNAcβ1**-3Galβ1-4GlcNAcβ1-3Galβ1-4Glcβ1-1C

Table 1 (cont.)

	Ref.	Structure
.mniotic	(9)	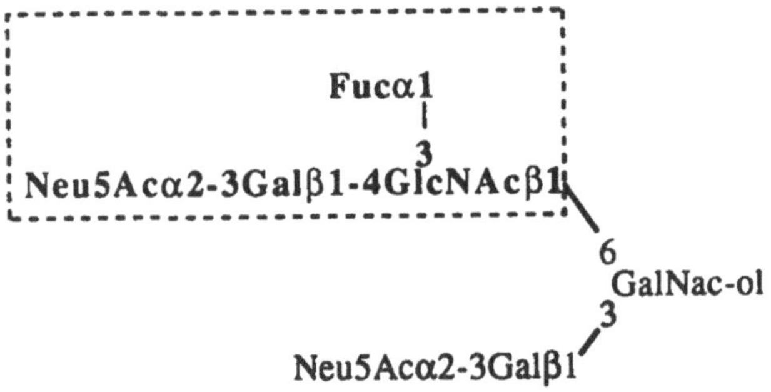
n teins	(10)	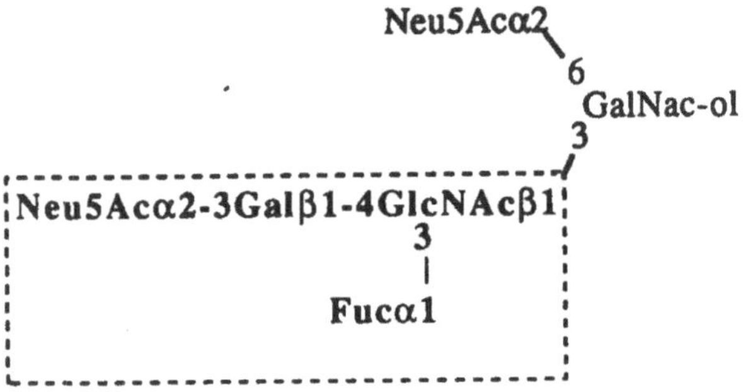

coprotrein
atic breast
oma

(11)

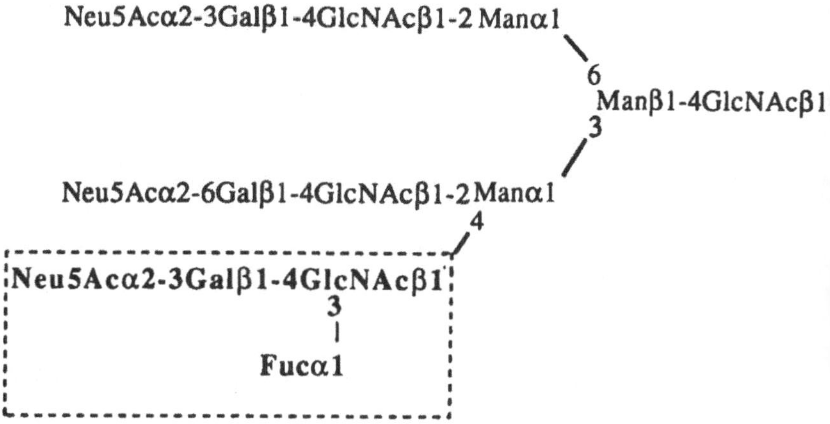

Table 1 (cont.)

Ref.	Structure
(12)	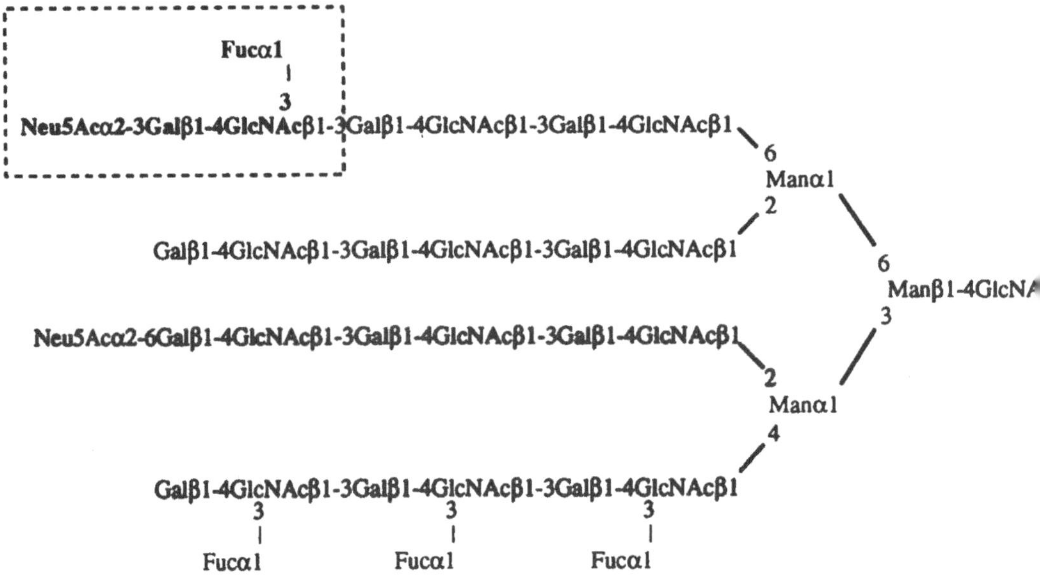

III. THE POTENTIAL FOR CARBOHYDRATE PHARMACEUTICALS

The mechanisms for diverse cellular adhesive interactions involve molecular complementarity between surface proteins and oligosaccharides. This is a repeating recognition theme that occurs between many pathogens and their target host cells or tissues,[13] between white blood cells and vascular endothelia during appropriate and inappropriate inflammation,[14] among cancer cells during metastases,[15] and among embryonic cells during normal and abnormal morphogenesis.[16] The control of undesirable cell adhesions, therefore, rests with the specific proteins involved and their cognate oligosaccharides. In many cases, the oligosaccharides are the inhibitory drug of choice.

A. ANTI-INFECTIVE OLIGOSACCHARIDES

The first step in most infectious diseases is the attachment of the bacterium, virus, protozoan, or fungus to its target. Subsequent phenomena are complex and may include multiplication, colonization, encystment, parasitism, invasion, cytolysis, and toxin production by the pathogen in question. In most cases where the biochemistry of pathogen attachment mechanisms is understood, they involve highly specific interactions between pathogen surface proteins (often called lectins or adhesins) and target cell surface oligosaccharides.

Much *in vitro* data show that the attachment of pathogens to cell surfaces can be inhibited by soluble forms of the target oligosaccharide. Indeed, soluble oligosaccharides (like those found in milk, saliva, tears, and sweat), and epithelial mucus layers are probably natural anti-infectives. Ontogenetically, oligosaccharides protect newborns before their immune systems mature. Phylogenetically, they are anti-infectives in invertebrates, none of which have immune systems.

At least in mammals, therefore, oligosaccharides are likely to be the first line of defense against a host of pathogenic organisms, including those that cause pneumonia,[17] diarrhea,[18] gastritis and ulcers,[19] periodontal disease,[20] candidiasis,[21] and sexually transmitted diseases caused, at least, by gonococcus[22] and chlamydia.[23]

Critical issues remain concerning the pharmaceutical potential for specific, anti-infective oligosaccharides. Will they be safe? Will they be effective prophylactics *in vivo?* Might they be therapeutic agents, as well?

The first question cannot be answered definitively until large amounts of specific complex carbohydrates are synthesized or isolated and administered to animals and, ultimately, humans. Although such tests have not been done, it is difficult to imagine why oral ingestion of such compounds will prove toxic at reasonable concentrations. The human airway and gastrointestinal systems deal daily with large amounts of heterologous complex carbohydrates from many sources. The oligosaccharide pharmaceuticals under discussion here would, of course, be autologous compounds. Even parenteral administration of specific, autologous oligosaccharides and their derivatives should be nontoxic and nonimmunogenic. These suppositions, however, require experimental testing before they can begin to be accepted.

As to the question of *in vivo* efficacy, observations suggest that oligosaccharides will be useful. Coppa et al.[24] have shown that the urine of breast-fed babies contains oligosaccharides similar to those found in their mothers' milk. These oligosaccharides inhibit the attachment of *Escherichia coli* (isolated from urinary tract infections) to urinary epithelial cells from the infants themselves. Urine from formula-fed infants contains no oligosaccharides and has no similar anti-infective properties. The ability of urinary oligosaccharides to prevent urinary tract infections could explain why pregnant women rarely have urinary tract infections despite the almost constant presence of bacteria in their urine. Pregnant women secrete many oligosaccharides into their urine beginning in the second trimester and dwindling at birth. In nonpregnant women, who do not secrete urinary oligosaccharides, bacteriuria is almost always associated with urinary tract infections.

In a more quantitative study, Mouricout et al.[25] administered orally as many as 10^{10} enterotoxic *E. coli* to newborn calves. Of the calves that were not further treated, all died from diarrhea. Experimental calves, however, were spared by the near-simultaneous, oral administration of 250-mg doses of bovine oligosaccharides prepared from blood glycoconjugates. Although it is not clear what fraction of the administered oligosaccharides was active against the *E. coli,* it is clear that at least some of the compounds were effective. Assuming that a human infant is one tenth the weight of a newborn calf, and that one tenth of the administered oligosaccharides was specific for the toxic bacteria, then it is possible that 2.5 mg of one oligosaccharide could protect an infant from a massive bacterial challenge.

There are, therefore, many experiments showing that oligosaccharides can prevent pathogen attachment to cells *in vitro,* and a smattering that suggest *in vivo* efficacy, as well.

A remaining question pertains to the ability of oligosaccharides to detach pathogens after they have attached to target tissues. From a purely theoretical view, detachment by soluble competitors of attached ligands will occur when the concentration of the competitor is sufficiently high; that is, above the association constant of the ligand for its substrate. This, after all, is how soluble competitors detach ligands during the specific elution phase of affinity chromatography. Consistent with this principle, Ofek et al.[26] have shown that the same oligosaccharides that inhibit *E. coli* attachment to cultured epithelial cells also effect the release, in minutes, of previously attached bacteria.

The degree to which these results will be applicable to *in vivo* situations will depend on many factors, including the rate with which attached pathogens become unavailable to diffusing, soluble inhibitors, however small. Clearly, much experimentation is required before any of these questions can be answered with great confidence.

For the moment, however, all indications suggest that oligosaccharides should be pursued vigorously as a potentially new class of anti-infectives that could be used alone, prophylactically and therapeutically, or with other, standard antibiotics. Such combination therapies might increase the therapeutic efficiencies of both agents by yielding equivalent clinical improvement at lower antibiotic concentrations, or by increasing the susceptible pathogen spectrum at standard concentrations.

B. ANTI-INFLAMMATORY OLIGOSACCHARIDES

Much early excitement has been stimulated by reports[27,28] that describe protein-carbohydrate interactions as mediators of white blood cell attachment to blood vessel endothelia, the first in a cascade of events that lead to local inflammation. Although many of these early descriptions suggested specific oligosaccharide structures (such as the Lewis X and sialylated Lewis X antigens) as molecular complements to the leukocyte adhesion proteins, or selectins, more recent results[29,30] suggest that these assignments may have been premature.

In the search for anti-inflammatory agents, nevertheless, the focus should remain strongly positive. Adhesive interactions among white cells, endothelial cells, and platelets are involved generally in the initiation, at least, of many inflammatory reactions. Further, such adhesive interactions are caused by molecular recognition between proteins and oligosaccharides. Eventually, many more selectins will no doubt be described, and the precise structures of the natural oligosaccharidic ligands for each of these selectins will emerge. As these molecular interactions become more and more clear, their uses as anti-inflammatory drugs will become equally straightforward.

Currently, the most prudent path is the one that seeks ever newer selectins, perhaps with specificities that are related to anatomic and pathologic variables, and then strives to find those carbohydrates that best associate with the proteins. Obviously these oligosaccharides should occur naturally in the time and place typical of the selectin and the inflammation under study.

For example, consider a particular yeast glucomannan that binds with a significant avidity to a human lymphocyte selectin. Even if the avidity of the selectin/glucomannan binding is greater than that between the selectin and a dozen mammalian oligosaccharides, tested systematically and rigorously, it would be incorrect to conclude that the glucomannan is the selectin's natural ligand, unless, and for the first time, the presence of that particular glucomannan is demonstrated in the system under study. In the absence of such a demonstration, one must conclude either that the natural ligand has not yet been found and tested, or that the natural ligand has a lower affinity for its selectin than do other oligosaccharides.

Once described, both the selectins and the carbohydrate ligands become candidates for anti-inflammatory drug testing. In theory, and on a molar basis, both the proteins and the oligosaccharides will be equally effective at inhibiting the initial adhesive interactions that are mediated by the particular, membrane-bound components in question. Molar potency is only one criterion, however, for overall drug desirability. For any selectin/oligosaccharide pair, the oligosaccharide moiety will be more stable (typical oligosaccharides can withstand temperature and pH extremes that will denature typical proteins) and more potent (with necessarily identical association constants, a tetrasaccharide with a molecular weight of, for example, 800 Da, will be ten times more potent, on a weight basis, than its selectin, with a molecular weight of 80,000 Da).

Another possible advantage of sugar-based anti-inflammatory agents, compared with their proteinaceous counterparts, is absorbability. Because proteins are not absorbed intact across the intestinal boundary, selectins, and even selectin fragments, will have to be administered parenterally. There are data,[31] however, suggesting that oligosaccharides at least as large as tetrasaccharides are absorbed in significant amounts after oral ingestion. If subsequent experimentation with a variety of oligosaccharides yields similar results, then it is likely that anti-inflammatory oligosaccharides could be administered orally.

C. DIAGNOSTICS

Specific oligosaccharides prevent attachment of pathogens to target cells and tissues because they bind to the pathogen adhesins, the carbohydrate-binding proteins on the bacteria, fungi, viruses, or protozoans. This same molecular complementarity can be utilized to create an entirely new class of diagnostics that could be used alone, or, more likely, to supplement antibody-based diagnostics, which are the dominant form today. Matrix-bound oligosaccharides would act as affinity substrates for those bacteria, e.g., with adhesins specific for the carbohydrate. Although individual oligosaccharide:adhesin affinities might be weak, the combined effects of thousands of bound ligands will firmly attach any pathogen to an appropriately derivatized matrix.

This approach could be used alone or with an antibody-based diagnostic test. Because it is extremely unlikely that a pathogen-specific antibody will be directed against that pathogen's carbohydrate-recognizing adhesin, a diagnostic assay with both oligosaccharidic and immunologic bases will necessarily have lower false-positive and false-negative rates than the assay with the immunologic base alone.

Oligosaccharide-based diagnostic methods have an added advantage in that the assay is detecting not merely a specific cell wall epitope, but a surface function that is required for virulence. Typical diagnostics in use today do not distinguish between virulent and avirulent forms of the pathogen in question. By contrast, a test that uses, even in part, an adhesin-specific oligosaccharide will react less avidly with a pathogen that has lost normal adhesin function.

D. MOLECULAR MAIL USING GLYCO-ADDRESSING

Two kinds of drug targeting are useful, and both of these could be aided significantly by specific oligosaccharides. The first is getting particular drugs only to particular parts of the body, the second is delivering antibiotics to particular pathogens.

A good deal of current research in glycobiology is aimed at defining the degree to which individual organs, tissues, and perhaps even cells, possess unique oligosaccharides and proteins that recognize unique oligosaccharides. Already, different carbohydrate-binding proteins with restricted tissue distributions can be localized to the liver, lymph nodes, and blood vessels. Therefore, specific oligosaccharides that bind to the target protein, when attached to a contrasting or visualizing agent, should increase enormously the eventual concentration of that agent in the organ or tissue that contains the target protein.

For pathogens with carbohydrate-binding proteins, a similar strategy could be used. Here, specific oligosaccharides would be attached not to visualizing agents, but to appropriate antibiotics.

The oligosaccharide portion of the chimeric molecule should increase the local concentration of the antibiotic around the pathogen by binding to the pathogen's carbohydrate-recognizing protein. Such an oligosaccharidically addressed antibiotic might be effective against bacteria at doses that are much lower than those necessary for the antibiotic alone. Furthermore, by using the chimeric compound at dose levels that are standard for the antibiotic alone, it is likely that the increased efficacy of the new drug will allow it to affect additional types of bacteria that otherwise would not be affected. By glyco-addressing antibiotics, therefore, they could be made effective at lower concentrations. Alternatively, at concentrations closer to those typical of standard antibiotics, these new, glyco-addressed antibiotics could enjoy a broader spectrum of susceptible bacterial species.

IV. OBSTACLES

A. OBTAINING SPECIFIC HUMAN OLIGOSACCHARIDES

With a potential for therapy and prophylaxis against infectious diseases caused by bacteria, viruses, and fungi, in addition to novel diagnostic and imaging uses, why are there are no data in humans that show the efficacy of specific oligosaccharides in any of these situations? The answer to this important question is quite clear — until recently, there has been no way to synthesize particular human oligosaccharides in large amounts and at reasonable costs. The absence of specific, pure, complex oligosaccharides in 100 g to kilogram quantities has made it impossible even to conduct toxicity tests in small mammals. Without toxicity data, safety and pharmacokinetic analyses in humans are not possible. And, needless to say, without toxicity, safety, and pharmacokinetic information, clinical efficacy studies cannot be initiated.

In years past, the inability to synthesize oligosaccharides in significant amounts led to three alternative approaches. The first alternative was to accumulate natural oligosaccharides by purifying them from natural sources, like human milk; the second was to use repeating oligosaccharidic polymers that are easily obtained from plants, yeast, or bacteria; the third is to attempt to design molecular analogs of naturally occurring oligosaccharides.

The main drawback associated with purifying human oligosaccharides from natural sources is, of course, the severely limited amount of raw material. Although most secreted human fluids contain some oligosaccharides, the amounts of these fluids available are insufficient for typical commercial applications. Unfortunately, the fluid most easily available, urine, possesses the smallest concentration of oligosaccharides. Other fluids, with much higher concentrations, like tears, seminal fluid, and milk, are also much less easily obtained.

Another drawback associated with purification of oligosaccharides from human fluids is the risk of contamination by viruses and other potential pathogens. For oligosaccharides, however, this risk can be minimized, or even eliminated completely, by taking advantage of the stability of complex sugars. Oligosaccharides can withstand pH and temperature extremes that would denature most proteins. Most oligosaccharides in aqueous solutions close to neutral pH can even be autoclaved, and many of these polymers are soluble in alcohol solutions that destroy all known infectious agents.

The therapeutic use of carbohydrate polymers that are isolated from plants, bacteria, or yeasts is effective in direct proportion to the molecular similarity between the isolated analogous polymer and its human homologue. Many such polymers, especially anionically charged polymers, such as the dextran sulfates, have antiviral and antibacterial properties *in vitro*. Disadvantages associated with these polymers include their lack of specificity and their potential as immunogens.

B. OLIGOSACCHARIDE ANALOGS BY RATIONAL DRUG DESIGN

The third alternative to the direct synthesis of natural, human cell surface oligosaccharides as therapeutic or diagnostic agents is the synthesis of oligosaccharide analogs, or rational drug design. Here, with the aid of computers, the three-dimensional structure of an oligosaccharide is determined, and that structure is then imitated with molecules more easily manipulated. The clay from which these sculptures can be created could be peptides, other organic molecules, inorganic compounds, or any combination thereof. One reason that this experimental feat has not yet been achieved could be the difficulties associated with the unequivocal determination of the tertiary, and even secondary, structures of an oligosaccharide, given complete knowledge of its primary structure. Because of the relatively high freedom of rotation of glycosidic bonds, especially compared with peptide bonds, the number of stable configurations even for a tetrasaccharide[32] is much larger than for a known tetrapeptide.

A more rational approach to rational drug design of complex carbohydrates might be the anti-idiotype or peptide library methods (see Chapters 7 and 10). That is, the fine structure of the active site of a known carbohydrate-binding protein[33,34] should be a valid indicator of at least one particular configuration of the oligosaccharide that is recognized by that carbohydrate-binding protein.

Within the limited framework of a particular carbohydrate-binding protein, therefore, an analog that results from rational drug design and synthesis may be a perfect representation of the target oligosaccharidic homologue. Nevertheless, it may be toxic in its interactions with other molecules, or immunogenic. For example, it may be possible to sculpt chemically a replica of the sialyl Lewis^x epitope that binds to E-selectin with exactly the affinity of the natural tetrasaccharide that defines this antigen. If, however, the sculpture is produced from nonhuman material, this material might itself interact undesirably with other receptors, or might trigger an immune response.

C. DIRECT SYNTHESIS OF NATURAL OLIGOSACCHARIDES

Much progress is being made on the direct synthesis of complex carbohydrates, and most of this progress currently is occurring in small, corporate laboratories. Synthetic methods fall into three classes: chemical, enzymatic, and a combination of both.

Chemical synthesis of oligosaccharides is difficult because of the exquisite specificities that lie within the anomeric and isomeric variations of the glycosidic bond, and because of the repeated protections and deprotection required by almost all of the hydroxyl groups, which are otherwise fairly reactive. As synthesis proceeds from a trisaccharide to a tetrasaccharide to a pentasaccharide, protection and deprotection become more and more difficult, and overall yields suffer. Despite these difficulties, several groups have chemically synthesized nonrepeating polymers as large as hexasaccharides, albeit in relatively small amounts.

At present, enzymatic synthesis shows the most promise for large-scale, cost-efficient manufacture of specific oligosaccharides. The enzymes most commonly used for this purpose are the anabolic glycosyltransferases and the catabolic glycosidases. The glycosyltransferases are the enzymes that *in vivo* catalyze the synthesis of all complex carbohydrates in nature. They are highly specific, and, with two possible exceptions, each enzyme forms a single glycosidic bond. Very few of these enzymes are commercially available, however, and for monosaccharide donors, they require sugar nucleotides, which are prohibitively expensive if purchased from typical suppliers of fine chemicals. The glycosyltransferase availability hurdle is now being overcome by recombinant methodologies, and, as in our own manufacturing operations, by iterative affinity purification of the enzymes from inexpensive, natural sources. The sugar nucleotide problem can be eliminated by direct self-manufacture.

The utilization of glycosidases as synthetic enzymes is not likely to be competitive with the glycosyltransferase-based methods for two reasons. First, to force the enzymes to synthesize glycosides, concentrations of acceptor molecules must be sufficiently high to compete with water molecules, which are the usual acceptors for the hydrolases. Second, the hydrolases are not nearly as specific as the transferases. Thus, a rather loose specificity in cleaving glycosidic bonds is reflected in the equally loose specificity apparent when the glycosidases are forced to work in reverse.

V. CONCLUSIONS

With the ability for large-scale, efficient synthesis of complex human oligosaccharides upon us, it will shortly be possible for the first time to test these long-studied molecules in clinical trials. As anti-infectives, a wealth of *in vitro* and physiological data suggests that oligosaccharides are effective inhibitors of bacterial and viral attachment processes, and that, in the form of respiratory and gastrointestinal mucins, they are, indeed, the first line of defense against entering pathogens. Because they represent an entirely new way to combat a host of infectious diseases, oligosaccharides could be used alone or with standard antibiotic therapies.

Free oligosaccharides complementary to the endothelial selectins might also be effective against excessive inflammatory reactions, although most such uses will require systemic administration methods (unless the oligosaccharides are efficiently absorbed in adults, as human milk oligosaccharides are absorbed by the gut of newborns).

For diagnostic and imaging processes, there can be little doubt that specific oligosaccharides will find their way into many products and procedures.

Because so many cases of intercellular adhesive recognition during embryogenesis and during metastasis are mediated by protein-carbohydrate interactions, oligosaccharide pharmacology may ultimately have its greatest impact on the early detection and treatment of birth defects and malignancies. These applications must remain on the horizon for now. Nevertheless, for oligosaccharides, that horizon is exceptionally vast, promising, and exciting.

REFERENCES

1. **Ashwell, G. and Morell, A.G.,** Role of surface carbohydrates in hepatic recognition and transport of circulating glycoproteins, *Adv. Enzymol.*, 41, 99, 1974.
2. **Taylor, M., Conary, J.T., Lennartz, M., Stahl, P., and Drickamer, K.,** Primary structure of the mannose receptor contains multiple motifs resembling carbohydrate-recognition domains, *J. Biochem.*, 265, 12156, 1990.
3. **Smith, P.L. and Baenziger, J.U.,** Molecular basis of recognition by the glycoprotein hormore-specific N-acetylgalactosamine-transferase, *Science*, 89, 329, 1992.
4. **McGuire, E.J., Kerlin, R., Cebra, J.J., and Roth, S.,** Human milk galactosyltransferase is specific for secreted, but not plasma IgA, *J. Immunol.*, 143, 2933, 1989.
5. **Roth, S., McGuire, E.J. et al.,** Evidence for cell-surface glycosyltransferases and their role in intercellular adhesive specificity, *J. Cell Biol.*, 15, 525, 1971.
6. **Lasky, L.,** Selectins: interpreters of cell-specific carbohydrate information during inflammation, *Science*, 258, 964, 1992.
7. **Grönberg, G., Lipniunas, P., and Lundgren, T.,** Isolation of monosialylated oligosaccharides from human milk and structural analysis of three new compounds, *Carbohydr. Res.*, 191, 261, 1989.
8. **Fukushi, Y. et al.,** Novel fucolipids accumulating in human adenocarcinoma, *J. Biochem.*, 259, 10511, 1984.
9. **Hanisch, F., Egge, H., Peter-Katalinic, J., and Uhlenbruck, G.,** Primary structure of a major sialylsaccharide alditol from human amniotic mucins expressing the tumor-associated sialyl-X antigenic determinant, *FEBS Lett.*, 200, 42, 1986.

10. **Capon, C., Leroy, Y., Wieruszeski, J.M., Ricart, G., Strecker, G., Montreuil, J., and Fournet, B.,** Structures of *O*-glycosidically linked oligosaccharides isolated from human meconium glycoproteins, *Eur. J. Biochem.*, 182, 139, 1989.
11. **Chandreasekaran, V., Davila, M., Nixon, D., and Mendicino, J.,** Structures of the oligosaccharide chains of two forms of α1-acid glycoprotein purified from liver mestases of lung, colon, and breast tumors, *Cancer Res.*, 44, 1557, 1984.
12. **Fukuda, M., Spooncer, E., Oates, J., Dell, A., and Klock, J.,** Structure of sialylated fucosyl lactosaminoglycan isolated from human granulocytes, *J. Biochem.*, 259, 10925, 1984.
13. **Elliott, K., O'Connor, M., and Whelan, J., Eds.,** *Proc. Symp. on Adhesion and Microorganism Pathogenicity*, Pitman Press, Bath, U.K., 1981.
14. **Walz, G., Aruffo, A., Kolanus, W., Bevilacqua, M., and Seed, B.,** Recognition by ELAM-1 of the Sialyl Le^x determinant on myeloid and tumor cells, *Science*, 250, 1132, 1990.
15. **Roth, S. and White, D.,** Intercellular contact and cell surface galactosyltransferase activity, *Proc. Natl. Acad. Sci., U.S.A.*, 69, 485, 1972.
16. **Roth, S.,** Glycosyltransferases as effectors of cell recognition, in *Molecular Approaches to Supracellular Phenomena*, (Roth, S.,) Ed., (Developmental Biology Series), University of Pennsylvania Press) Philadelphia, 1990, 201.
17. **Krivan, H., Roberts, D., and Ginsburg, V.,** Many pulmonary pathogenic bacteria bind specifically to the carbohydrate sequence GalNAcβ1-4Gal found in some glycolipids, *Proc. Natl. Acad. Sci. U.S.A.*, 85, 6157, 1988.
18. **Ashkenazi, S. and Mirelman, D.,** Nonimmunoglobulin fraction of human milk inhibits the adherence of certain enterotoxigenic *Escherichia coli* strains to guinea pig intestinal tract, *Pediatr. Res.*, 22, 130, 1987.
19. **Graham, D., Lew, G., Klein, P., Evans, D., Evens, D., Saeed, Z., and Malaty, H.,** Effect of treatment of *Helicobacter pylori* infection on the long-term recurrence of gastric or duodenal ulcer, *Anal. Intern. Med.*, 116, 705, 1992.
20. **Gibbons, R.J.,** Bacterial adhesion to oral tissues: a model for infectious diseases, *J. Dent. Res.*, 68, 750, 1989.
21. **Jimenz-Lucho, V., Ginsburg, V., and Krivan, H.,** *Cryptococcus neoformans, Candida albicans*, and other fungi bind specifically to the glycosphingolipid lactosylceramide (Galβ1-4Glcβ1-1Cer), a possible adhesion receptor for yeasts, *Infect. Immun.*, 58, 2085, 1990.
22. **Stromberg, N., Deal, C., Nyberg, G., Normark, S., So, M., and Karlsson, K.,** Identification of carbohydrate structures that are possible receptor for *Neisseria gonorrhoae*, *Proc. Natl. Acad. Sci. U.S.A.*, 85, 4902, 1988.
23. **Krivan, H.C., Nilsson, B., Lingwood, C.A., and Ryu, H.,** *Chlamydia trachomatis* and *Chlamydia pneumoniae* bind specifically to phosphatidylethanolamine in hela cells and to GalNaCβ1-4Galβ1-4Glc sequences found in Asialo-GM_1 Asialo-GM_2, *Biochem. Biophys.*, 175, 1082, 1991.
24. **Coppa, G.V., Gabvrielli, O., Giogi, P. et al.,** Preliminary study of breastfeeding and bacterial adhesion to uroepithelial cells, *Lancet*, 335, 569, 1990.
25. **Mouricout, M., Petit, J.M., Carias, J.R., and Julien, R.,** Glycoprotein glycan that inhibit adhesion of *Escherichia coli* mediated by K99 fimbriae: treatment of experimental colibacillosis, *Infect. Immun.*, 58, 98, 1990.
26. **Ofek, I., Mirelman, D., and Sharon, N.,** Adherence of *Escherichia coli* to human mucosal cells mediated by mannose receptors, *Nature*, 265, 623, 1977.
27. **Picker, L., Kishimoto, T., Smith, C.W., Warnock, A., and Butcher, E.,** ELAM-1 is an adhesion molecule for skin-homing T cells, *Nature*, 349, 796, 1991.
28. **Larsen, E., Palabrica, T., Sajer, S., Gilbert, G., Wagner, D., and Furie, B.,** PADGEM-dependent adhesion of platelets to monocytes and neutrophils is mediated by a lineage-specific carbohydrate, LNF III (CD15), *Cell*, 63, 467, 1990.
29. **Green, P., Tamatani, T., Watanabe, T., Miyasaska, M., Hasegawa, A., Kiso, M., Yuen, C.-T., Stoll, M.S., and Feizi, T.,** High affinity binding of the leucocyte adhesion molecule L-selectin to 3′-sulphated-Le^a and Le^x oligosaccharides and the predominance of sulphate in this interaction demonstrated by binding studies with a series of lipid-linked oligosaccharides, *Biochem. Biophys.*, 188, 244, 1992.
30. **Berg, E., Robinson, M., Mansson, O., Butcher, E., and Magnani, J.,** A carbohydrate domain common to both sialyl Le^a and sialyl Le^x is recognized by the endothelial cell leukocyte adhesion molecule ELAM-1, *J. Biochem.*, 266, 14869, 1991.
31. **Kumlien, J., Chester, A., Lindberg, B., Pizzo, P., Zopf, D., and Lundblad, A.,** Urinary excretion of a glucose-containing tetrasaccharide, *Clin. Chim. Acta*, Ch. III, 1988.
32. **Carver, J.P., Michnick, S.W., Imberty, A., and Cumming, D.A.,** Oligosaccharide-protein interactions: a three dimensional view, *Carbohydr. Recognition Cell. Funct.*, 6-19, 1989.
33. **Weis, W.I., Drickamer, K., and Hendrickson, W.A.,** Structure of a C-type mannose-binding protein complexed with an oligosaccharide, *Nature*, 360, 127, 1992.
34. **Drickamer, K.,** Engineering a galactose-binding activity into a C-type mannose-binding protein, *Nature*, 360, 183, 1992.

Chapter 7

GENE THERAPY

Jean D. Boyer and David B. Weiner

CONTENTS

I. INTRODUCTION

Gene therapy has provided an opportunity to supply genetic material to individuals and possibly alleviate certain diseases. It encompasses a variety of technologies that seek to improve the human condition through manipulation and transfer of genetic material. Although

0-8493-9422-8/94/$0.00+$.50

TABLE 1
Approved Human Gene Transfer Trials

Gene Therapy	Principal Investigator
ADA gene transfer to lymphocytes from ADA-deficient patients	R.M. Blaese (NIH)
LDL receptor gene transfer to hepatocytes from LDL receptor-deficient patients	J.M. Wilson (University of Pennsylvania)
TNF gene transfer to tumor-infiltrating lymphocytes	S.A. Rosenberg (NIH)
IL-2 gene transfer to tumor cells	S.A. Rosenberg (NIH)
TNF to tumor cells	S.A. Rosenberg (NIH)
Antigen transfer to tumor cells *in situ* to stimulate immune rejection	G.J. Nabel (University of Michigan)
ADA gene transfer to peripheral blood stem cells from ADA-deficient patients	R.M. Blaese (NIH)
CFTR gene transfer to the respiratory tracks of patients	Ronald G. Crystal (Cornell University) James Wilson (University of Pennsylvania) Michael Welsh (University of Iowa)
Toxin gene transfer to ovarian carcinoma cells for treatment of ovarian cancer	S.M. Freeman (University of Rochester)

it is basically still a new approach to treatment of any condition, advances are being made at a rapid pace. Table 1 lists a number of gene therapy treatments that have already been approved for clinical trials. Among the many conditions targeted for gene therapy are cancer treatment, persistent viral infections, and dysfunctions associated with genetic deficiency.

A wide variety of tumor cells are clearly able to evade the immune response, which often results in fatal disease. However, advances in the mechanisms of cell transformation have made it possible for gene therapy to be applied to cancer treatment in various ways that may prove helpful. It has been observed that there is a decrease of functional class I major histocompatibility complex (MHC) molecules expressed on the surface of tumor cells. Whereas most tumor cells express normal surface antigens in an abnormal fashion, some tumor cells display viral surface antigens which could serve as "flags" to the immune system. Many current gene therapy approaches to cancer treatment, therefore, involve the manipulation of the immune response. A second approach that is being investigated with vigor involves the delivery of a toxin to the tumor cells. This tactic takes advantage of the promoters that are turned on during cell transformation.

Some inherited disorders do not have any known treatment, such as Alzheimer's disease, or involve therapies that must continue throughout the patient's lifetime. The genes for many such disorders, including familial Alzheimer's disease,[1] Huntington's disease,[2] amyotrophic lateral sclerosis or Lou Gehrig's disease,[3] adrenoleukodystrophy,[4] and colon cancer[5] have recently been discovered and have become likely targets for gene therapy. The method of transgene transfer is a critical issue: some methods may be transient when a stable transfer is better or some modes of transfer may be too invasive. It may be necessary to inject directly into the affected organ or target the injection such that systemic expression will result. There are a number of modes of transfer that can be considered to meet the clinical needs of the patients.

Finally, the etiological causes of certain viral diseases, such as acquired immune deficiency syndrome (AIDS), have proven to be difficult to develop a vaccine against and may need novel approaches to abrogate. An effective immune response involves the recognition of the infectious organism. Gene therapy provides that opportunity to present to the host functional proteins by transfer of their genes while also allowing researchers to delete any genes which code for proteins that may have deleterious effects.

There are a number of ways transgenes can be transferred to an individual. No specific gene transfer technique is currently adequate to treat all conditions. DNA can be delivered to cells that have been removed from a patient. The cells are transfected *in vitro* and transferred back into the patient. This procedure is also referred to as *ex vivo* transfection or transduction. The gene can also be transferred to the patient *in vivo* using either an altered viral particle as a mode of transport and delivery or direct injection of DNA molecules. When considering gene therapy as a choice of treatment there are some basic considerations: the transgene, the delivery package, target tissue, and the level of expression. This chapter will examine the different methods of gene transfer and various conditions under which they have been used.

II. RETROVIRUSES

The properties of retroviruses make them a natural choice as vectors for the transmission and expression of foreign genes. The retroviral vector host range can be made diverse or specific by taking advantage of the amphotropic or ecotropic nature of the wild-type retroviruses. Also, gene transfer by way of retroviral particles leads to stable transduction of the cells because the retroviral genome is integrated into the host genome. Further, they can be used to transfer genes to humans by *in vivo* or *ex vivo* methods, as long as the cells to be transfected are in a state of mitosis. In tissue culture retroviruses can be grown to high titers and efficiency of infection can be 100%. Finally, retroviruses have relatively small genomes that can easily be manipulated for the introduction of foreign genes. Of concern, however, is the chance that insertional mutagenesis will occur. For example, recent *in vivo* studies have shown that a replication competent virus based on the moloney murine leukemia virus can induce lymphoma in monkeys.[6] Retroviral particles can, however, be manipulated such that they are replication defective. While the probability that a virus will integrate into an oncogenic site is very low if it is rendered nonreplicating, the possibility of oncogenic transformation should be deliberated when considering this method of gene transfer.

A. LIFE CYCLE OF RETROVIRUSES

Retroviruses predominantly infect vertebrates and most have a similar structure, mechanism of replication, and genome organization (see Figures 1 and 2). The 100-nm virion contains two molecules of single-stranded RNA surrounded by a nucleocapsid and an envelope composed of a cellular lipid bilayer containing the retroviral envelope proteins. The envelope proteins are made up of two subunits which are responsible for receptor binding (tropism) and viral membrane fusion with the host cell membrane. The internal nucleocapsid is made up of the core proteins, which include products of the *gag* gene. Also included in the nucleocapsid are several proteins, products of the *pol* gene, containing enzymatic activity important for replication. These include the reverse transcriptase, which converts the genetic information from single-stranded RNA to double-stranded DNA, integrase, which is necessary for covalently joining the viral DNA to endogenous DNA to form the provirus, and protease, responsible for cleaving the core proteins from the products of the *pol* gene as well as further *gag/pol* processing. There are other proteins encoded for by retroviruses which are not universal to all retroviruses. These proteins seem to be responsible for up- or downregulating transcription and translation or facilitating virus adaption to the cell. An example is the rev protein in the human immunodeficiency virus (HIV). This small protein binds to a nucleotide sequence on the transcribed RNA, rev responsive element, and increases translation through transport from nucleus to cytoplasm where the virus message binds to ribosomes in the endoplasmic reticulum and is translated into proteins.

Retroviruses share a common genetic organization, illustrated in Figure 2. Long terminal repeats (LTRs) are formed at each end as the viral RNA is transformed to provirus. They are composed of the nucleotide sequences U5 and U3 separated by the short R region. The U5 region is necessary for reverse transcription, integration, and packaging of the viral RNA. The U3 region contains enhancers and promoters and is responsible for transcriptional control. Neighboring each LTR are primer binding sites involved in reverse transcription of the viral RNA. The structural, or *trans*-acting genes, and the *cis*-acting genes described here can be manipulated in such a way that the retrovirus can be rendered replication defective.

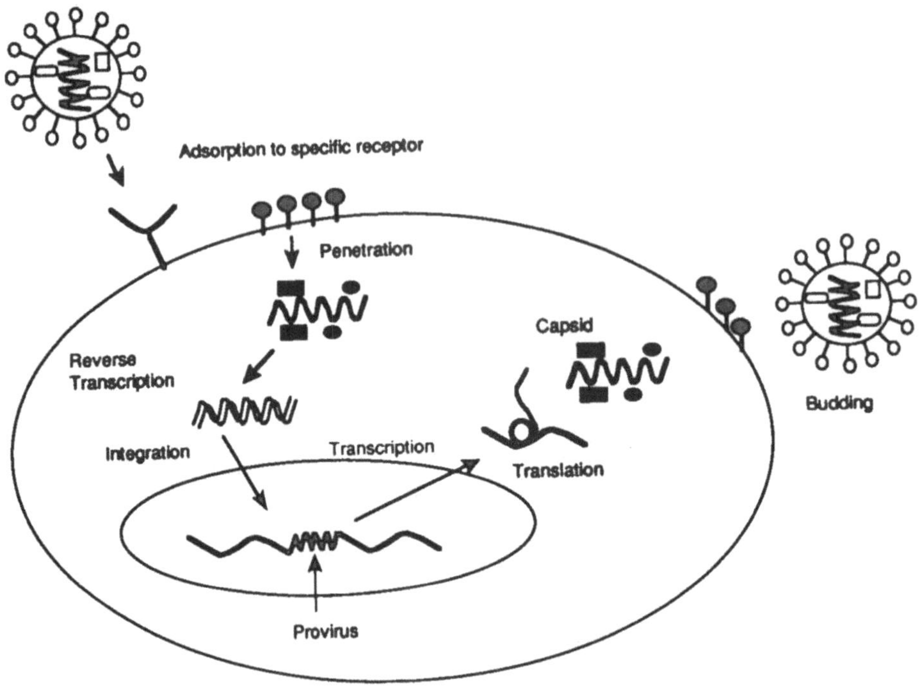

FIGURE 1. Mechanism of retroviral infection and replication. The retroviral particle binds to the cell receptor and penetrates the cell membrane. The reverse transcriptase is still complexed with the RNA and begins reverse transcription in the cytoplasm. The DNA, complexed with the integrase, then enters the nucleus and is integrated into the chromosomal DNA.

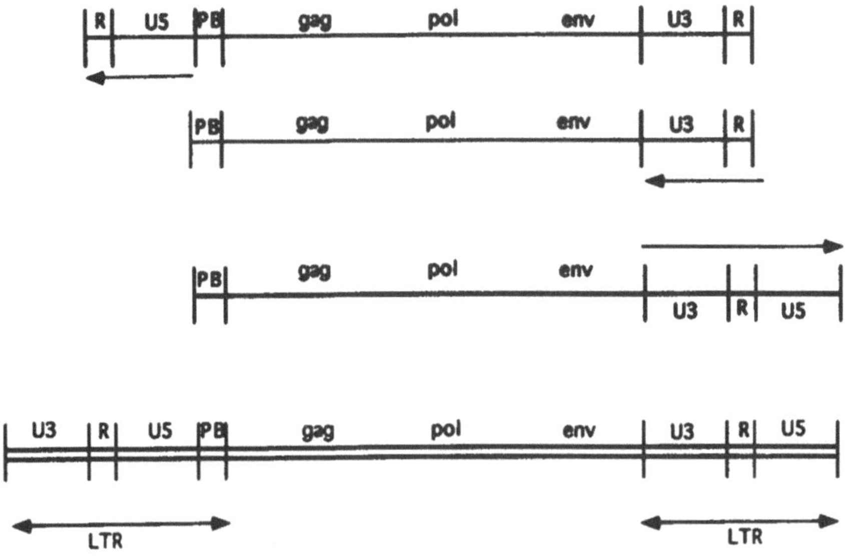

FIGURE 2. Schematic of retroviral organization and reverse transcription. The thin line represents RNA, the thick line represents DNA, and the single-headed arrow represents DNA synthesis. Reverse transcriptase initially binds to the U5 region and begins synthesis of the antisense strand of DNA. Once the U5 and R region is completed the DNA and enzyme move to the other strand of RNA, the R regions overlap, and reverse transcription continues. Next the sense strand is synthesized beginning at the U3 region. After PB is synthesized the antisense strand loops around so that the PB regions overlap and synthesis of the sense strand is completed.

B. REPLICATION DEFECTIVE RETROVIRUS VECTORS

By rendering retroviruses replication defective they become a safer option for gene transduction. A nonreplicating retroviral particle can be assembled using two plasmid vectors. One vector, or helper vector, provides the structural genes, which produces structural proteins for packaging, while a second vector provides the *cis*-acting sequences that enable the foreign gene to be packaged and delivered. The helper vector which is maintained in a helper cell line, also called a packaging cell line, provides the structural proteins needed for infection, reverse transcription, and integration. The *cis*-acting genes have been altered or removed from the helper vector. The second vector, containing the *cis*-acting genes, is then transfected into the packaging cell line. The *cis*-acting viral sequences must be retained by a vector if it is to be packaged efficiently. These sequences include the two LTRs, the priming sites for reverse transcription, and the packaging signal (Ψ signal) sequence, which is located close to the 5′ LTR. The Ψ signal is present in all retroviral genomes and is thought to be required for the viral RNA genome or foreign gene to be collected and folded within the nucleus core. This second vector, also of retroviral origin, does not contain the structural genes and is primarily responsible for encoding the genes which will be transferred to the patient.[7] Figure 3 illustrates the production of a replication defective retroviral particle.

C. TARGETS

A primary consideration for retroviral transduction is the inability of the virus to infect nonreplicating cells. However, this matter has made replication defective retroviruses an obvious choice for gene therapy of solid tumors *in vivo* or stable transduction of cells *in vitro* followed by transfer of the transduced cells into humans.

1. Transfected Stem Cells

The first human gene therapy clinical trials to be approved included *ex vivo* transfection of human lymphocytes with a retroviral vector containing the sequence for adenosine deaminase (ADA). Severe combined immunodeficiency disease (SCID) is the result of one or more defects in the lymphoid cell lineages. Among this group of congenital diseases is a deficiency in the production of ADA, an enzyme of the purine salvage pathway. High levels of 2′-deoxyadenosine result and lead to destruction of B and T cells. The disease is characterized by severe infections starting in early infancy. Bone marrow transplantation can be successful in correcting the disorder; however, only one third of the patients have matched donors. Patients have also responded to treatment with ADA conjugated to polyethylene glycol (PEG). Several groups began to investigate and subsequently showed stable expression of ADA in retroviral transduced murine hematopoietic stem cells.[8-10] The success of these studies eventually led to approval to replace the absent protein by transferring the gene to the lymphocytes of ADA-deficient patients.[11] Patients who were being treated with PEG-ADA had their T cells transduced with the retroviral vector containing the ADA gene and infused back into the patient (PEG-ADA treatment was not discontinued). Immune functions in the patients have improved. Further, a large number of corrected T cells have persisted for over 6 months.

2. Tumors

Retroviral vector transduction can take advantage of the proliferation of the tumor cells among the normal quiescence of most human cells. Rousculp et al.[12] evaluated the efficiency of gene transduction into a human lung cancer cell line. The recombinant retrovirus preparation was able to maintain infectibility *in vitro* after manipulations that would be seen normally under clinical conditions, such as lypholization. However, evidence was not presented that

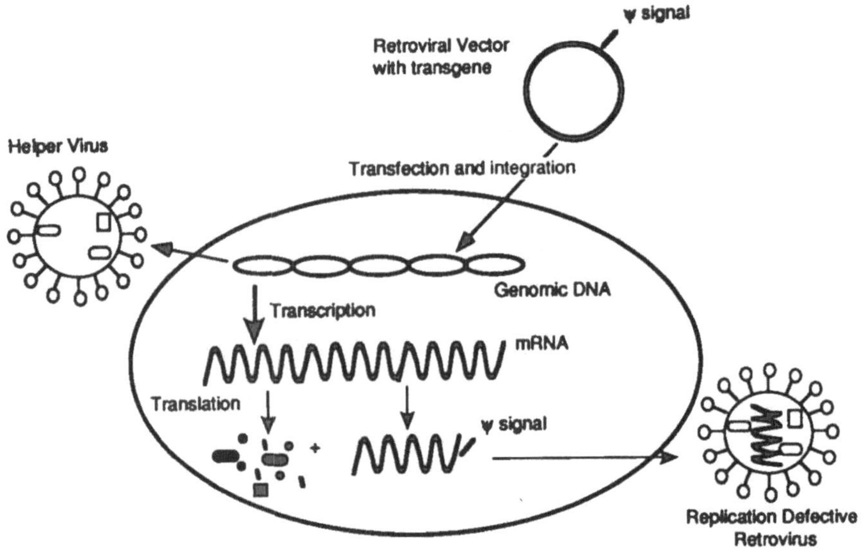

FIGURE 3. Producing a replication defective retrovirus. A cell line is initially transfected with a vector which contains the genes for proteins that are needed only in *trans* for a retroviral vector. This DNA is incorporated into the chromosome and maintained through selection. A retroviral vector that contains *cis*-acting genes and the transgene is than transfected into this helper cell line. This DNA is also incorporated into the chromosome and maintained with selection also. The mRNA from the vector containing the transgene is packaged into what is now a replication defective viral particle. This particle can infect cells but is not able to replicate. Also, a helper virus that does not contain any RNA is produced constitutively.

ensured the retroviral vector would not infect normal epithelial cells *in vivo*. While tumor cells would be the preferential target for infection, there are strategies that will further eliminate the possibility of gene transduction to normal cells.

The first strategy of treating cancer with retroviral vectors involves the delivery of a gene that encodes a toxin via a retroviral vector. The gene is under the control of a tumor specific promoter; thus, only the tumor cells would initiate translation if the vector happened to transduce a normal cell. Maxwell et al.[13] transduced B cell lymphoma, heptocellular carcinoma, and other normal cell lines with diphtheria toxin A that was under the control of promoters and enhancers from immunoglobulin heavy chain or κ-light chain genes. This strategy lead to cell death of B cells while sparing other cells *in vitro;* however, the technique needs to be cultivated such that diphtheria toxin A is activated in lymphoid cells only. A less volatile mechanism of destroying tumor cells that has been showing great success is virally directed enzyme prodrug therapy (VDEPT). VDEPT involves the transfer of a gene which encodes an activating enzyme that is capable of converting a prodrug to its destructive form. This method is more advantageous than the mechanism by which diphtheria toxin A destroys cells because there exists the ability to control the effects of the transduced gene. The activating enzyme is under the control of a tumor cell promoter, the patient is treated with a prodrug and the activating enzyme converts the prodrug to its toxic form which is harmful to the tumor cells only. At any time therapy can be discontinued.

A well-established VDEPT system involves hepatoma cells.[14] Hepatoma cells have been shown to express the thymidine kinase (TK) gene when the gene is under the control of the α-fetoprotein promoter, which is selectively activated in liver tumor cells. α-Fetoprotein is one of several tumor- or tissue-expressed genes that are not essential to the survival of the whole organism. TK was not expressed in normal liver cells when controlled by this same promoter. TK-transduced cells can then be negatively selected for by treatment with 6-methoxypurine arabinonucleoside (Ara-M). TK converts Ara-M to Ara-AMP, Ara-ADP, and Ara-ATP, which are cytotoxic to cells. Other tissue or tumor cell markers are listed in Table 2.

TABLE 2
Proteins that Have Specific Promoters for Gene Expression and their Respective Tissues or Tumors

Marker	Tissue or Tumor
Carcinoembryonic antigen	Gastrointestinal tract, lungs
α-Fetoprotein	Hepatoma, teratoma
DOPA decarboxylase	Small cell lung cancer, neuroectoderm
Neuron-specific enolase	Small cell lung cancer
Prostate-specific antigen	Prostate
Calcitonin	Thyroid (medullary)
Thyroglobulin	Thyroid
Polymorphic epithelial mucin	Breast, pancreas
Villin	Gastrointestinal tract, pancreas
erb-B2	Breast, gastrointestinal tract
erb-B3	Breast, gastrointestinal tract

Data from Reference 65.

A second strategy that has been employed with great success in tumor therapy is the delivery of cytokines that promote the development of cytotoxic immune responses against the malignant tumors. Recent studies demonstrate that engineered tumor cells which secrete cytokines did not form tumors in mice.[15,16] Gansbacher et al.[17] transduced CMS-5 cells via a retroviral vector containing the gene for human interleukin-2 (IL-2) under the transcriptional control of a cytomegalovirus promoter. CMS-5 are a weakly immunogenic mouse fibrosarcoma cell line of Balb/c origin. Following implantation *in vivo* the transduced fibrosarcomas did not form tumors. Further, when the treated mice were rechallenged with the parent cell line tumor-specific cytolytic activity persisted against the cytokine negative strain and the tumor cells were rejected. In similar studies ecotropic and amphotropic packaging cell lines both proved to be an efficient method of gene transfer *in vitro*. Lotze et al.[18] also investigated IL-2-producing tumor cell lines in an immunotherapy protocol. BL-6, a highly metastatic murine melanoma cell line, was transduced with the IL-2 gene and introduced into mice. The mean tumor size within mice after injection of the nontransfected cells compared with the transfected cells went from 220.0 to 3.4 mm. These reports indicate that local lymphokine production, imitating helper T cell function, can initiate an MHC class I restricted cytolytic T lymphocyte response against the same tumor cell lines *in vivo*. Further, these results suggest that once T cells have been developed against the tumor cell line this lymphocyte population remains and targets new tumors in the absence of tumor-initiated lymphokine stimulation.

Several important observations were made by Dranoff et al.[19] with regard to transfecting tumor cells with cytokine genes. An extensive library of cytokines was tested in a murine melanoma model. A melanoma cell line, B16, was transfected with a retroviral vector containing the moloney murine leukemia virus LTRs and a gene coding for one of the murine cytokines IL-2, IL-4, IL-5, IL-6, granulocyte-macrophage colony stimulating factor (GM-CSF), γ-interferon (γ-IFN), IL-1 receptor antagonist protein (IRAP), ICAM, CD2, or tumor necrosis factor-α (TNF-α). Only cells transduced with GM-CSF were able to induce an immune response that elicited protection against subsequent challenge with untransfected B16 cells. This study was followed by the transduction of several other tumor cell lines (that had previously shown positive results with various cytokines) with GM-CSF; CT-26,[15] a colon carcinoma, CMS-5,[17,20] Renca,[16] a renal carcinoma, and WP-4,[21] a fibrosarcoma. None of these GM-CSF-transfected cell lines were able to induce a protective immune response. These results suggest that the immunostimulatory effects induced by various cytokines is not consistent between tumor cell types; therefore, when developing a tumor vaccine the cell type must be considered. Two other observations that were made in these studies should be noted.

First, transduced irradiated cells induced a far higher protective response over nonirradiated transduced cells. This finding indicates that the more efficacious tumor vaccine is in fact safer. Second, and most importantly, Dranoff and coworkers found that transduced irradiated cells led to tumor regression of preexisting tumors.

3. Lymphocytes

Cytokines have also been transferred to tumor-infiltrating lymphocytes (TIL). TILs are lymphoid cells that infiltrate solid tumors and kill the tumor cells. They can be grown by culturing single-cell suspensions from tumors in IL-2. The TILs are transduced and expanded *in vitro* and administered back into the patient. TILs were transduced with IL-2 along with the neomycin gene as a marker by Rosenberg et al.[22] and infused back into the donors, who had metastatic melanoma. None of the patients showed any adverse side effects, and TILs were recovered 64 d after cell administration.

4. Other Tissues

In a model for hemophilia, mouse primary myoblasts were infected with replication defective retroviruses. The transduced myoblasts expressed biologically active canine factor IX for greater than 6 months after transplantation back into mice.[23] Canine and rabbit hepatocytes were also transfected *ex vivo* and produced proteins once transplanted back into the autologous animals.[24,25] Epithelial cells were transfected *in vitro* with the normal cystic fibrosis conductance regulator (CFTR) and exhibited properties similar to normal cells.[26] The above account of tissues that have had transgenes successfully incorporated into them illustrates the diversity of cell types retroviruses can infect.

These studies show successful transfection of quiescent cells with retroviruses: the cells were removed from the patient, transfected, cultured and later transplanted back into the patient. However, this procedure of incorporating a transgene in patients may be too invasive under some circumstances. Kay et al.[27,28] developed a method for hepatic gene transfer *in vivo* by infusing a recombinant retroviral vector into the portal vasculature of mice and dogs. The hemophilia B dog model displayed that canine factor IX could be expressed constitutively for more than 5 months. This work will advance retroviral gene transduction for the treatment of disorders that involve tissues not in a mitotic state.

D. VACCINES

Replication defective retroviruses are also being explored as a new approach to vaccination. Mice immunized with live Rauscher murine leukemia virus (RLV) that was disabled from replication by following immunizations with treatment of the animals with azidothymidine (AZT) and α-interferon, induced a T cell response capable of protecting against a lethal retrovirus-induced disease.[29,30] However, a live viral vaccine can be problematic, for example, HIV has certain epitopes that may lead to antibody-enhanced infection.[31] Further, it would be beneficial to generate a vector unable to replicate, as AZT is not capable of aborting HIV infection in humans. A recombinant replication defective retroviral vector can also be used to introduce a foreign gene which, when translated, will elicit an immune response against the target condition. Further, any genes that may pose potential hazards to the patient can be removed from the vector, thus increasing the safety of immunization with a recombinant retroviral vector over that of drug-induced abortive replication. This strategy is illustrated in Figure 4. The RNA is reverse transcribed to DNA and integrated into the chromosomal DNA. The genes are translated and either degraded intracellularly or secreted and are eventually expressed on the MHC class I and class II molecules.

Raun and Lilly[32] immunized adult mice with a replication defective friend murine leukemia virus (FMuLV). FMuLV was rendered replication defective by deleting a portion of the envelope gene. The replication defective virus was then transfected into several packaging cell lines: Ψ1, Ψ2, and PA12. After two immunizations BALB/c, BALB/b, BALB/k mice showed

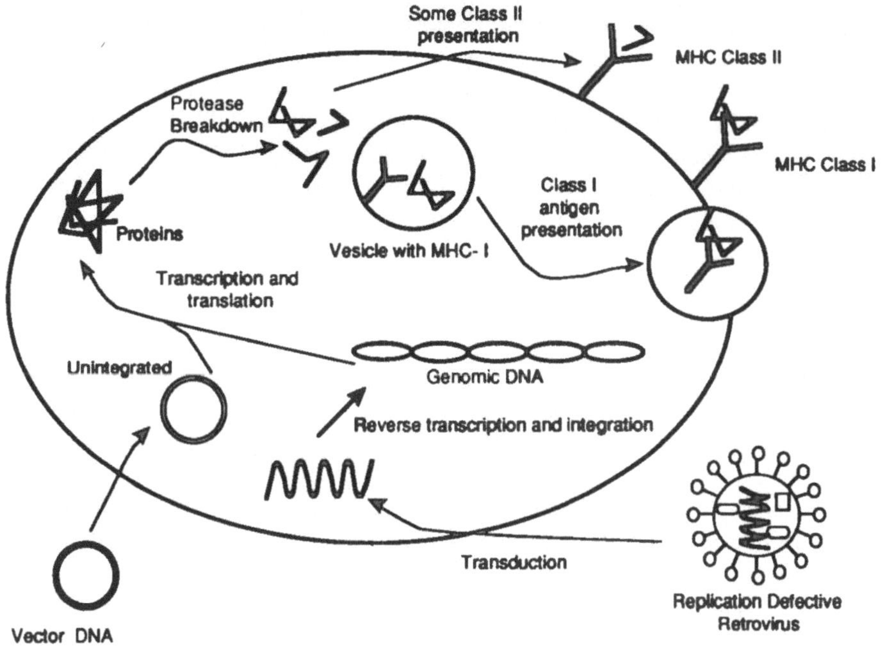

FIGURE 4. Transduction with replication defective retroviruses and vector DNA are used to illustrate how an immune response is elicited with gene therapy. Once the cell is infected the transgene is translated to proteins where some are broken down with proteases that exist within the cytoplasm. The protein particles are engulfed in vesicles that express the MHC-I where they are complexed. The vesicle migrates to the cell membrane. The MHC-antigen complex is then expressed on the cell surface, class I antigen presentation. Some of the protein particles are secreted by the cell and bind to MHC-II from class II presentation.

protection against challenge with friend virus (FV). FV is related to FMuLV and leads to erythroleukemia and immunosuppression in adult mice. Williams et al.[33] also tested the ability to immunize with a replication-defective retrovirus. They investigated the ability to elicit a "tumor antigen" specific immune response. This strategy employed an amphotropic retroviral packaging system containing the cDNA for the tumor antigen human CD4, common to T helper cell lymphocytes, under the control of a retroviral promoter. It is expected that intraperitoneal inoculation would result in diffuse tissue expression of the human CD4 antigen. There was evidence for a humoral response in these mice by both enzyme-linked immunosorbent assay (ELISA) and FACS analysis. Fifty percent of the mice immunized with the CD4-expressing retrovirus did not succumb to CD4-expressing tumors. These results are in contrast to reported strong cellular but very weak humoral immunity induced by vaccinia virus.[34] A possible explanation for this observed difference may be due to the ability of the retroviral vectors to incorporate surface glycoproteins (including CD4) into budding particles which could serve as humoral immunogens. As the CD4 antigen is a monomeric membrane protein, it would be expected to elicit a thymic-dependent antibody response.

Currently replication defective retroviral vectors are the choice of many companies: Genetic Therapy Inc., Viagene, and Transgene are investigating treatment of cancer, cardiovascular and genetic diseases, and AIDS, and Genzyme is researching treatment of cystic fibrosis.[35]

E. EXPRESSION

It is important that the level of expression of any transduced gene be adequate to either treat the disorder it was meant to or induce a protective immune response. A viral promoter alone is usually not sufficient for integrated transgene DNA expression. The location of integration can cause a variation in expression depending on the promoter's relationship to enhancers.

Dillon[36] suggests that the use of locus-control regions (LCRs) may be useful. LCRs are elements that give rise to gene expression that is insensitive to position of integration and activates transcription directly in a dominant positive manner. The β-globin LCR was the first to be isolated. LCR fragments were ligated together resulting in a fully active, 6-kb fragment.[37] Coupled with a globin promoter, LCRs can lead to a high level of gene expression. The integration of retroviral DNA leads to stable transfection and it is thus important that these genes be properly expressed regardless of chromosomal position. However, constitutive gene expression of some genes may be fatal to certain cells.

III. ADENOVIRUS

The adenovirus has the capacity for carrying large pieces of DNA, greater than 7.5 kb, has a large host range and low pathogenicity to humans. Adenoviral vectors are important when considering gene transfer to nonmitotic cells. The examples discussed in this section will highlight the reasoning for choosing adenoviruses. There are two major disadvantages to using recombinant adenoviruses, the inclusion of many adenovirus genes and transient transduction of cells. The adenovirus genome does not integrate into the host genome and transfection may be transient; however, this is currently being reconsidered. Possibly because the host cells are not dividing the cell is not given the opportunity to eliminate the episomal DNA.

A. LIFE CYCLE

Adenovirus replication can be described by an early and late phase, as illustrated in Figure 5. During infection the fiber of the virus attaches to a specific receptor on the cell membrane; there are 40 serotypes that vary in hemagglutinin group. The virus, bound to its receptor, migrates within the plasma membrane to clathrin-coated pits that form endocytic vesicles or receptosomes which are taken into the cell cytoplasm. A change in pH within the receptosome alters the vesicle causing it to lyse and releasing the virus into the cytoplasm. At this point the virus also sheds its capsid. The viral DNA is transported through the cytoplasm to the nucleus by microtubules and enters the nucleus through a nuclear pore.

E1A is the first gene to be transcribed and is needed for the transcription of E1B, E2A, E3, and E4. E1A and E1B proteins have been recognized as tumor antigens and are needed together for complete transformation of the infected cell. The ability to form tumors varies within the 40 different serotypes. Some strains such as type 5 do not lead to cell transformation. E2A codes for a protein that is a modulator of transcription and is a DNA-binding protein which is essential in DNA replication. E2B codes for two proteins that are also involved in DNA replication. E3 and E4 code for various proteins that have not been completely defined yet. After DNA replication begins there is a switch from early to late gene transcription. Late genes code for the structural proteins. See Figure 6 for an example of adenoviral genomic organization.

B. CONSTRUCTION OF ADENOVIRUS VECTOR

To disable an adenovirus from replication, portions of the E1 and E3 genes are deleted. A cassette containing the transgene, promoter, and polyadenylation is inserted into the replication defective adenoviral vector. The resulting construct is cotransfected into the 293 cell line which is a human embryonic-kidney cell line that expresses E1 constitutively. The adenoviral vector that is produced in the 293 cell line is infectious for the target cells but will only replicate in these target cells if the cells are incidentally infected with another adenovirus which will then furnish the E1 and E3 proteins.

C. TARGETS

1. Epithelia Cells

Cystic fibrosis (CF) is a lethal genetic disease common among Caucasians. The disease has an autosomal recessive pattern of inheritance and causes abnormal electrolyte transport in

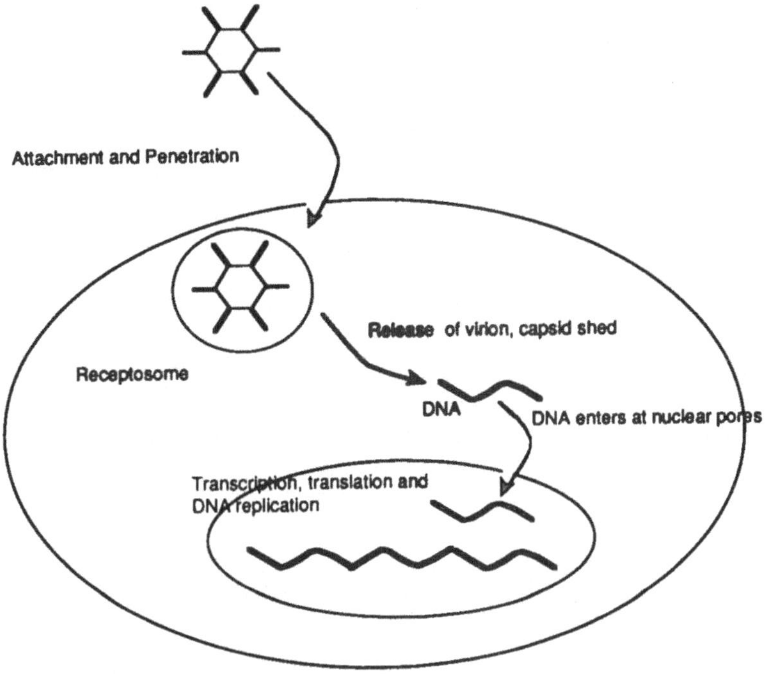

FIGURE 5. A schematic representation of the infection and replication of adenovirus. The adenovirus does not have an envelope but has a polypeptide fiber at each of its 12 vertices which attaches to a cell receptor. The virus becomes engulfed in a receptosome that is acidic at pH 5.5. The capsid is shed and the receptosome lyses. The viral particle migrates to the nucleus leaving many of its proteins behind in the cytoplasm. The viral DNA remains extrachromosomal.

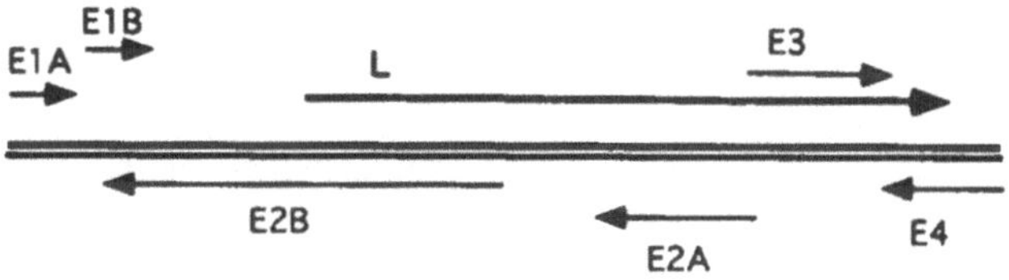

FIGURE 6. Genomic map of adenovirus type 2. The arrows indicate the general position of genes which encode the late and early proteins. The genes that are transcribed early are indicated with an E and the late genes are indicated by an L. There are several mRNAs that are spliced at different locations within each gene-coding region.

airway, intestinal, and pancreatic ductal epithelia. The discovery of the cystic fibrosis gene,[38-40] now called the cystic fibrosis transmembrane conductance regulator (CFTR),[41,42] led researchers to transfer a normal CFTR gene into CF cells.[43,44] Subsequently, correction of the Cl^- transport defect was accomplished. An adenoviral vector was an elegant choice by Englehardt et al.[45] for treatment of CF; adenovirus naturally infects airway passages in humans and epithelial cells are normally in a nonmitotic state. Xenografts were seeded with human bronchial epithelial cells in *nu/nu* mice to produce an epithelial organization similar to native airways. Infection with replication defective adenoviruses showed transgene expression for up to 5 weeks, in 5 to 20% of the surface epithelia. All cell types except basal cells were infected, the transduction of the genes appeared to be stable, and no pathology existed. This work has lead to the approval of phase I trial of Ad.CB-CFTR in patients. This vector is based on adenovirus type 5 with an E1 and E3 deletion and the human CFTR expressed from the cytomegalovirus enhancer and the β-actin promoter.

2. Muscles

Muscular dystrophy is also a likely candidate for gene transfer by recombinant adenovirus vectors. Muscular dystrophy is the progressive atrophy of skeletal muscles. Muscle cells are largely nonmitotic cells and treatment with retroviral vaccines may be difficult. *In vivo* transduction is not efficient and due to the large number of muscles that would need treatment *ex vivo*, transduction and transplantation of transfected cells would be a highly invasive procedure. A recombinant adenoviral vector will allow *in vivo* transduction of muscle cells and thus the need for transplantation is eliminated. The dystrophin gene is approximately 11,000 base pairs in length which also provides incentive for using recombinant adenoviral vectors. A type 5 adenovirus with deleted E1 and E3 regions was used to transfer β-galactosidase to muscle cells *in vivo*.[46] The β-gal gene was under the control of a mouse α-actin gene promoter and a murine muscle-specific enhancer. Muscles cells of mice were injected with the recombinant adenoviral vector that allowed muscle-specific expression of β-galactosidase. Expression was observed for up to 15 d after injection and unintegrated DNA was observed for up to 33 d.

3. Other Tissues

Transfer of genetic material to nerve cells is a consequential goal. There is considerably less exchange between capillaries and the brain compared to exchange between capillaries and other organs. This phenomenon, known as the blood-brain barrier, has made treatment of neurological disorders difficult at times. La Salle et al.[47] showed that a recombinant adenovirus containing the β-gal gene has the ability to infect nerve cells *in vitro* and *in vivo*. Another likely target for adenoviral gene therapy are hepatocytes. While previous studies show *in vitro* manipulation of hepatocytes, they are in general difficult to cultivate in tissue culture. Gomez-Foix et al.[48] showed adenovirus-mediated gene transfer into primary hepatocytes. The demonstration of altered regulation of glycogen metabolism as a consequence of expression of a noncognate phosphorylase isozyme may have implications for gene therapy of glycogen storage diseases.

IV. HERPES VIRUS

Vectors derived from herpes simplex-1 have been able to deliver transgenes to postmitotic neurons. DNA-delivered herpes virus vectors, like adenovirus vectors, remain as episomes and therefore reduce the possibility of insertional mutagenesis. Transfer of genetic material is transient in dividing cells. Herpes can infect a wide range of host cells. However, the disadvantage is herpes can be pathogenic.

Herpes virus consists of a core, capsid, tegument, and envelope. The core contains the linear double-stranded DNA suspended in what may be a proteinaceous substance. The capsid, which is approximately 100 nm in size and has 162 pentameric capsomeres, is icosadeltahedron in shape and is surrounded by an asymmetric tegument which can vary in thickness. The envelope is made up of lipids most likely from cell membranes and has an abundance of extended glycoprotein spikes.

All herpes viruses have numerous enzymes that are responsible for viral processing such as DNA synthesis and nucleic acid metabolism. Three other characteristics that all herpes viral strains have in common include DNA synthesis and capsid assembly within the nucleus, irreversible destruction of the host cell, and the ability to remain latent. Some strains can infect various cells and remain latent for longer periods while others have a more rigid tropism, replicating and destroying the host cell more efficiently.

Some work has been done with replication defective herpes simplex virus vectors.[49,50] Specifically, herpes has shown promise in transfecting nerve cells and may be an alternative to adenovirus gene transfer when studying brain functions. It is not clear at this point whether herpes will be a good vector for gene transfection.

V. DIRECT DNA INJECTIONS

Nucleic acid inoculation *in vivo* has been utilized as a research tool for a number of years. More recently, Wolff et al.[51,52] reported that when pRSVL plasmid DNA, which contains the gene that encodes for luciferase, was injected into mouse muscle, luciferase was expressed for a minimum of 2 months. A dose-response curve showed the level of luciferase expression increased linearly with the amount of injected DNA. The advantages to using direct DNA injection into the muscles of living animals are the complete elimination of any reversion back to an infectious virus and the coding region that is of interest can be selected for specifically while eliminating any extraneous viral coding regions.

An obvious choice for treatment of intramuscular injection of DNA is Duchennes' muscular dystrophy, which leads to myopathy of skeletal and cardiac muscles and premature death. As was discussed in the section on adenovirus gene transfer, retroviral gene transduction would involve a highly invasive transplantation procedure. Direct DNA injection, like adenovirus transfer, could be performed *in vivo* to the nonmitotic cells. The advantage to using direct gene transfer would be the elimination of the extraneous adenoviral proteins. However, when human dystrophin complementary DNA genes were injected into mdx mice, the human dystrophin proteins were present in the cytoplasm and sarcolemma of only 1% of the myofibers.[53] A higher percentage of myofibers must be transfected and express human dystrophin.

Much work done with DNA injections involves intramuscular injections. However, it has been shown that the capability exists for systemic gene expression after intravenous (i.v.) DNA delivery.[54] A number of important findings were observed that should be investigated in much greater detail. A mixture of an expression vector containing the chloramphenicol acetyltranserase (CAT) gene and DOTMA:dioleoylphosphatidyl-ethanolamine (DOPE) liposome was injected i.v. into mice. A ratio of 1 μg DNA to 8 nmol DOPE showed the highest level of expression in lung, heart, and lymph node tissues. It was concluded that DNA liposomes were primarily concentrated in the extravascular parenchymal cells in the spleen, liver, lymph nodes, and bone marrow and confined to the vascular compartment of the heart and kidney. While no toxic side effects existed, further work must be done to understand the therapeutic importance of systemic delivery of a gene.

A. NUCLEIC ACID VACCINATION AGAINST VIRUSES

As mentioned earlier some viruses have proved difficult to develop vaccines against, such as influenza A and HIV, which have a high envelope diversity among strains. Recent efforts have been made to create vaccines that will be cross-reactive. It is generally considered that a CTL response will lead to a high level of protection. A CTL response *in vivo* requires endogenous expression of the antigen, analogous to virus infection. To generate a viral antigen for presentation to the immune system plasmid DNA encoding influenza A nucleoprotein was injected into the quadriceps of BALB/c mice. This resulted in the generation of nucleoprotein-specific CTLs and protection from a subsequent challenge with a heterologous strain of influenza A virus, as measured by decreased viral lung titers, inhibition of mass loss, and decreased mortality.[55]

Wang et al.[56,57] also demonstrated that plasmid DNA, encoding HIV-1 gp160, pM160, injected into muscles of mice, elicited a protective immune response. Mice were initially injected with bupivacaine hydrochloride followed up by injection of pM160. After four inoculations the sera from mice injected with pM160 reacted with recombinant gp160 as shown by ELISA. T cell proliferation and cytotoxic T lymphocyte assays showed splenocytes from mice injected with pM160 responded to stimulation by gp120. Finally, the sera also exhibited neutralization and anti-syncytium capabilities in both mice and nonhuman primates. These results indicate that gene inoculation can possibly induce a protective immune response.

B. TUMOR THERAPY

Raz et al.[58] demonstrated that intramuscular injection of cytokine genes, in the absence of infectious viral vectors, can regulate humoral and cellular immune responses *in vivo*. Genes for IL-2, IL-4, and type β1 transforming growth factor (TGF-β1) were injected intramuscularly. IL-2 enhanced humoral and cellular immune responses to an exogenous antigen, transferrin, while IL-4 increased IgG1 levels but did not alter the cellular immune response to transferrin, and finally TGF-β1 depressed the anti-transferrin antibody response when coinjected with IL-2. These results indicate that active cytokines can be translated *in vivo*. Plautz et al.[59] reported use of a method to induce tumor regression by transfer and expression of a recombinant gene directly to tumors *in vivo*. The murine colon adenocarcinoma line CT26 was transduced *in vivo* with a foreign MHC molecule, H-$2K^S$. Using polymerase chain reaction (PCR) analysis the construct was shown to be present within the tumor cells. Lymphocytes from these mice demonstrated a cytolytic response to H-$2K^S$. They further recognized and lysed unmodified CT26 cell suggesting the initiation of an antitumor response to the parental cell line. Antibodies to H-$2K^S$ were not detected. Unfortunately preimmunization with H-$2K^S$ was required for tumor regression of the transduced CT26 cell line *in vivo*.

C. EXPRESSION

The studies done so far in this area have only begun to provide solutions to the questions needed to be answered. The immune responses that are elicited must be studied more thoroughly to draw a parallel between the animal models and the immune response that might be seen in humans. Sites of injection and the vectors that might be used are also being studied and will provide some vital information. In cases where genes remain extrachromosomal, the highest level of gene expression may be obtained by using viral promoters as they have evolved to function extrachromosomally.

The relative strengths of five viral and five cellular promoters controlling the production of the luciferase protein were quantitatively determined in five different rat tissues: skin epidermis, dermis, muscle, liver, and pancreas. The data include results from the cytomegalovirus (CMV) immediate enhancer/promoter, Rous sarcoma virus LTR, Simian virus 40 early enhancer/promoter, the U3 region of murine leukemia virus LTR, the mouse metallothionein gene promoter, and mouse phosphenol pyruvate carboxykinase gene promoter, bovine β-lactoglobulin gene promoter and bovine prolactic PL gene promoter. Cytomegalovirus immediate enhancer/promoter activity was consistently the highest in each tissue. The other promoter activities displayed tissue-specific preferences.[60] It should not be concluded from these studies that the CMV enhancer and promoter will always give the highest level of expression, due to effects of different genes and animal species.

VI. ANIMAL MODELS

Many of the animal models currently being used in gene therapy were bred for a given condition, such as the Watanabe rabbit, which has extremely high cholesterol. When considering gene therapy it is important that the animal phenotype and genotype relate to the human phenotype and genotype. An animal which shows a similar phenotype to humans can have a different biochemical basis. Because mice are inexpensive, small, and multiply at a high rate they are the species of choice for many initial scientific studies. In addition the mouse genome has been mapped extensively and most of the genetic mutations are known. Further, the development of the transgenic mouse will expedite the development of animal models for gene therapy. An example is sickle cell anemia, in which case the human β-globin Hbs transgene was injected into murine oocytes. The cells from the transgenic mice show typical red cell sickling when induced *in vitro* under conditions of low oxygen tension.[61]

VII. CONCLUSION

The National Institutes of Health's Recombinant DNA Advisory Committee (RAC) was established to consider the science and ethics of gene therapy. The *Points to Consider* is the principal document used by the RAC in considering human gene research proposals and from 1982 to 1992 42 protocols have been approved.[62,63] The document states that the RAC and its subcommittee will not consider germline gene transfer, but will consider somatic cell gene transfer. However, it must be ensured that there is no possibility of vertical transmission of any transgenic DNA or the chance of infection to another individual. The Food and Drug Administration (FDA) also has a *Points to Consider* document. The FDA, however, is more concerned with quality control during production. It has set up a series of tests that must be carried out on each batch or lot that is produced.[64]

At what point does gene manipulation become immoral? This is certainly a subjective question; Jean's grandmother felt that having a pacemaker was taking medical advances beyond their ethical limitations. There are two separate situations that must be considered. The first such situation includes treatment of a condition in which the patient is an adult. The second situation involves gene transfer to infants or children. It seems only logical to correct a disease such as cystic fibrosis, and certainly uncovering possible causes of disease is a top priority for scientists involved in the Human Genome Project and gene therapy. But researchers will certainly continue to probe the human genome and uncover the genes for eye color, height, and other physical attributes, because it is illogical to think that mankind will stop learning. What we will do with the knowledge is the dilemma. For now, there is adequate guidance through the regulatory committees so that gene therapy will continue to advance and provide new therapies. People have a right to the best possible medical care doctors and science can provide, and gene therapy has entered this domain and cannot be dismissed.

VIII. ACKNOWLEDGMENTS

We would like to acknowledge Drs. Bin Wang, Lori Gilbert, Emily Russo, and Elizabeth Hanna for their critical discussions. JDB is an NIH Post Doctoral Fellow. DBW is supported in part by grants from NIH.

REFERENCES

1. **Schellenberg, G.D., Bird, T.D., Wijsman, E.M., Orr, H.T., Anderson, L., Nemens, E., White, J.A., Bonnycastle, L., Weber, J.L., Alonso, M.E., Potter, H., Heston, L.L., and Martin, G.M.,** Genetic linkage evidence for a familial Alzheimer's disease locus on chromosome 14, *Science*, 258, 668, 1992.
2. The Huntington's Disease Collaborative Research Group, A novel gene containing a trinucleotide repeat that is expanded and unstable on Huntington's disease chromosomes, *Cell*, 72, 971, 1993.
3. **Rosen, D.R., Teepu, S., Patterson, D., Figlewicz, D.A., Sapp, P., Hentati, A., Donaldson, D., Goto, J., O'Regan, J.P., Deng, H., Rahmani, Z., Krizus, A., McKenna-Yasek, D., Cayabyab, A., Gaston, S.M., Berger, R., Tanzi, R.E., Halperin, J.J., Herzfeldt, B., Van der Bergh, R., Hung, W., Bird, T., Deng, G., Mulder, D.W., Smyth, C., Laing, N.G., Soriano, E., Pericak-Vance, M.A., Haines, J., Rouleau, H.R., Gusella, J.S., Hortvitz, H.R., and Brown, R.H.,** Mutations in Cu/Zn superoxide dismutase gene are associated with familial amyotrophic lateral sclerosis, *Nature*, 362, 59, 1993.
4. **Mosser, J., Douar, A., Sarde, C., Kioschis, P., Feil, R., Moser, H., Poustka, A., Mandel, J., and Aubourg, P.,** Putative X-linked adrenoleukodystrophy gene shares unexpected homology with ABC transporters, *Nature*, 361, 726, 1993.
5. **Peltomaki, P., Aaltonen, L.A., Sistonen, P., Pylkkanen, L., Mecklin, J., Jarvinen, H., Green, J.S., Jass, J.R., Weber, J.L., Leach, F.S., Petersen, G.M., Hamilton, S.R., Chapelle, A., and Vogelstein, B.,** Genetic mapping of a locus predisposing to human colorectal cancer, *Science*, 260, 810, 1993.

6. **Donahue, R.E., Kessler, S.W., Bodine, D., McDonagh, K., Dunbar, C., Goodman, S., Agricola, B., Byrne, E., Raffield, M., Moen, R., Bacher, J., Zsebo, K.M., and Nienhius, A.W.,** Helper virus induced T cell lymphoma in nonhuman primates after retroviral mediated gene transfer, *J. Exp. Med.*, 176, 1125, 1992.
7. **Scott, M.R.D. and Brown, A.M.C.,** *Retroviral Vectors, DNA Cloning*, Vol. 3, Glover, B.M., Ed., IRL Press, Washington, D.C., 1987.
8. **Lim, B., Apperley, J.F., Orkin, S.H., and Williams, D.A.,** Long-term expression of human adenosine deaminase in mice transplanted with retrovirus-infected hematopoietic stem cells, *Proc. Natl. Acad. Sci. U.S.A.*, 86, 8892, 1989.
9. **Van Beusechem, V.W., Kukler, A., Heid, P.J., and Valerio, D.,** Long-term expression of human adenosine deaminase in monkeys transplanted with retrovirus-infected bone-marrow cells, *Proc. Natl. Acad. Sci. U.S.A.*, 89, 7640, 1992.
10. **Wilson, J.M., Danos, O., Grossman, M., Raulet, D.H., and Mulligan, R.C.,** Expression of human deaminase in mice reconstituted with retrovirus-transduced hematopoietic stem cells, *Proc. Natl. Acad. Sci. U.S.A.*, 87, 439, 1990.
11. **Miller, D.A.,** Human gene therapy comes of age, *Nature*, 357, 455, 1992.
12. **Rousculp, M.D., Goldsmith, K.T., and Garver, R.I.,** Quantitative evaluations of retroviral gene transduction efficiency in human lung cancer cells, *Hum. Gene Ther.*, 3, 471, 1992.
13. **Maxwell, I.H., Glode, L.M., and Maxwell, F.,** Expression of diphtheria toxin A-chain coding sequence under the control of promoters and enhancers from immunoglobulin genes as a means of directing toxicity to B-lymphoid cells, *Cancer Res.*, 51, 4299, 1991.
14. **Huber, B.E., Richards, C.A., and Krenitsk, T.A.,** Retroviral-mediated gene therapy for the treatment of heptocellular carcinoma: an innovative approach for cancer therapy, *Proc. Natl. Acad. Sci. U.S.A.*, 88, 8039, 1991.
15. **Fearon, E.R., Pardoll, D.M., Itaya, T., Golumbek, P., Levitsky, H.I., Simons, J.W., Karasuyama, H., Vogelstein, B., and Frost, P.,** Interleukin 2 production by tumor cells bypasses T helper function in the generation of an antitumor response, *Cell*, 60, 397, 1990.
16. **Golumbek, P.T., Lazenby, A.J., Levitsky, H.I., Jaffee, L.M., Karasuyama, H., Baker, M., and Pardoll, D.M.,** Treatment of established renal cancer by tumor cells engineered to secrete interleukin 4, *Science*, 254, 713, 1991.
17. **Gansbacher, B., Zier, K., Daniels, B., Cronin, K., Bannerji, R., and Gilboa, E.,** Interleukin 2 gene transfer into tumor cells abrogates tumorigenicity and induces protective immunity, *J. Exp. Med.*, 172, 1217, 1990.
18. **Lotze, M.T., Zeh, H.J., Elder, E.M., Cai, Q., Pippin, B.A., Rosenstein, M.M., Whiteside, T.L., and Heberman, R.,** Use of T-cell growth factors (interleukins 2, 4, 7, 10, and 12) in the evaluation of T-cell reactivity to melanoma, *J. Immunol.*, 12, 212, 1992.
19. **Dranoff, G., Jaffee, E., Lazenby, A., Golumbek, P., Levitsky, H., Brose, K., Jackson, V., Hamada, H., Pardoll, D., and Mulligan, R.C.,** Vaccination with irradiated tumor cells engineered to secrete murine granulocyte-macrophage colony-stimulating factor stimulates potent, specific and long-lasting anti-tumor immunity, *Proc. Natl. Acad. Sci. U.S.A.*, 90, 3539, 1993.
20. **Gansbacher, B., Bannerji, R., Daniels, B., Zier, K., Cronin, D., and Gilboa, E.,** Retroviral vector-mediated γ-interferon gene transfer into tumor cells generates potent and long lasting antitumor immunity, *Cancer Res.*, 50, 7820, 1990.
21. **Asher, A.L., Mule, J.J., Kasid, A., Restifo, N.P., Salo, J.C., Reihert, C.M., Jaffe, G., Fendly, B., Kriegler, M., and Rosenberg, S.A.,** Murine tumor cells transduced with the gene for tumor necrosis factor-α, *J. Immunol.*, 146, 3227, 1991.
22. **Rosenberg, S.A., Aebersold, P., Cornetta, K., Kasid, A., Morgan, R.A., Moen, R., Karson, E.M., Lotze, M.T., Yang, J.C., Topalian, S.L., Merino, M.J., Culver, K., Miller, A.D., Blaese, R.M., and Anderson, W.F.,** Gene transfer into humans; immunotherapy of patients with advanced melanoma, using tumor-infiltrating lymphocytes modified by retroviral gene transduction, *N. Engl. J. Med.*, 323, 570, 1990.
23. **Dai, Y., Roman, M., Naviaux, R.K., and Verma, I.M.,** Gene therapy via primary myoblasts: long-term expression of factor IX protein following transplantation in vivo, *Proc. Natl. Acad. Sci. U.S.A.*, 89, 10892, 1992.
24. **Kay, M.A., Baley, P., Rothenberg, S., Leland, F., Fleming, L., Ponder, K.P., Liu, T., Finegold, M., Darlington, G., Pokorny, W., and Woo, S.L.C.,** Expression of human α_1-antitrypsin in dogs after autologous transplantation of retroviral transduced hepatocytes, *Proc. Natl. Acad. Sci. U.S.A.*, 89, 89, 1992.
25. **Chowdhury, J.R., Grossman, M., Gupta, S., Chowdhury, N.R., Baker, J.R., and Wilson, J.M.,** Long-term improvement of hypercholesterolemia after ex vivo gene therapy in LDLR-deficient rabbits, *Science*, 254, 1802, 1991.
26. **Johnson, L.G., Olsen, J.C., Sarkadi, B., Moore, K.L., Swanstrom, R., and Boucher, R.C.,** Efficiency of gene transfer for restoration of normal airway epithelial function in cystic fibrosis, *Nature Genet.*, 2, 21, 1993.
27. **Kay, M.A., Rothenberg, S., Landen, C.N., Bellinger, D.A., Leland, F., Toman, C., Finegold, M., Thompson, A.R., Read, M.S., Brinkhous, K.M., and Woo, S.L.C.,** In vivo gene therapy of hemophilia: sustained partial correction in factor IX-deficient dogs, *Science*, 262, 117, 1993.

28. **Kay, M.A., Li, Q., Liu, T., Leland, F., Toman, C., Finegold, M., and Woo, S.L.C.,** Hepatic gene therapy: persistent expression of human α1-antitrypsin in mice after direct gene delivery *in vivo*, *Hum. Gene Ther.*, 3, 641, 1992.
29. **Hom, R.C., Finberg, R.W., Mullaney, S., and Ruprecht, R.M.,** Protective cellular retroviral immunity requires both CD4⁺ and CD8⁺ immune T cells, *J. Virol.*, 65, 220, 1991.
30. **Ruprecht, R.M., Mullaney, S., Bernard, L.D., Sosa, M.A.G., Hom, R.C., and Finberg, R.W.,** Vaccination with a live retrovirus: the nature of the protective immune response, *Proc. Natl. Acad. Sci. U.S.A.*, 87, 5558, 1990.
31. **Berzofsky, J.A.,** Development of artificial vaccines against HIV using defined epitopes, *FASEB J.*, 5, 2412, 1991.
32. **Raun, K. and Lilly, F.,** Approach to a retrovirus vaccine: immunization of mice against friend virus disease with a replication-defective friend murine leukemia virus, *Proc. Natl. Acad. Sci. U.S.A.*, 89, 12202, 1992.
33. **Williams, W.V., Boyer, J.D., Merva, M., Livolsi, V., Wilson, D., Wang, B., and Weiner, D.B.,** Genetic infection induces protective in vivo immune responses, *DNA Cell Biol.*, 12, 675, 1993.
34. **Bernards, R., Destree, A., McKenzie, S., Gordon, E., Weinberg, R.A., and Pencali, D.,** Effective tumor immunotherapy directed against an oncogene-encoded product using vaccinia virus vector, *Proc. Natl. Acad. Sci. U.S.A.*, 84, 6854, 1987.
35. **Dodet, B.,** Commercial prospects for gene therapy — a company survey, *TIBTECH*, 11, 182, 1993.
36. **Dillon, N.,** Regulating gene expression in gene therapy, *TIBTECH*, 11, 167, 1993.
37. **Talbot, D., Collis, P., Antoniou, M.,** A dominant control region from the human β-globin locus conferring integration site-independent gene expression, *Nature*, 338, 352, 1989.
38. **Rommens, J.M., Iannuzzi, M.C., Kerem, B., Drumm, M.L., Melmer, G., Dean, M., Rozmahel, R., Cole, J.L., Kennedy, D., Hidaka, N., Zsiga, M., Buchwald, M., Riordan, J.R., Tsui, L., and Collins, F.S.,** Identification of the cystic fibrosis gene: chromosome walking and jumping, *Science*, 245, 1059, 1989.
39. **Riordan, J.R., Rommens, J.M., Kerem, B., Alon, N., Rozmahel, R., Grzelczak, Z., Zielenski, J., Lok, S., Plavsic, N., Chou, J., Drumm, M.L., Iannuzzi, M.C., Collins, F.S., and Tsui, L.,** Identification of the cystic fibrosis gene: cloning and characterization of complementary DNA, *Science*, 245, 1066, 1989.
40. **Kerem, B., Rommens, J.M., Buchanan, J.A., Markiewicz, D., Cox, T.K., Chakravarti, A., Buchwald, M., and Tsui, L.,** Identification of the cystic fibrosis gene: genetic analysis, *Science*, 245, 1073, 1989.
41. **Gregory, R.J., Cheng, S.H., Rich, D.P., Marshall, J., Paul, S., Hehir, K., Ostedgaard, L., Klinger, K.W., Welsh, M.J., and Smith, A.E.,** Expression and characterization of the cystic fibrosis transmembrane conductance regulator, *Nature*, 347, 382, 1990.
42. **Bear, C.D., Li, C., Kartner, N., Bridges, R.J., Jensen, T.J., Ramjeesingh, M., and Riordan, J.R.,** Purification and functional reconstitution of the cystic fibrosis transmembrane conductance regulator, *Cell*, 68, 809, 1992.
43. **Rich, D.P., Anderson, M.P., Gregory, R.J., Cheng, S.H., Paul, S., Jefferson, D.M., McCann, J.D., Klinger, K.W., Smith, A.E., and Welsh, M.J.,** Expression of cystic fibrosis transmembrane conductance regulator corrects defective chloride channel regulation in cystic fibrosis airway epithelial cells, *Nature*, 347, 358, 1990.
44. **Drumm, M.T., Pope, H.A., Cliff, W.H., Rommens, J.M., Marvin, S.A., Tsui, L., Collins, F.S., Frizzel, R.A., and Wilson, J.M.,** Correction of the cystic fibrosis defect in vitro by retrovirus-mediated gene transfer, *Cell*, 62, 1227, 1990.
45. **Englehardt, J.F., Yang, Y., Stratford-Perricaudet, L.D., Allen, E.D., Kozarsky, K., Perricaudet, M., Yankaskas, J.R., and Wilson, J.M.,** Direct gene transfer of human CFTR into human bronchial epithelia of xenografts with E1-deleted adenoviruses, *Nature Genet.*, 4, 27, 1993.
46. **Quantin, B., Perricaudet, L.D., Tajbakhsh, S., and Mandel, J.,** Adenovirus as an expression vector in muscle cells in vivo, *Proc. Natl. Acad. Sci. U.S.A.*, 89, 2581, 1992.
47. **La Salle, G.L.G., Robert, J.J., Berrard, S., Ridoux, V., Stratford-Perricaudet, L.D., Perricaudet, M., and Mallet, J.,** An adenovirus vector for gene transfer into neurons and glia in the brain, *Science*, 259, 988, 1993.
48. **Gomez-Foix, A.M., Coats, W.S., Baques, S., Alam, T., Gerard, R., and Newgard, C.B.,** Adenovirus-mediated transfer of the muscle glycogen phosphorylase gene into hepatocytes confers altered regulation of glycogen metabolism, *J. Biol. Chem.*, 267, 25129, 1992.
49. **Geller, A.I. and Freese, A.,** Infection of cultured central nervous system neurons with a defective herpes simplex virus 1 vector results in stable expression of Escherichia coli β-galactosidase, *Proc. Natl. Acad. Sci. U.S.A.*, 87, 1149, 1990.
50. **Geller, A.I. and Breakefield, X.O.,** A defective HSV-1 vector expresses Escherichia coli β-galactosidase in cultured peripheral neurons, *Science*, 241, 1667, 1988.
51. **Wolff, J.A., Williams, P., Acsadi, G., Jiao, S., Jani, A., and Chong, W.,** Conditions affecting direct gene transfer into rodent muscle *in vivo*, *Biotechniques*, 11, 474, 1991.
52. **Wolff, J.A., Malone, R.W., Williams, P., Chong, W., Acsadi, G., Jani, A., and Flegner, P.L.,** Direct gene transfer into mouse muscle *in vivo*, *Science*, 247, 1465, 1990.

53. **Acsadi, G., Dickson, G., Love, D.R., Jani, A., Walsh, F.S., Gurusinghe, A., Wolff, J.A., and Davies, K.E.,** Human dystrophin expression in mdx mice after intramuscular injection of DNA constructs, *Nature*, 352, 815, 1991.
54. **Zhu, N., Liggit, D., Liu, Y., and Debs, R.,** Systemic gene expression after intravenous DNA delivery into adult mice, *Science*, 261, 209, 1993.
55. **Ulmer, J.B., Donnelly, J.J., Parker, S.E., Rhodes, G.H., Felgner, P.L., Dwarki, V.J., Gromkowski, S.H., Deck, R.R., DeWitt, C.M., Friedman, A., Hawe, L.A., Leander, K.R., Martinez, D., Perry, H.C., Shiver, J.W., Montgomery, D.L., and Liu, M.A.,** Heterologous protection against influenza by injection of DNA encoding a viral protein, *Science*, 259, 1745, 1993.
56. **Wang, B., Ugen, K.E., Srikantan, V., Agadjanyan, M.G., Dang, K., Rafaeli, Y., Sato, A.I., Boyer, J.D., Williams, W.V., and Weiner, D.B.,** Gene inoculation generates immune responses against human immunodeficiency virus type 1, *Proc. Natl. Acad. Sci. U.S.A.*, 90, 4156, 1993.
57. **Wang, B., Boyer, J.D., Srikantan, V., Coney, L., Carrano, R., Phan, C., Merva, M., Dang, K., Gilbert, L., Ugen, K.E., Williams, W.V., and Weiner, D.B.,** DNA inoculation induces neutralizing immune responses against human immunodeficiency virus type 1 in mice and nonhuman primates, *DNA Cell Biol.*, 12, 799, 1993.
58. **Raz, E., Wantanabe, A., Baird, S.M., Eisenberg, R.A., Park, T.B., Lotz, M., Kipps, T.J., and Carson, D.A.,** Systemic immunological effects of cytokine genes injected into skeletal muscle, *Proc. Natl. Acad. Sci. U.S.A.*, 90, 4523, 1993.
59. **Plautz, G.E., Yang, Z., Wu, B., Gao, X., and Huang, L.,** Immunotherapy of malignancy by in vivo gene transfer into tumors, *Proc. Natl. Acad. Sci. U.S.A.*, 90, 4645, 1993.
60. **Cheng, L., Ziegelhoffer, P.R., and Yang, N.,** In vivo promoter activity and transgene expression in mammalian somatic tissues evaluated by using particle bombardment, *Proc. Natl. Acad. Sci. U.S.A.*, 90, 4455, 1992.
61. **Greaves, D.R., Fraser, P., Vidal, M.A., Hedges, M.J., Ropers, D., Luzzatto, L., and Grovsveld, F.,** A transgenic mouse model of sickle cell disorder, *Nature*, 343, 183, 1990.
62. N.I.H. and F.D.A., The revised "Points to Consider" document, *Hum. Gene Ther.*, 1, 93, 1990.
63. **Wivel, N.A.,** Regulatory consideration for gene-therapy strategies and products, *TIBTECH*, 11, 189, 1993.
64. N.I.H. and F.D.A., Points to consider in human somatic cell therapy and gene therapy, *Hum. Gene Ther.*, 2, 251, 1991.
65. **Sikora, K.,** Gene therapy for cancer, *TIBTECH*, 11, 197, 1993.

Chapter 8

ANTISENSE DEOXYNUCLEOTIDES AND RIBOZYMES: MECHANISMS OF ACTION AND POTENTIAL IN GENE THERAPY

Scott K. Shore and E. Premkumar Reddy

CONTENTS

I. INTRODUCTION

The controlled expression of genes is the cornerstone in the regulation of growth and development of cells and organisms. The copying of DNA into RNA and the translation of the messenger RNA (mRNA) into a polypeptide is a fundamental tenet in all living organisms. The controlled progression from one step to the other means that the interruption or modification of any of these steps can result in dramatic consequences that affect cellular metabolism. For example, the destruction of DNA by chemicals or radiation can be fatal to the cell because of the break in this chain of events. Similarly, prevention of the translation of a protein may prove fatal or can produce subtle phenotypic alterations to the cell or organism. As the understanding of the processes that control the proliferation and differentiation of cells increases we can begin to identify the genes (and their encoded proteins) that are a part of these pathways. Once identified, these become putative targets for interruption by modulation of their expression. For example, the cellular response to growth factor-induced proliferation begins with the ligand-receptor binding, proceeds through an intricate pathway of signaling, and results in the activation of specific gene expression in the nucleus. An interruption of the pathway by elimination of components in this process will prevent the signal that leads to the proliferation of the cell. One of the more novel means of accomplishing this is to specifically target an RNA molecule and destroy it, thereby preventing the expression of its encoded

0-8493-9422-8/94/$0.00+$.50

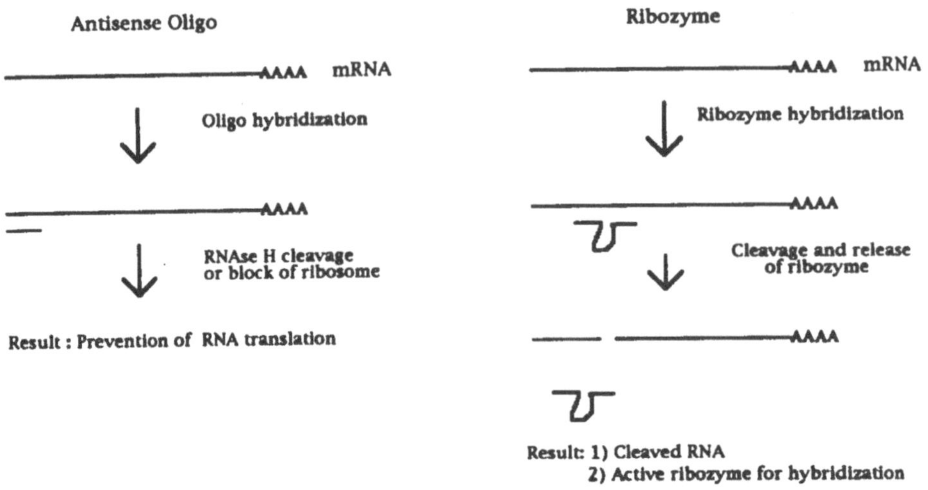

FIGURE 1. Depiction of the mechanisms for inhibiting gene expression by antisense oligodeoxynucleotides and ribozymes in cells. The net result of each agent is the inhibition of gene expression by the prevention of translation of the mRNA transcript.

protein but leaving other RNA molecules and the DNA unaffected (see Figure 1). This chapter describes two means of accomplishing this: antisense molecules and ribozymes. A few years ago this would have been predominately conjecture. But today with the dramatic progress in molecular genetics, the identification, isolation, cloning, and sequencing of genes, these techniques have acquired great importance in therapy and several of the antisense molecules have entered phase I clinical trials.

II. ANTISENSE MOLECULES: HISTORICAL PERSPECTIVE

Antisense-based inhibition of gene expression occurs following the annealing of either DNA or RNA molecules that are complementary to a mRNA molecule. The duplex regions that form from the complementary sequences prevent translation either by precluding the movement of the ribosomal complex or by creating a substrate for RNAse H cleavage. Bacterial genetics provided the basis for the use of antisense molecules to inhibit gene expression. It had been demonstrated that bacterial Tn10 transposase gene expression was regulated by an antisense RNA transcript transcribed from its own promoter. When the antisense was present it could base-pair with the Tn10 transposase mRNA and prevent its translation.[1] The first study to use this prokaryotic means of regulation and demonstrate the inhibition of eukaryotic gene expression by an antisense RNA was conducted by Izant and Weintraub in 1984.[2] They expressed the full-length antisense transcript of the thymidine kinase gene and demonstrated that they could attenuate the biological effect of a transfected thymidine kinase gene in mouse cells. It has since been shown that the inhibitory effect of antisense molecules is not limited to full-length complementary RNA, but also results following the introduction of oligodeoxynucleotides complementary to small stretches of the RNA transcript. Small oligodeoxynucleotides, added to the culture medium, were first shown to elicit a biological effect *in vivo* by limiting the transformation of cells by v-src.[3]

III. ANTISENSE MOLECULES AS REGULATORS OF GENE EXPRESSION

Early studies on gene inhibition by oligodeoxynucleotides indicated that the stability of these molecules in the cell was critical for their effective inhibition of expression. It was observed that oligodeoxynucleotides were degraded in both culture medium and plasma.[4,5] Therefore, the modification of oligodeoxynucleotides to enhance their stability and penetration into the cell was explored. By altering the phosphodiester bond an increase in both nuclease resistance and the effective intracellular concentration of the oligodeoxynucleotides was observed. A phosphorothioate linkage was found to be more effective than either methyl phosphonate or the unmodified phosphodiester bond.[6,7] The actual mechanism for the uptake of oligodeoxynucleotides by cells is unclear. Since these molecules are highly charged, it is somewhat surprising to find that they are effectively taken up by mammalian cells. This phenomenon led to suggestions that receptors that mediate this uptake may exist on cell surfaces. There have been two reports in the literature of a receptor-mediated endocytosis, but a receptor has yet to be cloned and the exact mechanism remains to be determined.[8,9]

The specificity of the antisense molecule to a single mRNA transcript is dependent on its length and ability to hybridize to its target. Full-length RNA antisense transcripts will be the most specific, since they represent an exact mirror image of the targeted strand. However, with long antisense RNA molecules, the chance of intramolecular folding and possible inactivity due to secondary structure increases. With shorter synthetic oligodeoxynucleotides it has been found that they can exhibit specificity that can be disrupted by single base mismatches[10,11] or they can have very general effects because of their interference with cellular metabolism.[12,13]

The mechanism of antisense-mediated inhibition of gene expression is based upon the ability of RNA or DNA to form duplexes by Watson-Crick base pairing. RNA can hybridize to form duplexes with other RNA molecules or with DNA as long as the complementary bases are present. Similarly, a single-stranded DNA molecule can hybridize with both single-stranded DNA and RNA. Studies by Paterson et al.[14] demonstrated that antisense oligodeoxynucleotides could inhibit the translation of RNA transcripts in cellular extracts. This inhibition of translation was found to result from the cleavage of the RNA in a RNA:DNA duplex by RNAse H[15] and therefore could be relieved by depleting the RNAse H activity by the addition of an excess of a RNA:DNA duplex as a competitor.[16] A similar mechanism has been shown to occur in *Xenopus* oocytes.[17,18]

RNA-based inhibition cannot proceed via RNAse H since RNA:RNA duplexes are not substrates for cleavage by RNAse H. The prevention of RNA splicing and processing, the steric interference of ribosome attachment, or the inhibition of the ribosome complex from processing the RNA appear to be the mechanism for inhibition. Experimentally antisense inhibition is usually reported as a biological phenotype and the mechanism is disregarded. However, early experiments on inhibition of translation in *Xenopus* oocytes following the microinjection of full-length complementary RNA detected RNA:RNA duplexes.[19,20] Surprisingly, shorter antisense RNA that hybridizes exclusively to the 3′ end of a mRNA transcript has also been shown to inhibit translation,[21] although no effect on posttranscriptional modification or transport of the mRNA sense strand to the cytoplasm was observed. These experiments included antisense transcripts against the last exon and flanking untranslated sequences of the creatine kinase gene.[22] The common observation in these experiments is an inhibition of translation that appears to result independently of the location of duplex formation.

IV. ANTISENSE MOLECULES AS THERAPEUTIC AGENTS

Antisense targeting has been found to be highly flexible and has been used to inhibit expression of a variety of cellular genes. Antisense molecules frequently were made against (1) the 5′ cap site,[23,24] (2) the initiation codon and adjacent 3′ sequences,[11,25] (3) the codons immediately downstream of the initiation codon,[26] and (4) 3′ codons including sequences that are in the untranslated flanking region of the gene.[22,27] For viral inhibition the sequences that constitute 5′ splice donor-acceptor sites have been successfully targeted.[28,29] In general, the use of oligodeoxynucleotides complementary to the cap site or the initiation codon appears to be used most frequently.

The first indication of demonstrable inhibition by antisense was against viral genes. In 1978 the inhibition of Rous sarcoma viral replication in infected chicken cells was reported following the addition of oligodeoxynucleotide 13-mers to the culture.[3] Later the antisense inhibition of other viral RNAs was demonstrated by reductions, to varying degrees, of infectivity in cultured cells. These included herpes simplex virus,[30] human immunodeficiency virus (HIV),[31,32] influenza virus,[33] and vesicular stomatitis virus.[34]

With the accessibility of automated DNA synthesizers, the field of antisense inhibition has grown. This is a result of the virtually limitless exploitation of this technology. These areas include understanding the role that protooncogenes play in cellular growth and development. Antisense studies have confirmed biologically what were previously only descriptive results based on the examination of RNA expression. Such studies have demonstrated the critical role these genes play in proliferation and differentiation by silencing their expression. The *myc* gene has been extensively manipulated because of its high level of expression during proliferation and its subsequent downregulation during chemically induced differentiation, in a variety of cells. Studies using antisense *myc* oligodeoxynucleotides have generated diverse results for reasons that are unclear. Treatment of HL-60 myeloid leukemia cells has been reported to result in a decrease in myc protein and non-cell cycle-specific decrease in proliferation at 4 μM,[11] while others required 10 μM[25] or 50 μM for a similar effect.[35] Treatment of HL-60 cells with antisense oligodeoxynucleotides directed against the *myb* oncogene resulted in blocking their entry into S phase. This, in turn, results in the inhibition of proliferation by a mechanism different from induction of terminal differentiation. This inhibition of proliferation also appears to be different from that seen with antisense inhibition of *myc* expression, indicating the usefulness of antisense oligodeoxynucleotides in the dissection of cellular processes.[36]

Based on these and other experiments that have detailed the potential specificity of antisense inhibition by oligodeoxynucleotides, the potential use of antisense as a treatment for cancer has been explored. Chronic myelogenous leukemia (CML) is the result of a chromosomal translocation that generates a novel fusion gene, *BCRABL*. Since this gene is only present in leukemia cells it constitutes a cancer-specific target. The cancer cell-specific *BCRABL* gene that is the etiologic agent in CML has been targeted by antisense as well as the common cellular gene c-*myb*. These studies have indicated the effect on proliferation of blastic CML cells by treatment with both the antisense *myb* and *BCRABL* oligodeoxynucleotides.[37-39] The use of antisense *myb* to eliminate leukemic cells has the potential of affecting normal cells as well; for example, during a bone marrow purge.[40,41] However, a differing sensitivity between normal, chronic, and blastic leukemia cells has been reported which indicates that the degree of malignancy corresponds to the requirement for *c-myb* expression.[36,42]

Oligodeoxynucleotides may also be used as a component of a therapeutic regime to sensitize the cell to conventional therapies. Non-Hodgkin's lymphoma often contains a t(14;18) chromosomal translocation that causes an over-expression of the *bcl-2* gene, resulting in an increased resistance to chemotherapy and irradiation. By decreasing *bcl-2* expression by antisense oligonucleotide treatment cells may become more sensitive to treatment by conventional therapies.[43]

V. RIBOZYME MOLECULES: HISTORICAL PERSPECTIVE

RNA molecules that are able to specifically cleave other RNA molecules or form chemical bonds are called ribozymes and fall into three categories. The first observation of a reactive RNA ribozyme was made in *Tetrahymena* by the Cech group in 1982.[44] They described the intramolecular removal of an intervening sequence by a mechanism dependent on RNA secondary structure, a divalent cation, and GTP, while being independent of any protein. The discovery that bacterial RNAse P was cleavage competent even in the absence of its associated protein subunit, identified yet another ribozyme. This reaction removes 5′ sequences in precursor tRNA molecules and each RNAse P molecule is capable of multiple turnover resulting in catalytic reactivity *in vivo*.[45] These two cleavage reactions produce products containing 2′-,3′-OH and 5′-PO_4 ends, and share the need for complementary sequences for the identification of the reactive site (reviewed in References 46 and 47). A third category of ribozyme molecule is the self-cleaving species present in a wide variety of plant pathogens and plays a crucial role in the replication of their genomes. This cleavage is dependent only on divalent cations, a specific cleavage sequence (originally identified as GUC), and a highly conserved secondary structure. The termini of the cleaved products differ from the *Tetrahymena* and RNAse P cleavage products and consist of a 2′,3′-cyclic phosphate and a 5′-hydroxyl.

The discovery of this third group of ribozymes was a result of studies with avocado sun blotch viroid (ASBV) and tobacco ringspot satellite virus (sTRSV) infected plants.[48,49] The infected leaves were found to contain oligomers of the (+) RNA strand but only monomeric and dimeric (-) strands. These viruses replicate by a rolling circle, whereby a concatameric transcript results from the polymerase continually copying the genome. These concatameric transcripts must be modified to yield the circular monomeric RNA. Following *in vitro* transcription of cDNA clones of the ASBV (-) strand, self-cleavage of the oligomeric transcript was observed, resulting in multiple monomers that could be ligated into circular molecules. Self-cleavage resulted from the folding of the viral RNAs into a distinctive secondary structure that resembled the head of a hammer and was dubbed the "hammerhead".[50]

Based on sequence analysis from RNA molecules known to self-cleave, a consensus sequence for the self-catalytic cleavage motif was determined.[51] The structure of a typical hammerhead ribozyme is shown in Figure 2. Self-cleavage required the presence of 3 highly conserved helices, 13 unpaired bases, and a cleavage-specific sequence consisting of the 3 ribonucleotides GUX, where X can be C, A, or U. This folding into a reactive configuration occurs within contiguous bases in many virusoid plant pathogens.[50] However, the ASBV catalytic configuration can result from the folding of either two separate RNA molecules or from a single RNA that looped out the bases not involved in the catalytic structure.[50] This observation raised the possibility that *trans*-cleavage of an RNA molecule was possible following the correct folding of two separate RNA molecules. The first experimental evidence to support the idea that the ribozyme could be assembled from different RNA molecules was provided by Uhlenbeck in 1987,[51] when he separated the ribozyme into two independent molecules, each containing consensus catalytic domain sequences and complementary sequences flanking the catalytic domain. When the arms annealed by Watson-Crick base pairing the catalytic sequences were brought into an active configuration and cleavage resulted. The cleavage was demonstrated to be dependent on the presence of the GUC cleavage sequence, exhibited first-order kinetics, and required the addition of a divalent cation. One year later Haseloff and Gerlach,[52] using a ribozyme mutated by linker insertion, further separated the self-cleavage reaction into two distinct components, substrate and the catalytic ribozyme. The ribozyme supplied the catalytic domain while the substrate contained the GUC cleavage sequence. By complementary base pairing they could be brought together into a cleavage competent molecule. This observation found immediate application since any RNA molecule could be targeted by appropriate designing of the cleavage component. This was first demonstrated by synthesizing ribozymes targeted for GUC sequences present in the bacterial chloramphenicol acetyl transferase gene (CAT). The CAT-encoded RNA has no natural self-cleaving ability, but following incubation of the CAT RNA with the synthetic ribozymes in the presence of Mg^{2+}, they were able to show that site-specific cleavage of the CAT RNA occurred specifically at the GUC target sequence.

The replicative life cycle of the tobacco ringspot virus (TRSV) appears to involve cleavage of both the (+) and (-) strands, yet sequences that would result in a hammerhead structure could only be found in the (+) strand. A novel cleavage motif for the (-) strand was proposed by Hampel and Tritz[53] based on computer modeling that generated a secondary structure that

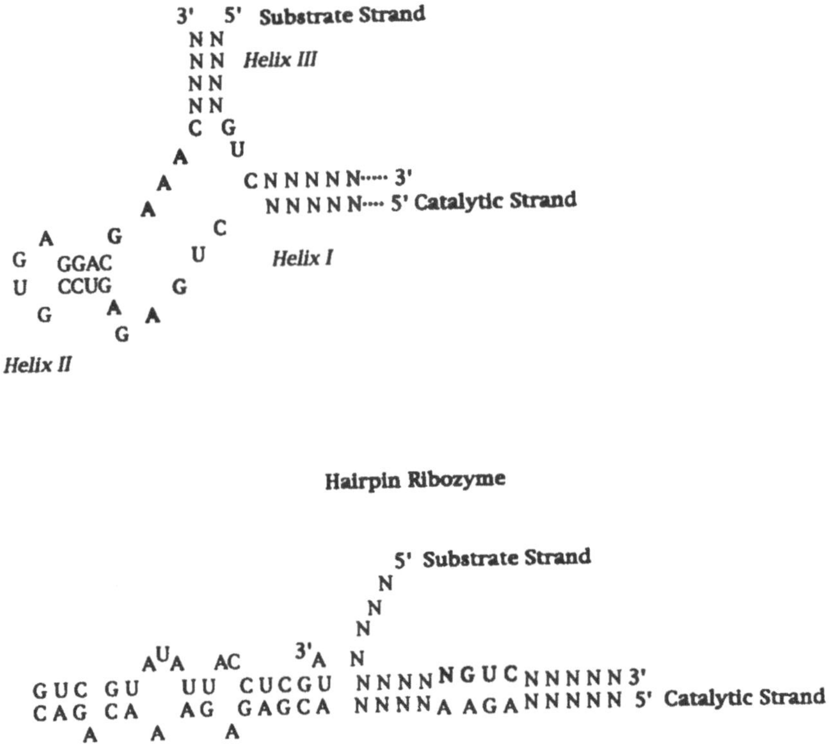

FIGURE 2. Consensus hammerhead secondary structures are shown for both the hammerhead and hairpin configurations. In each example the catalytic strand is separated from the substrate strand. The three helices of the hammerhead are identified and the conserved single-stranded region is indicated with the bold type. Cleavage by the hammerhead occurs 3′ to the GUC sequence shown in bold type on the substrate RNA strand. For the hairpin ribozyme the cleavage site NGUC in the substrate strand is indicated in bold and cleavage occurs 5′ of the N in this sequence.

resembled a hairpin. This ribozyme is shown in Figure 2. The reaction products of this hairpin ribozyme cleavage are 2′,3′-cyclic phosphate and 5′-hydroxyl, identical to the hammerhead products. Similar to the hammerhead ribozymes, the reaction proceeds enzymatically and requires divalent cations. The differences lie in the conserved sequences that form the catalytic domain that fold to form a more reactive molecule at lower temperatures than the hammerhead. Also, the (-) strand is cleaved at the 5′ side of G in the sequence NGUC (N is G or C).[53,54] Similarly, this ribozyme also can be targeted to substrates by virtue of two helices that form between the target molecule and the catalytic strand. By changing these sequences in TRSV it has been demonstrated that the exact TRSV nucleotide sequence is not essential, only that complementary sequences are present that can anneal to form the requisite helix.[54] Therefore, these may be modified to allow for the targeting of a hairpin ribozyme similar to the hammerhead.

VI. COMMON, NATURALLY OCCURRING SELF-CLEAVING RNA MOLECULES

Self-cleaving RNA exists in a variety of plant and animal virus-like genomes (Table 1). The products of this cleavage all share the 2′,3′-cyclic phosphate and 5′-hydroxyl termini, but the structure of the catalytic domains may vary. The hammerhead-type domain is found in the majority of the self-cleaving RNAs currently known. These include not only plant viruses and virusoids,[55] but also a newt RNA transcript of satellite 2 DNA.[56] Additional self-cleaving

TABLE 1
Natural Self-Cleaving Reactions Yielding Common Products

	Rolling Circle Replication	2′,3′-Cyclic Phosphate and 5′-Hydroxyl Termini
1. Hammerhead 2° structure (strand cleaved)		
Newt satellite 2 DNA (RNA transcript)	-	+
Avocado sunblotch viroid (plus and minus)	+	+
Encapsidated linear satellite RNA		
Tobacco ringspot virus (plus)	+	+
Barley yellow dwarf virus (plus and minus)	+	+
Encapsidated circular satellite RNA		
Velvet tobacco mottle virus (plus)	+	+
Subterranean clover mottle virus (plus)	+	+
Solanum nodiflorum mottle virus (plus)	+	+
Lucerne transient streak virus (plus and minus)	+	+
2. Hairpin 2° structure (strand cleaved)		
Encapsidated linear satellite RNA		
Tobacco ringspot virus (minus)	+	+
3. Axhead potential 2° structure (strand cleaved)		
Hepatitis delta virus RNA (plus and minus)	+	+
4. Unknown mechanism (strand cleaved)		
RNA transcript of *Neurospora* mitochondrial DNA plasmid (plus)	-	+

domains have been identified in the animal virus hepatitis delta virus,[57,58] in which both the (+) and (-) strands of RNA cleave to generate products with 2′,3′-cyclic phosphate and 5′-hydroxyl termini but the actual mechanism of cleavage is not known, although an ax head structure has been proposed. *Neurospora* strain Varkud-1c mitochondria (+) strand RNA was shown to self-cleave following *in vitro* transcription.[59] The RNA cleavage products contain the common 2′,3′-cyclic phosphate and 5′-hydroxyl termini but the sequence of this RNA shows no homology to known self-cleaving structures. It has been estimated that in every 1.1 $\times 10^3$ bases a hammerhead-like structure will exist;[60] therefore, it is likely that these structures will continue to be found in diverse organisms.

VII. CHEMISTRY OF GENE INACTIVATION BY HAMMERHEAD RIBOZYMES

Studies with ASBV synthetic transcripts clearly distinguished the differences between the self-cleavage reactions of *Tetrahymena* and the hammerhead ribozymes. The hammerhead-mediated cleavage did not require a nucleotide cofacter such as GTP or guanosine, but did require a divalent cation such as Mg^{2+} or Ca^{2+}. By directly sequencing the products, the exact site of cleavage was determined to be immediately 3′ of the sequence GUC. The 5′-terminus of the product is a hydroxyl group, as shown by its ability to be phosphorylated following incubation with ^{32}P-ATP and polynucleotide kinase. The 3′-terminus could not be kinased even with extensive alkaline phosphatase treatment, indicating that it was unique from the 5′-terminus. The 3′-terminus could be phosphorylated, however, after treatment first with HCl followed by dephosphorylation. This indicated that although this terminus was neither a monophosphate ester or a hydroxyl, it could be a 2′,3′-cyclic phosphate. This was confirmed enzymatically using wheat germ ligase, which is known to ligate a 2′,3′-cyclic phosphate end to 5′-OH or 5′-PO_4 ends. The successful self-ligation of the cleaved ASBV (+) strand to a circular species by wheat germ ligase confirmed the nature of the 3′-terminus to be a 2′,3′-cyclic phosphate.[49]

The cleavage reaction (substrate binding-cleavage-product release) appears to be strongly influenced by the formation of the secondary structure (see Figure 2). For example, a study comparing four ribozymes that cleaved at the same site-specific sequence (GUC) in the substrate but differed in the complementary base-pairing in helices 1 and 3 found that the differences in the catalytic efficiencies were due to differences in the K_m.[61] This suggested that the folding of the ribozyme and substrate played a crucial role in determining the steady-state kinetics of cleavage. Since all the ribozymes showed a similar K_{cat} the conserved sequences are sufficient for the cleavage reaction. The helices 1 and 3 are the major sites that can be modified to enhance the efficiency of cleavage.

Mutagenesis experiments on the hammerhead motif (see Figure 2) have mapped the essential bases for cleavage as those strictly conserved among the naturally occurring ribozymes. Deletion analysis has indicated that helix 2 is not essential for activity and as a result the minimally active ribozyme is one that eliminates helix 2 but retains the consensus unpaired sequences.[62] The mutagenesis of bases that constitute the consensus sequences result in either the loss of activity or the drastic reduction in the kinetics of the cleavage rates, effectively rendering the ribozyme nonfunctional. A mutational analysis of the cleavage site in the satellite RNA of tobacco ringspot virus revealed a much greater diversity in target-site cleavage than had been found in naturally occurring ribozymes.[63] Comparable cleavage rates based on $T_{1/2}$ kinetics occurred at the 3′ end of the following triplets: GUC, GUA, GUU, UUC, and CUC, although only GUC and GUA have been found naturally.[50,64]

The cleavage reaction is an acid-base mechanism involving the movement of a proton from the 2′-OH and the acceptance of a proton at the 5′ cleavage site. But by its very nature it is difficult to study since as soon as the RNA molecule assumes the reactive conformation it is cleaved. In an effort to spectroscopically examine the ribozyme reaction, a proton nuclear magnetic resonance (NMR) study was performed using a catalytically active ribozyme and a deoxyribonucleotide noncleavable substrate. The resulting spectra confirmed the presence of the three helices, as was initially proposed based on Watson-Crick base pairing. The addition of Mg^{2+} made little difference spectrally, indicating that it is not involved conformationally but as a catalyst.[65] Studies using phosphothioate substitutions show that several phosphates are critical to the cleavage reaction other than that at the target site. These groups are most likely to be involved in the Mg^{2+} coordination.[66] Substitution of deoxyribonucleotides for ribonucleotides in a ribozyme showed that an all-deoxyribonucleotide ribozyme is inactive,[67,68] whereas individual substitutions in the conserved nucleotides result in decreases in activity. The 2′-OH groups in the GAAAC single-stranded region have specifically been shown to be important for activity.[69] The substitution of deoxyribonucleotides for all of the nonconserved bases in a ribozyme has been reported to increase the amount of product of the ribozyme reaction when compared to an all-ribonucleotide ribozyme.[62]

These studies have provided useful information for modifying the ribozyme in an effort to optimize its biological activity. It will be important to determine if any of these modifications will show effectiveness *in vivo*.

VIII. RIBOZYMES AS THERAPEUTIC AGENTS

By utilizing Watson-Crick base pairing, theoretically a hammerhead-type ribozyme may be targeted to any potential RNA substrate where a cleavage target site sequence is present. The demonstration that the hammerhead's catalytic function and substrate cleavage site can exist on independent molecules[51] showed that ribozymes had a potentially universal application. The small size, multiple turnover, and lack of modification during the cleavage reaction suggested that the ribozyme may be more effective at inhibition of gene expression than antisense molecules.

The first example of the application of ribozyme technology for *trans*-cleavage was with the *Tetrahymena* ribozyme.[70] The first two reports of a targeted hammerhead ribozyme were by Haseloff and Gerlach[52] and Koizumi et al.,[71] both published in 1988. The use of a catalytic hammerhead RNA molecule to cleave the CAT gene, as described by Haseloff and Gerlach,[52] was to become the model for future experiments. Until this time all reactions utilized purified RNA samples in a Tris buffer with 10 m*M* Mg^{2+}, and it was uncertain if ribozymes would function similarly in the cellular milieu. The ability of a ribozyme to cleave RNA in mammalian nuclear extracts was shown by Cotten et al.[72] with a ribozyme designed to inhibit the *in vitro* small nuclear ribonucleoprotein U7-dependent histone pre-mRNA processing. The experiments showed that there was a vast difference between *in vitro* cleavage and cleavage in the extracts, with cleavage being much less effective in the presence of the added extract. Additionally when compared to antisense DNA and RNA oligodeoxynucleotide-mers, the ribozyme was the least effective inhibitor of U7 mRNA processing, requiring a 10^3-fold excess over the substrate. To overcome problems such as concentration and stability, the same U7 ribozyme was inserted into a tRNA expression cassette and microinjected into the nucleus of *Xenopus* oocytes.[73] The ribozyme was constitutively expressed from the tRNA pol III promoter and was capable of intracellular cleavage of a microinjected substrate. This suggested that a ribozyme may be targeted to an exogenous substrate and could be expressed intracellularly from an expression vector while still retaining its catalytic activity. The intracellular inhibition of gene expression by a ribozyme was reported by Cameron and Jennings,[74] who extended the CAT ribozyme experiments of Haseloff and Gerlach[52] using COS cells in transient transfection studies. A CAT-specific ribozyme expressed at a 10^3 *M* excess over the CAT substrate RNA was shown to inhibit the acetylation of chloramphenicol by COS cell extracts with 60% efficiency.

Initial cellular experiments with targeted ribozymes were conducted on transcripts not endogenous to the cell, such as infectious viral RNA. The HIV genome has been targeted by hammerhead ribozymes to a number of sites, including *gag*, the long terminal repeat (LTR), the U5 region of the LTR, the 5′ leader sequences, integrase, and the *env* gene.[75-81] Most of these reports indicate that the ribozyme is capable of *in vitro* cleavage of RNA fragments at the expected GUX site. Differing degrees of success at inhibiting HIV replication are reported, though. Expression of the *gag* ribozyme in $CD4^+$ Hela cells was shown to reduce the amount of secreted gag (p24) antigen 50-fold compared to nontransfected controls.[75] The detection of p24 HIV protein released into the culture medium by enzyme-linked immunosorbent assay (ELISA) is a common means of measuring the replication of HIV. The ribozyme targeted to the 5′ leader sequence was shown to delay viral production in some MT4 cells that were stable expressors of ribozyme from times that varied from 4 to 20 d, depending upon the promoter used.[76] In one of the more thoroughly executed studies it was found that the best effect of the ribozyme was in MT4 cells that were first infected with the ribozyme-expressing retrovirus and then challenged with HIV rather than introducing the ribozyme into cells chronically infected with HIV. The ribozyme-infected cells exhibited a two- to threefold decrease in reverse transcriptase activity following the infection with HIV.[77] By targeting multiple cleavage sites along the HIV *env* RNA with a single ribozyme molecule, the ability of the virus to evolve by mutation to a cleavage-resistant mutant can be greatly diminished. *In vitro* cleavage reactions demonstrated an improved efficiency of a multiunit molecule (nonaribozyme) compared to single ribozymes added individually or together.[81] When these *env* ribozymes were cotransfected with vectors into $CD4^+$ Hela cells, the protection from syncitia formation and the release of p24 was dependent not only on the modality of the ribozyme but also the promoter used in the ribozyme expression vector. The best combination nonaribozyme with SV40 promoter resulted in a 10-fold decrease in p24 release. The targeting of multiple sites may prove to be crucial in the successful cleavage of a dynamic target such as HIV that has the ability to mutate its sequences which would generate a resistant strain. Recently, a hairpin ribozyme was described that was directed to the 5′ leader sequences of HIV strain HXB2 that was shown to have an inhibitory effect on the replication of HXB2 as well as other strains. These studies also indicated the importance of the promoter selected to express the ribozyme in cells. Using a pol III expression cassette Yu et al. were able to inhibit 95% of p24 expression in a transient cotransfection assay in Hela cells.[82]

The inhibition of endogenously expressed genes by ribozyme-mediated cleavage has also been reported. A ribozyme was designed to cleave within the first exon of the *fos* gene and transfected as a fos-ribozyme expression vector into the ovarian carcinoma line A2780S. The effect of *fos* inhibition was an increase in sensitivity to chemotherapeutic agents and a decreased expression of genes involved in DNA synthesis.[83] One of the problems in targeting endogenously expressed genes is the role they may play in normal cellular growth, which may make their inhibition deleterious to normal cells. Therefore, the ability to target phenotypically specific transcripts is desirable. These transcripts can be the result of point mutations that would introduce a cleavage site as well as activate the oncogenicity of the gene, or they may result from chromosomal translocations that result in the generation of a new gene specific to the malignant phenotype. CML is the result of a chromosomal translocation that generates a novel fusion gene, *BCRABL*. To assess the applicability of ribozyme-based reactions as a potential therapy for CML, we designed a ribozyme that can cleave specifically *BCRABL* RNA, thereby blocking the synthesis of BCRABL protein, the primary cause of this leukemia.[84] To assay the effect of this ribozyme on *BCRABL* RNA we expressed the ribozyme sequences constitutively by inserting the appropriate nucleotide sequence into retroviral expression vectors. This approach allowed determination of the effect of ribozyme expression in CML cells and assay for the loss of the BCRABL P210 protein kinase. The results show that high-level expression of such ribozymes incorporated into retroviral vectors introduced into Ph+ human CML cell lines results in the loss of BCRABL-associated protein kinase activity.[84] Similar results have been reported with the introduction of a ribozyme introduced into cells by lipofection.[85] In addition we have recently constructed a multiunit ribozyme that targets additional cleavage sites flanking the break point and have demonstrated this ribozyme cleaves *BCRABL* transcripts 10 times more efficiently than the single unit ribozyme (manuscript in preparation).

Efforts to improve the efficacy of ribozymes have included altering the length of the complementary sequences in helices 1 and 3.[77] These experiments show an optimization of *in vitro* turnover in ribozymes with a 12-base flanking sequence. The derivatization of chemical groups in the ribozyme has been shown to increase its stability without altering catalytic activity[69] and should therefore increase the intracellular half-life. Experiments do show that the presence of flanking sequences adjacent to the ribozyme unit do not inhibit cleavage, since cleavage active ribozymes are expressed constitutively in cells by both RNA polymerase II and RNA polymerase III promoters, and the success of *in vitro* cleavage is not a reliable indicator of *in vivo* activity. In many reports it is unclear if the biological effects observed are due to actual ribozyme cleavage or an antisense inhibition due to the complementary sequences in helices 1 and 3. Although the targeting of ribozymes is relatively simple, the efficacy of this technology as a basis for gene therapy is still uncertain.

In order to utilize the potential of ribozymes in a therapeutic sense a critical step will be the delivery of the ribozyme to the cells. The goal in delivery is the achievement of efficacious concentrations of functionally competent ribozyme molecules into the proper cellular compartment. Two methods of delivery, exogenous and endogenous, are currently being used and, as can be expected, each has advantages and disadvantages. rNTP ribozyme is degraded by ribonucleases in the medium; therefore, the simple addition of the RNA ribozyme to cells is not possible. The encapsulation of a synthesized ribozyme in a liposome is one means of exogenous delivery. Using this means of delivery the ribozyme introduced may be synthesized with modified bases or as a dNTP/rNTP hybrid molecule. These modifications may play important roles in increasing the stability of the ribozyme intracellularly. However, liposomes show no preference for the cells to which they fuse and the content of liposomes are processed via the endosomal pathway where the contents tend to be degraded.[86] To overcome these limitations the liposome may include on its surface antibodies or ligands that would specifically target the delivery of the ribozyme to a desired cell. This may also prevent the trafficking of the liposome to the lyzosome. The successful targeting and delivery by an exogenous method of delivery will only supply a finite amount of material that will eventually degrade and its effect will stop. By expressing the ribozyme as a part of an RNA transcript from within the cell, a continual concentration may be maintained. It has been shown both experimentally and naturally that ribozymes function even when they are flanked by nonspecific sequences, and functional ribozymes may be transcribed from both vectors with either RNA polymerase II- or RNA polymerase III-based promoters. The transcripts are naturally modified by 5′ capping and polyadenylation in the case of pol II transcription, while the tRNA-based pol III transcripts fold into a specific secondary structure. These modifications may increase the half-life of the ribozymes.

The introduction of these expression cassettes is generally done by including them in retroviral vectors and infecting cells with replication-defective retroviruses. The infection efficiency of cells is high and most replicating cells are susceptible to infection and integration of the retrovirus into the cell's genome. However, the retroviral delivery system is hampered by an important shortcoming, as the insertion of the retroviral genome may act as a mutagenic event to the cell and prove deleterious. In addition the expression of the genes from retroviral LTRs has been shown to decrease over time, which could seriously affect the efficacy of ribozyme-based treatments. Major challenges in this field reside in developing methods that result in efficient cleavage of substrate RNAs by ribozymes *in vivo* and in the development of tissue-specific delivery systems. While these two subjects are being pursued with vigor, it is becoming clear that ribozymes have little or no cytotoxic effects and exhibit a great degree of specificity in their ability to cleave the target molecules.

IX. CONCLUSIONS

Ribozyme and antisense-based inhibition of gene expression can be targeted specifically to any mRNA. Each requires a series of nucleotides that are complementary to the targeted gene, though the ribozyme has an additional need of a GUN sequence in the substrate mRNA. A direct comparison between ribozymes and oligodeoxynucleotides has been reported for the gene encoding the U7 small nuclear ribonucleoprotein that processes histone pre-mRNA. These studies were performed *in vitro* using nuclear extracts with antisense RNA, antisense DNA of varying lengths, and a ribozyme molecule. The antisense molecules were compared to determine the amount of antisense compared to mRNA template necessary to achieve similar levels of inhibition of U7-mediated processing. A 6-fold excess concentration of antisense RNA, a 600-fold excess of an 18-mer oligodeoxynucleotide, and a 60-fold excess of full-length antisense DNA would specifically inhibit the processing >90%. However, to achieve this level of inhibition it was necessary to have a 1000-fold excess of ribozyme.[72] Whether this difference is indicative of a general property or specific to this substrate is uncertain. More comparisons will be necessary in order to evaluate the efficaciousness of these methods of gene inhibition.

Theoretically, these approaches allow inactivation of a single gene transcript out of the thousands of RNAs present in the cell at any given time. However, theory and practicality still are not hand in hand. Issues that must be understood in order to present these as viable treatments in the clinic include efficient and effective introduction into cells, effects of secondary structure in the targeted RNA on the annealing of the inhibitor molecule, stability in the cellular milieu, duration of gene inactivation and dosing, and toxicity to cells that do not express the target. While these parameters need to be determined, the vast amount of work carried out in this area suggests that many of these issues will soon be addressed and the antisense and ribozyme therapy will soon be a reality.

REFERENCES

1. Simons, R. and Kleckner, N., *Cell*, 34, 683, 1983.
2. Izant, J.G. and Weintraub, H., *Cell*, 36, 1007, 1984.
3. Zamecnik, P.C. and Stephenson, M.L., *Proc. Natl. Acad. U.S.A.*, 75, 280, 1978.
4. Wickstrom, E., *J. Biochem. Biophys. Methods*, 13, 97, 1986.
5. Eder, P., DeVine, R., Dagle, J., and Walder, J., *Antisense Res. Dev.*, 1, 141, 1991.
6. Marcus-Sekura, C., Woerner, A., Shinozuka, K., Zon, G., and Quinnan, G., *Nucleic Acids Res.*, 15, 5749, 1987.
7. Reed, J.C., Stein, C.A., Subasinghe, C., Halder, S., Croce, C., Yum, S., and Cihen, J., *Cancer Res.*, 50, 6565, 1990.
8. Loke, S.L., Stein, C.A., Zhang, X.H., Mori, K., Nakanashi, M., Subasinghe, C., Cohen, J., and Neckers, L.M., *Proc. Natl. Acad. Sci. U.S.A.*, 86, 3474, 1989.
9. Yakubov, L.A., Deeva, E., Zarytova, V., Ivanova, E., Ryte, A., Yurchenko, L., and Vlassov, V., *Proc. Natl. Acad. Sci. U.S.A.*, 86, 6454, 1989.
10. Wang, A.M., Creasy, A., Ladner, M.B., Lin, L.S., Strickler, J., Van Ardsell, J.N., Yamamoto, R., and Marks, D.F., *Science*, 228, 149, 1985.
11. Holt, J.T., Redner, R.L., and Nienhius, *Mol. Cell. Biol.*, 8, 963, 1988.
12. Majumdar, C., Stein, C., Cohen, J., Broder, S., and Wilson, S., *Biochemistry*, 28, 1340, 1989.
13. Stein, C., Neckers, L., Mumbauer, S., Hoke, G., and Pal, R., *J. AIDS*, 4, 686, 1991.
14. Paterson, B.M., Roberts, B.E., and Kuff, E., *Proc. Natl. Acad. Sci. U.S.A.*, 74, 4370, 1977.
15. Minshull, J. and Hunt, T., *Nucleic Acids Res.*, 16, 6433, 1986.
16. Walder, R.Y. and Walder, J.A., *Proc. Natl. Acad. Sci. U.S.A.*, 85, 5011, 1988.
17. Kawasaki, E., *Nucleic Acids Res.*, 13, 4991, 1985.
18. Shuttleworth, J. and Coleman, A., *EMBO J.*, 7, 427, 1988.
19. Melton, D., *Proc. Natl. Acad. Sci. U.S.A.*, 82, 144, 1985.
20. Harland, R. and Weintraub, H., *J. Cell. Biol.*, 101, 1094, 1985.
21. Wormington, M., *Proc. Natl. Acad. Sci. U.S.A.*, 83, 8639, 1986.
22. Ch'ng, J., Mulligan, R., Schimmel, P., and Holmes, E., *Proc. Natl. Acad. Sci. U.S.A.*, 86, 10006, 1989.
23. Bacon, T. and Wickstrom, E., *Oncogene Res.*, 6, 13, 1990.
24. Daaka, Y. and Wickstrom, E., *Oncogene Res.*, 5, 267, 1990.
25. Wickstrom, E.L., Bacon, T.A., Gonzales, A., Freeman, D.L., Lyman, G.H., and Wickstrom, E., *Proc. Natl. Acad. Sci. U.S.A.*, 85, 1028,
26. Anfossi, G., Gewirtz, A.M., and Calabretta, B., *Proc. Natl. Acad. Sci. U.S.A.*, 86, 3379, 1989.
27. Chiang, M., Chan, H., Freir, S., Lima, W., Bennett, C., and Zounes, M.A., *J. Biol. Chem.*, 266, 18162, 1991.
28. Goodchild, J., Agrawal, S., Civeria, M., Sarin, P., Sun, D., and Zamecnik, P., *Proc. Natl. Acad. Sci. U.S.A.*, 85, 5507, 1988.
29. Zamecnik, P., *Proc. Natl. Acad. Sci. U.S.A.*, 85, 5507, 1988.
30. Smith, C., Aurelin, L., Reddy, M., Miller, P., and Ts'o, P., *Proc. Natl. Acad. Sci. U.S.A.*, 83, 2787, 1986.
31. Zamecnik, P.C., Goodchild, J., Yagushi, Y., and Sarin, V., *Proc. Natl. Acad. Sci. U.S.A.*, 83, 4143, 1986.
32. Matsukura, M., Shinozuka, K., Zon, G., Mitsuya, H., Reitz, M., Cohen, J., and Broder, S., *Proc. Natl. Acad. Sci. U.S.A.*, 84, 7706, 1987.
33. Zerial, A., Thoung, N.T., and Helene, C., *Nucleic Acids Res.*, 15, 9909, 1987.
34. Agris, C.H., Blake, K., Miller, P., Reddy, M., and Ts'o, P., *Biochemistry*, 25, 6268, 1986.
35. Loke, S.L., Zhang, X.H., Avigan, M., Cohen, J., and Neckers, L.M., *Curr. Top. Microbiol. Immunol.*, 141, 282, 1988.
36. Calabretta, B., Sims, R.B., Valtieri, M., Caracciolo, D., Szczylik, C., Venturelli, D., Beran, M., and Gewirtz, A.M., *Proc. Natl. Acad. Sci. U.S.A.*, 88, 2351, 1991.
37. Ratajzak, M.Z., Hijiya, N., Catani, L., DeRiel, K., Luger, S.M., McClave, P., and Gewirtz, A.M., *Blood*, 79, 1, 1992.
38. Calabretta, B., Sims, R.B., Valtieri, M., Caracciolo, D., Szczylik, C., Venturelli, D., Beran, M., and Gewirtz, A.M., *Proc. Natl. Acad. Sci. U.S.A.*, 88, 2351, 1991.
39. Szyczylik, C., Skorski, T., Nicolaides, N.C., Manzella, L., Malaguarnera, L., Venturelli, D., Gewirtz, A.M., and Calabretta, B., *Science*, 253, 562, 1991.
40. Gewirtz, A. and Calabretta, B., *Science*, 242, 1303, 1988.
41. Gewirtz, A.M., Anfossi, G., Venturelli, D., Valpreda, S., Sims, R., and Calabretta, B., *Science*, 245, 180, 1989.
42. Ratajzak, M.Z., Hijiya, N., Catani, L., DeRiel, K., Luger, S.M., McClave, P., and Gewirtz, A.M., *Blood*, 79, 1, 1992.

43. Kitchada, S., Miyashita, S., and Reed, J.C., *Antisense Res. Dev.*, 3, 157, 1993.
44. Kruger, K., Grabowski, P.J., Zaug, A.J., Sands, J., Gottschling, D.E., and Cech, T.R., *Cell*, 31, 147, 1982.
45. Guerrier-Takada, C., Gardiner, K., Marsh, T., Pace, N., and Altman, S., *Cell*, 35, 849, 1983.
46. Cech, T.R. and Bass, B.L., *Annu. Rev. Biochem.*, 55, 599, 1986.
47. Altman, S., *Adv. Enzymol.*, 62, 1, 1987.
48. Buzayan, J.M., Hampel, A., and Bruening, G., *Nucleic Acids Res.*, 14, 9729, 1986.
49. Hutchins, C.J., Rathjen, P., Forster, A.C., and Symons, R.H., *Nucleic Acids Res.*, 14, 3627, 1986.
50. Forster, A.C. and Symons, R.H., *Cell*, 49, 211, 1987.
51. Uhlenbeck, O.C., *Nature*, 328, 596, 1987.
52. Haseloff, J. and Gerlach, W.L., *Nature*, 334, 585, 1988.
53. Hampel, A. and Tritz, R., *Biochemistry*, 28, 4929, 1989.
54. Hampel, A., Tritz, R., Hicks, M., and Cruz, P., *Nucleic Acids Res.*, 18, 299, 1990.
55. Symons, R.H., *Trends Biochem. Sci.*, 14, 445, 1989.
56. Epstein, L.M. and Gall, J.G., *Cell*, 48, 535, 1987.
57. Kuo, M.Y.-P., Sharmeen, L., Dinter-Gottlieb, G., and Taylor, J., *J. Virol.*, 62, 4439, 1988.
58. Branch, A.D. and Robertson, H.D., *Proc. Natl. Acad. Sci. U.S.A.*, 88, 10163, 1991.
59. Saville, B.J. and Collins, R.A., *Cell*, 61, 685, 1990.
60. Ruffner, D.E., Stormo, G.D., and Uhlenbeck, O.C., *Biochemistry*, 29, 10695, 1990.
61. Fedor, M.J. and Uhelenbeck, O.C., *Proc. Natl. Acad. Sci. U.S.A.*, 87, 1668, 1990.
62. McCall, M.J., Hendry, P., and Jennings, P.A., *Proc. Natl. Acad. Sci. U.S.A.*, 89, 5710, 1992.
63. Perriman, R., Davis, A., and Gerlach, W.L., *Gene*, 85, 157, 1992.
64. Bruening, G., *Methods Enzymol.*, 180, 546, 1990.
65. Heus, H.A. and Pardi, A., *J. Mol. Biol.*, 217, 113, 1991.
66. Ruffner, D.E., Dahm, S.-A.C., and Uhlenbeck, O.C., *Gene*, 82, 31, 1989.
67. Jeffries, A.C. and Symons, R.H., *Nucleic Acids Res.*, 17, 1371, 1989.
68. Perreault, J.-P., Wu, T., Cousineau, B., Ogilvie, K.K., and Cedergren, R., *Nature*, 344, 565, 1990.
69. Pieken, W.A., Olsen, D.B., Bensler, F., Aurup, H., and Eckstein, F., *Science*, 253, 314, 1991.
70. Zaug, A.J., Been, M.D., and Cech, T.R., *Nature*, 324, 429, 1986.
71. Koizumi, M., Iwai, S., and Ohtsuka, E., *FEBS Lett.*, 239, 285, 1988.
72. Cotten, M., Schaffer, G., and Birnstiel, M.L., *Mol. Cell. Biol.*, 9, 4479, 1989.
73. Cotten, M. and Birnstiel, M.L., *EMBO J.*, 8, 3861, 1989.
74. Cameron, F.H. and Jennings, P.A., *Proc. Natl. Acad. Sci. U.S.A.*, 86, 9139, 1989.
75. Sarver, N., Cantin, E.M., Chang, P.S., Zaia, J.A., Ladne, P.A., Stephens, D.A., and Rossi, J.J., *Science*, 247, 1222, 1990.
76. Sioud, M. and Drlica, K., *Proc. Natl. Acad. Sci. U.S.A.*, 88, 7303, 1991.
77. Goodchild, J. and Kohli, V., *Arch. Biochem. Biophys.*, 284, 386, 1991.
78. Weerasinghe, M., Liem, S.E., Asad, S., Read, S.E., and Joshi, S., *J. Virol.*, 65, 5531, 1991.
79. Heidenreich, O. and Eckstein, F., *J. Biol. Chem.*, 267, 1904, 1992.
80. Dropulic, B., Lin, N.H., Martin, M., and Jeang, K.-T., *J. Virol.*, 66, 1432, 1992.
81. Chen, C.-J., Banerjea, A.C., Harmison, G.G., Haglund, K., and Schubert, M., *Nucleic Acids Res.*, 20, 4581, 1992.
82. Yu, M., Ojwang, J., Yamada, O., Hampel, A., Rapapport, J., Looney, D., and Wong-Staal, F., *Proc. Natl. Acad. Sci. U.S.A.*, 90, 6340, 1993.
83. Scanlon, K.J., Jiao, L., Wang, W., Tone, T., Rossi, J.J., and Kashini-Sabet, M., *Proc. Natl. Acad. Sci. U.S.A.*, 88, 10591, 1991.
84. Shore, S.K., Nabissa, P.M., and Reddy, E.P., *Oncogene*, 8, 3183, 1993.
85. Snyder, D.S., Wu, Y., Wang, J.L., Rossi, J.J., Swiderski, P., Kaplan, B.E., and Forman, S.J., *Blood*, 82, 600, 1993.
86. Huang, A., Kennel, S.J., and Huang, L., *J. Biol. Chem.*, 258, 14034, 1983.

INDEX

A

B

C

H

I

K

L

N

O

P

R

S